FUNDAMENTALS OF OBSTETRICS AND GYNAECOLOGY

Volume II: **GYNAECOLOGY**

FUNDAMENTALS OF OBSTETRICS AND GYNAECOLOGY

Volume II

GYNAECOLOGY

Derek Llewellyn-Jones OBE, MD, MAO, FRCOG, FRACOG

Associate Professor of Obstetrics and Gynaecology,
* University of Sydney, New South Wales, Australia*
Visiting Obstetrician and Gynaecologist,
* St Margaret's Hospital, Sydney*

Illustrations by Audrey Besterman

FIFTH EDITION

faber and faber
LONDON·BOSTON

First published in 1970
by Faber and Faber Limited
3 Queen Square London WC1N 3AU

Reprinted 1972, 1973 and 1975
Second edition 1978
Reprinted 1980
Third edition 1982
Fourth edition 1986
Fifth edition 1990
Printed and bound in Great Britain
by Richard Clay Ltd
Bungay, Suffolk
All rights reserved

British Library Cataloguing in Publication Data

Llewellyn-Jones, Derek
    Fundamentals of obstetrics and gynaecology.—
    5th ed.
    Vol.2: Gynaecology
    1. Gynecology   2. Obstetrics
    I. Title
    618   RG101
ISBN 0–571–14228–1

Library of Congress Cataloguing in Publication Data

Llewellyn-Jones, Derek
    Fundamentals of obstetrics and gynaecology.

    Includes bibliographies and index.
    Contents: v. 2. Gynaecology
    1. Obstetrics   2. Gynecology   I. Title [DNLM:
    1. Genital Diseases, female.   2. Obstetrics. WQ 100
    L791f]
    RG101.L542   1986   618   85–6846

ISBN 0 571 14228 3 (pbk.: v. 2)

Contents

Preface

This book, which is the second volume of *Fundamentals of Obstetrics and Gynaecology*, deals specifically with matters which are considered conventionally to constitute gynaecology. Although most teachers today agree that obstetrics and gynaecology form two intertwined branches of a single discipline, a combined textbook in 'gyniatrics' would be too bulky for convenient handling. I believe it important that a book should not only be clear, informative and stimulating to read, but it should be pleasant to handle. However, so that this book on gynaecology may stand on its own, two chapters from the volume on obstetrics have been included, with only slight modification; these are the chapters on Abortion and Ectopic Gestation.

This book is intended primarily for undergraduates and for those graduates spending a six months' residency in obstetrics and gynaecology. In the latter period, reading should be supplemented by reference to recent articles and to specialist monographs. However, the heavy 'work load' in the undergraduate period has the effect of precluding this approach, and consequently it is suggested that if a student wishes for more detailed information on a particular subject, he will be able to find the appropriate references in the larger textbooks recommended later in the Bibliography, or preferably will seek the advice of his tutors and study the specialist journals.

My conviction that the medical and psychosomatic aspects of gynaecology are of considerably greater importance than the mechanical-surgical approach which was common until recently, will be observed by the discerning reader. For this I make no apology. Today over 80 per cent of gynaecological complaints require thoughtful analysis and critical assessment by the physician, and only 20 per cent require surgical intervention. All too often the doctrine of 'if in doubt, cut it out' prevails, and the amount of unnecessary, and often harmful, gynaecological surgery performed in all countries, and under a variety of medical philosophies, is distressing to observe. This observation in no way diminishes the need for well-trained, highly qualified, surgically expert gynaecologists within the community, but it emphasizes that their numbers need not be great, and that much gynaecology will continue to be performed by the patient's personal physician.

The value of the personal physician is of particular importance as in no specialty is the influence of the mind upon the body of greater consequence, and the neglect of this aspect in the past is a discredit to our chosen profession. It is hoped that in stressing this aspect of gynaecology, the student will be persuaded to continue to retain an enquiring mind in his graduate years.

The need for a Fifth Edition has enabled me to revise the book considerably. The sexually transmissible diseases, particularly those due to *Chlamydia trachomatis* and the human papillomavirus, are causing increased concern. These two infections receive extensive attention. In the case of the human papillomavirus infection it has meant that the section on cervical neoplasia has been rewritten. The chapter about amenorrhoea has required considerable revision with the information that weight loss is an important factor in the onset and continuation of amenorrhoea. The new reproductive technologies (IVF and GIFT) are discussed although they only benefit a tiny minority of women and their partners. Urinary incontinence continues to pose problems in diagnosis and in management and is discussed. The prevention of osteoporosis is an important health issue which should be of concern to gynaecologists, and new information about this degenerative condition is included.

Surgical techniques are not discussed in this text, as I believe that these craft aspects of gynaecology are better learnt in the graduate years by assisting at operations, and by supplementing this activity with reading during the period of specialist training. Nor do I believe that a knowledge of surgical techniques forms a proper part of undergraduate training in gynaecology, the aim of which is surely to stimulate the student's enquiring mind regarding disorders peculiar to women, and to stress the influence of the psyche on the soma, and the soma on the psyche in this discipline.

If this text achieves at least part of this aim, I shall be well satisfied.

DEREK LLEWELLYN-JONES *Sydney*, 1990

Chapter 1

Gynaecological Examination

The word gynaecology is from the Greek words gynē (woman) and logos (science; discourse), and implies a study of womankind; although in recent years gynaecology has been restricted to a study of disorders of the female genital organs. There is much merit today in broadening the scope of gynaecology to encompass its original definition, for it is increasingly realized that the control and functions of the genital organs are intimately bound up with the endocrine system, and that this, to some extent, is manipulated by the psyche. In the early part of this century, operative expertise separated the surgeon-specialists who believed that diseases of the female genital tract were surgical problems, and the physician-accoucheurs who dealt with obstetrical problems; whereas, of course, obstetrics is but a part of gynaecology. This false division has now been repaired, but the cumbersome term, 'obstetrician and gynaecologist' still describes specialists in diseases of women. Perhaps a better, more precise, term would be to call such physicians 'gyniatricians', for today, as 80 per cent of gynaecology is of medical or psychosomatic origin, the medical care of women should only be in the hands of physicians who have been trained in the biology of woman. They should have a knowledge of human reproductive processes and the social and psychological effects of femininity. Surgical technique of a high order will continue to be required by the gyniatrician, but he must be mainly a physician skilled in women's diseases. In determining the cause of the disease, the gyniatrician must consider the whole woman, not just her pelvic organs, and in obtaining the history of her complaint and in examining her subsequently, this concept must be kept constantly in the front of his mind.

THE HISTORY

The importance in gynaecology of obtaining an accurate history of the complaint and of recording this concisely, cannot be overstressed. Once the trust of the patient has been obtained and she has been put at ease, the physician should include questions relating to her social and sexual background, as psychosomatic disorders predominate in over one-third of all patients with gynaecological complaints. The way in which the patient answers the questions often gives a clue to the origin of the complaint. The patient whose complaints are of psychological origin, induced perhaps by unhappiness, inadequacy or frustration, tends to delay in seeking medical aid, to have used a variety of self-medicaments, and to answer the questions evasively and with little clarity, often introducing irrelevant facts, and interpreting her symptoms. Yet this patient requires as much help as one with an organic lesion, and the time spent in disentangling the story and obtaining the confidence of the patient, is time well spent.

In obtaining the history, the cultural reluctance of many women, of all social classes, to discuss gynaecological and sexual matters must be recognized. The physician must therefore be tactful, courteous, gentle and unhurried in his approach. So that the patient may become accustomed to him, it is well to start by obtaining general information (name, address, age, marital status), and enquiring about past illnesses and operations before discussing the main complaint. The account of the patient's symptoms should be recorded, and the history of each delineated (time of onset, duration, previous treatment, apparent cause). If pain is a main symptom, the nature of its onset and its duration should be determined, and its exact site and radiation delineated. Uterine pain is deep seated and midline (hypogastric) in site, radiating occasionally down the inner aspects of the thighs. The pain distribution from lesions of the oviducts or ovaries is felt low in the abdomen on one or both sides, and its radiation is to the back. The menstrual history (age of onset, regularity, duration, amount, clots, pain and other associated symptoms, and the dates of the last two menstrual periods) and the sexual history (pregnancies and outcome; contraceptive measures; frequency of coitus; pain during coitus) are next obtained. In this regard it is well to remember that women often find it difficult to describe their menstrual cycle. The physician should explain that the menstrual cycle starts on the first day of menstruation (day 1), and includes both the period of bleeding and the interval between bleedings. For example, if a woman says she bleeds for 5 days every 22 days, she may mean that the *interval* is 22 days, and in fact the cycle is normal. The patient should also be interrogated to determine if she is taking a drug, particularly hormone pills.

Once the history has been taken, and before examining the patient, the physician must fix in his mind the main symptoms, so that whilst the physical examination is in progress the history is constantly related to the complaints.

Community studies show that about 10 per cent of British and Australian women have psychiatric morbidity (as detected by the Present State Examination). Two studies noted a significant relationship between gynaecological symptoms, psychiatric morbidity and adverse life-events. The relationship is particularly marked in women who present with menstrual cramps [dysmenorrhoea] and the premenstrual syndrome, but no relationship is found in women who present with other menstrual disturbances. If a woman presents with a gynaecological complaint, particularly if no organic cause is readily apparent, a brief psychological history should be taken. General psychological adjustment is assessed by asking about irritability, poor concentration and fatigue. Depressive symptoms are elicited by asking about depressed mood, self-blame, tearfulness, sadness, early morning waking, mood disturbance, loss of appetite, weight, and libido. Anxiety is assessed by asking about 'tension', phobias and persistent worrying thoughts.

The interplay between psychological and physical causes of gynaecological complaints must be borne in mind, and both must receive attention. The provision of information, talking *with* the patient, discussion of her problems and reassurance are important ingredients in the management of gynaecological disorders.

THE EXAMINATION

Unless the patient has been seen before, a general examination should be made, as the gynaecological complaint may only be a local manifestation of a general disorder. This examination, which can be performed quite quickly, should include inspection of the head and neck, palpation of the supraclavicular areas for enlarged lymph nodes, auscultation of the heart and determination of the pulse rate and blood pressure.

The gynaecological portion of the examination should include (1) a breast examination, (2) an abdominal examination, (3) an inspection of the external genitalia, (4) a pelvic examination, by speculum and then digitally as a bimanual vaginoabdominal examination, and (5) a rectal examination in certain instances.

Breast examination (Fig. 1/1)

With the patient sitting facing the examiner, the breasts are inspected, first with the patient's arms at her sides and then with her arms raised above her head. The shape, contour and size of the breasts, their height on the chest wall, and the position of the nipples are compared, any nipple retraction being noted. The supraclavicular regions and axillae are next palpated. The latter can only be palpated satisfactorily if the pectoral muscles are relaxed. This relaxation can be obtained if the physician supports the patient's arm whilst palpating the axilla. Palpation is then performed with the patient lying supine, her shoulders elevated on a small pillow. Palpation should be gentle and orderly, using the flat of the fingers of one hand. Each portion of the breast should be palpated systematically beginning at the upper, inner quadrant, and palpating each portion sequentially until the upper, outer quadrant is finally palpated.

Abdominal examination

The examination is conducted with the patient lying comfortably on her back, *having emptied her bladder immediately before*. Inspection of the abdomen will show its contour, the presence of striae and scars, or of dilated veins. If the patient raises her head and coughs, hernias and divarication of the recti abdominis muscles will be evident. Palpation systematically of the viscera is performed; the liver, the gall bladder, the spleen and the kidneys being palpated in turn. The caecum and colon are next palpated, and finally the lower abdomen is palpated, the hand pressing down gently as the patient breathes out. Percussion may be required if free fluid is suspected.

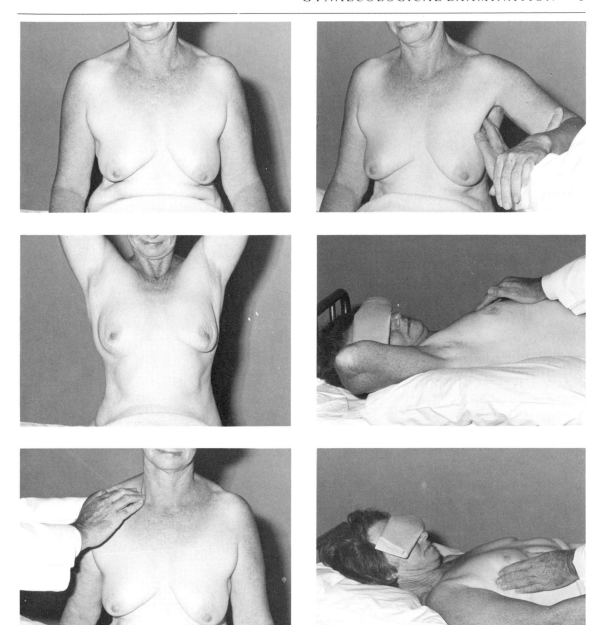

Fig. 1/1 Sequence of examination of the breast

(1) Inspection of the breasts – the patient's arms at her side

(2) Inspection of the breasts – the patient's arms raised above her head. During the inspection, the contour of the breasts, the size and shape of the areolae, and the condition of the nipples are examined. An indentation, or a bulge in the contour may indicate a lesion

(3) Supraclavicular palpation

(4) Axillary palpation. Note that the patient's arm is supported on the gynaecologists's left forearm

(5) Palpation of the inner half of the breast. Note the pillow under the patient's shoulder, and the position of her arms

(6) Palpation of the outer half of the breast

Conditions of the abdominal wall
    Obesity
    Tumours (rare)
    Inflammatory area
    Ventral hernia
    Divarication of the recti muscles

Conditions of the intestines
    Flatus
    Faecal impaction

Conditions of the peritoneal cavity
    Ascites

Conditions of abdominal organs
    Distended bladder
    Pregnant uterus
    Enlarged liver or spleen
    Ovarian or uterine tumour

Table 1/1 Causes of abdominal prominence

Pelvic examination

The pelvic examination should follow the abdominal examination, and never be omitted unless the patient is a virgin. The external genitalia are first inspected under a good light with the patient in the dorsal position, the hips flexed and abducted, and knees flexed (Fig. **1/2**). If she or the doctor prefer, she may lie in the left lateral position (Fig. **1/3**). Some women are more comfortable and feel less exposed in the latter position. The patient must have voided just before the examination (unless stress incontinence is complained of), and should preferably have defaecated that morning. If urinary infection is suspected, a mid-stream specimen of urine may be obtained at this time.

The patient is asked to strain down to detect any evidence of prolapse, after which a bivalve speculum is inserted and the cervix visualized. If the physician intends to take a cervical smear to examine the exfoliated cells, *no lubricant apart from water* should be used on the speculum. The vagina and cervix are inspected by opening the bivalve speculum (Fig. **1/2**). If the patient has a prolapse, the degree of the vaginal wall or uterine descent can be best assessed if a Sims speculum is used with the patient in the left lateral position (Fig. **1/3**).

Digital examination follows, one or two fingers of the gloved hand being introduced. In most countries, apart from the USA, it is usual to use the right hand as the fingers of this hand in a right-handed person are more 'educated'. After the labia minora have

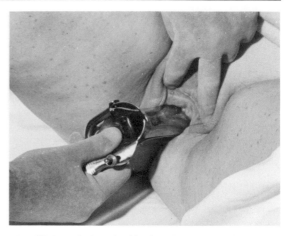

Fig. 1/2 Introducing the bivalve (Cusco) speculum. Note the oblique position of the instrument; this avoids painful pressure on the urethra

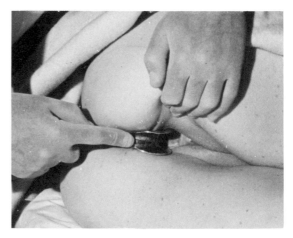

Fig. 1/3 The patient in the left lateral position, a Sims speculum has been inserted into the vagina

been separated with the left hand to expose the vestibule, the fingers are introduced passing *upwards and backwards* to palpate the cervix. The left hand palpates the pelvis through the abdominal wall simultaneously so that the uterus and ovaries may be palpated. Normal oviducts are never palpable. As the intravaginal fingers push the cervix backwards, the abdominal hand is placed just below the umbilicus and the fingers reach down into the pelvis, slowly and smoothly, until the fundus is caught between them and the fingers of the right hand in the anterior vaginal fornix (Fig. **1/4**).

The information obtained by bimanual examination includes:

1. *By palpation of the uterus.* Position, size, shape,

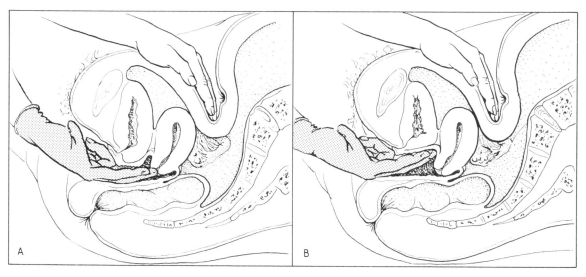

Fig. 1/4 Bimanual examination of the uterus. Note that the bladder is empty, the patient having voided just before the pelvic examination. (A) The vaginal fingers push the cervix back and upward so that the fundus can be reached by the abdominal fingers; (B) The vaginal fingers now palpate the anterior surface of the uterus which is held in position by the abdominal fingers

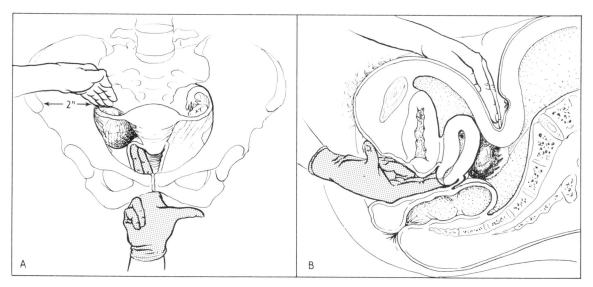

Fig. 1/5 Bimanual palpation of the adnexal area. Note the position of the fingers; normally the ovary cannot be felt. In this case a cystic mass lying in the position of the ovary can be identified

consistency, mobility, tenderness, attachments. The normal uterus is either in the anterior or posterior position, and is about 9cm long. It is pear-shaped and of firm consistency, and can be moved in all directions. It is normally tender when squeezed between the two hands.

2. *By palpation of the ovaries and oviducts.* The tips of the vaginal fingers are placed in each lateral fornix in turn and then pushed backwards and upwards as far as possible without causing pain. The abdominal fingers simultaneously press backwards about 5cm (2in) medial and parallel to the superior iliac spine (Fig. **1/5**). The normal oviduct cannot be palpated, and the normal ovary may or may not be

felt. If it is palpable, it is extremely tender on bi-manual pressure.

Rectal examination

A rectal examination, or a recto-abdominal bi-manual examination, may replace a vaginal examination in children and in virgin adults, but the examination is less efficient and more painful than the vaginal examination. A rectal examination is a useful adjunct to a vaginal examination, when either the outer parts of the broad ligaments, or the utero-sacral ligaments, require to be palpated. On occasions a rectovaginal examination, the index finger in the vagina and the middle finger in the rectum, may help to determine if a lesion is in the bowel or between the rectum and the vagina.

ANCILLARY AIDS TO DIAGNOSIS

1. *Anaesthesia*. In obese patients, or when the delineation of the genital organs is obscure, examination under anaesthesia may be of great help, particularly if a short-acting muscle relaxant is used. However, it is an ancillary aid, and should only be used in difficult cases after attempting a bimanual pelvic examination. Often the opportunity is taken to perform a diagnostic curettage, or to obtain an endometrial biopsy.

2. *Endometrial biopsy*. Information regarding the state of the uterine endometrium may be obtained by using a narrow, sharp curette to take a strip of endometrium. The procedure requires no an-aesthetic, but it is inadequate for the exclusion of endometrial carcinoma.

3. *Cytodiagnosis*. Smears from the lateral vaginal wall may give some indication of the hormonal status of the patient, whilst cervical smears should be made routinely to detect, or exclude, the presence of pre-clinical malignancy of the cervix.

4. *Ultrasound*. The increasing development of ultrasound has added considerably to the diagnostic accuracy in many gynaecological conditions. Ultra-sound can identify if an abortion has occurred, detect a benign or a malignant ovarian tumour, detect some uterine tumours, and is useful in identifying ectopic gestation. Ultrasound is a valuable tool which increases the clinician's decision-making powers but does not supersede them.

SPECIAL INVESTIGATIONS

Occasionally special investigations are required. These investigations require considerable expertise which can only be obtained by regular practice. They include (1) inspection and magnification of the cervix with a colposcope, (2) radiography of the uterus and tubes using a water-soluble contrast medium, and image-intensity screening (hystero-salpingography), (3) direct inspection of the pelvic organs, through a tiny subumbilical stab wound (laparoscopy) or rarely through the posterior vaginal fornix (culdoscopy).

These investigations should only be attempted by specialists, and, apart from hysterosalpingography, only specially interested and trained gyniatricians.

Chapter 2

The Anatomy of the Female Genital Tract

By the time the student studies gynaecology, he has been well grounded in the disciplines of anatomy and physiology, and only a brief review of the anatomy of the female genital tract will be made here.

THE VULVA (Fig. 2/1)

The *labia majora* are two large folds containing sebaceous and sweat glands embedded in adipose and connective tissue and covered by skin. They form the lateral boundaries of the vulval cleft, and are the homologues of the scrotum. Anteriorly they unite in

an adipose pad over the symphysis pubis, to form the mons veneris. In the adult female the mons is covered with hair, which terminates cephalically in a horizontal upper border. Hair also grows on the outer, but not the inner, surface of the labia majora. Posteriorly the labia majora unite to form the posterior commissure. In childhood the labia majora contain little adipose tissue, and in age the adipose tissue disappears. At the extremes of life, therefore, the labia majora are relatively small.

The *labia minora* are flat, delicate folds of skin containing connective tissue and some sebaceous glands, but no adipose tissue. On their medial aspect the keratinized epithelium of the skin changes into

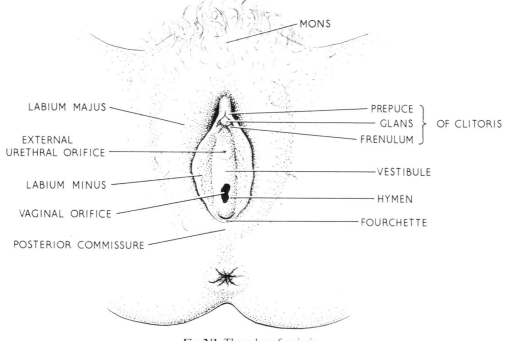

Fig. 2/1 The vulva of a virgin

poorly keratinized squamous epithelium, containing many sebaceous glands. Anteriorly the labia minora split into two parts, one passing over the clitoris to form the prepuce of the organ, the other passing beneath to form the homologue of the frenulum of the male. Posteriorly they fuse to form the four-chette, which is always torn during parturition. In the reproductive years the labia minora are hidden by the labia majora, but in childhood and old age they appear to be more prominent as the labia majora are relatively small. The size of the labia minora varies considerably in different women, but this is of little clinical importance.

The cleft between the labia minora is called the *vestibule*, and contains the *external urethral meatus* and the *hymen*, which lies just inside and surrounds the vaginal orifice. The vestibule is surmounted by the *clitoris*, which is the homologue of the penis, and is composed of erectile tissue. As with the penis, it becomes enlarged and stiffens during sexual excitement. The clitoris is one of the major erotic zones of the female. Only the glans and prepuce of the clitoris are normally visible, but the corpus can be palpated along the lower surface of the symphysis pubis as a cord-like structure.

The *hymen* is a thin, incomplete membrane surrounding the vaginal orifice, and has one or more apertures in it, which allow menstrual blood to escape. The apertures are of various shapes and sizes. The hymen varies considerably in elasticity, but is generally torn during a first coitus. An 'intact' hymen is considered a sign of virginity, but this is not reliable as in some cases coitus fails to cause a tear, and in others the hymen may be torn by digital interference. In attempting to make a decision regarding virginity, palpation to feel a circular ridge of hymenal tissue is more accurate than inspection. Although the hymen is relatively avascular, tearing at first coitus may be accompanied by a small amount of bleeding, which ceases rapidly. Childbirth causes a much greater tearing of the hymen, and after parturition only a few tags remain. These are called carunculae myrtiformes (Fig. **2/2**). Just lateral to the hymen, surrounding the vaginal orifice on each side, and deep to the bulbocavernosus muscle (the sphincter vaginae), are two collections of erectile tissue – the *vestibular bulbs*. Embedded in the posterolateral parts of the bulbs, on each side is Bartholin's gland (Fig. **2/3**), which is the homologue of Cowper's gland in the male. The gland is pea-sized and not palpable unless infected. It is connected to the posterior part of the vestibule, between the hymen and the four-chette, by a duct some 2cm in length. It is lined by columnar cells, which secrete a mucoid substance during sexual excitement.

Vascular supply of the vulva

Arteries
The external genitalia are very vascular, and are supplied by branches of the internal pudendal arteries, which originate from the internal iliac arteries, and by the external pudendal arteries, deriving from the femoral arteries.

Veins
The veins of the vulva form large venous plexuses, which become dilated during sexual excitement, and to an even greater degree during pregnancy, when varicosities are not uncommon. Most of the veins accompany the corresponding arteries, but those draining the clitoris join the vaginal and vesical venous plexuses.

Lymphatics
Lymphatic vessels form an interconnecting meshwork which extends through the labia minora, the prepuce, the fourchette and the vaginal introitus. These vessels join to form 'trunks'. The anterior

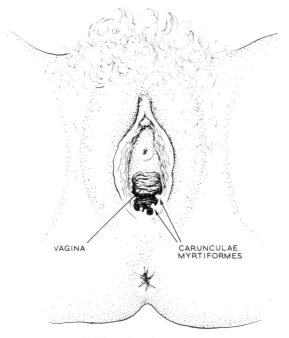

VAGINA   CARUNCULAE
                          MYRTIFORMES

Fig. 2/2 The vulva of a parous woman

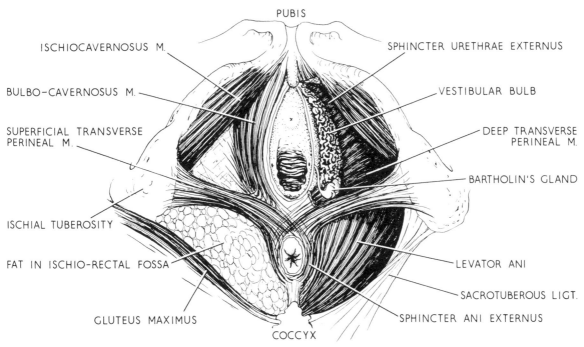

PUBIS

ISCHIOCAVERNOSUS M.

BULBO-CAVERNOSUS M.

SUPERFICIAL TRANSVERSE
PERINEAL M.

ISCHIAL TUBEROSITY

FAT IN ISCHIO-RECTAL FOSSA

GLUTEUS MAXIMUS

COCCYX

SPHINCTER URETHRAE EXTERNUS

VESTIBULAR BULB

DEEP TRANSVERSE
PERINEAL M.

BARTHOLIN'S GLAND

LEVATOR ANI

SACROTUBEROUS LIGT.

SPHINCTER ANI EXTERNUS

Fig. 2/3 Dissection of the perineum to show the superficial muscles, the position of Bartholin's gland and the vestibular bulb

trunks join with a lymphatic meshwork over the mons (which also drains the glans of the clitoris). The anterior collecting trunks pass to reach the ipsilateral and contralateral superficial femoral nodes. The lymphatics from the labia majora also form trunks and pass to the superficial femoral nodes. There are connections between the superficial and the deep femoral nodes, which then connect with the nodes along the external iliac vessels.

The lymphatics from the clitoral shaft (which interconnect with those of the glans) pass directly to interiliac nodes in the pelvis (Fig. **2/4**). The lymphatics anastomose with those of the opposite side, and consequently bilateral or contralateral involvement is not uncommon in malignant tumours of the vulva. The vulval lymphatics also anastomose with the lymphatics of the lower third of the vagina, which drain into the external iliac nodes.

THE VAGINA

The vagina is a fibromuscular sheath, extending upwards and backwards from the vestibule, at an angle

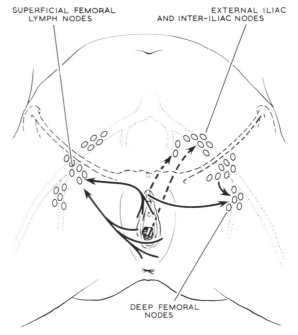

SUPERFICIAL FEMORAL
LYMPH NODES

EXTERNAL ILIAC
AND INTER-ILIAC NODES

DEEP FEMORAL
NODES

Fig. 2/4 Schematic diagram showing the distribution of the lymphatics of the vulva. It shows that an extensive intercommunication exists between the lymphatics of each side

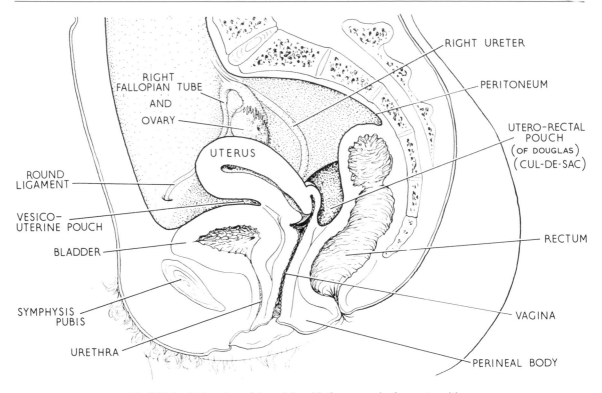

Fig. 2/5 Sagittal section of the pelvis, with the woman in the erect position

of about 85° to the horizontal, and parallel with the plane of the pelvic brim when the woman is erect (Fig. **2/5**). The walls of the vagina, as well as being muscular, contain a well-developed venous plexus. Normally the walls are in apposition, the vagina being a potential cavity, and having an H-shape in cross-section in the middle third (Fig. **2/6**). In the lower third, the widest diameter of the vagina is the anteroposterior diameter, but above this the widest diameter is the transverse diameter. Knowledge of this is of importance when introducing a vaginal bivalve speculum. Because of the well-developed walls, the lining epithelium tends to be lifted into ridges, or rugae, which run in a circumferential manner from two longitudinal columns running sagittally the length of the anterior and posterior vaginal walls. The formation of the rugae in this manner permits the great distension without damage of which the vagina is capable. The length of the anterior vaginal wall is 7cm, and its upper end is invaginated by the cervix. Because of this, the posterior vaginal wall, which ends blindly, is 2cm longer. The vaginal vault is divided into four areas, which are related to the projecting cervix. These are the

shallow *anterior fornix*, the capacious *posterior fornix* and the shallow *lateral fornices*. Although the vagina varies considerably in length and width, its functional size is largely determined by the tone in its muscular wall and the contractions of the surrounding muscles. These are under voluntary control. Unless the vagina has been injured or shortened at operation, anatomical variations in size do not cause difficulty or pain (dyspareunia) during coitus; and most cases of dyspareunia are psychosomatic in origin.

The vagina is surrounded by several important structures. The anterior wall is in contact with the urethra, to which it is closely bound, and above this with the base of the bladder. Posteriorly the lower one-third is separated from the rectum by the complex of muscles and fascia which constitutes the perineal body, but above is in direct contact with the rectum. The upper one-quarter, including the posterior fornix, is covered by the peritoneum of the utero-rectal pouch (pouch of Douglas or cul-de-sac). The upper third of the lateral walls are in intimate contact with the pelvic connective tissue, and the fornices abut the parametrium which contains a rich

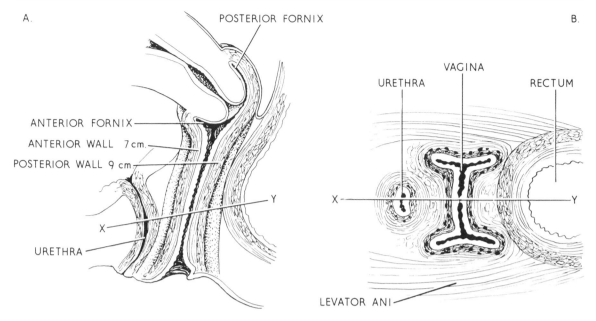

Fig. 2/6 The vagina in cross-section. Note the greater length of the posterior wall and the 'H' shape on cross-section. It can be seen that the vaginal walls are normally in apposition

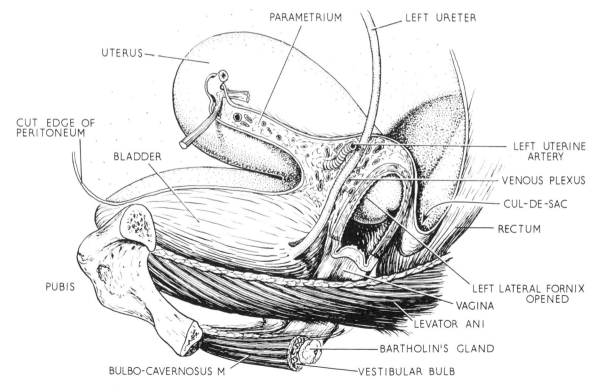

Fig. 2/7 The relationship of the parametrium to the vagina and other pelvic organs

venous plexus. Lying about 1cm above each lateral fornix are the uterine artery and the ureter (Fig. 2/7). In the middle third, the lateral wall blends with the levator ani muscles, which together with the muscular vagina form one of the supports of the uterus. In the lower third the walls are related to the bulbocavernosus muscle, the bulb of the vestibule and Bartholin's glands.

Histology of the vagina

The vagina is lined with stratified, squamous, non-keratinized epithelium, some 10 to 30 cells deep, which rests upon a basement membrane and is continuous at the upper end with an identical epithelium covering the vaginal portion of the cervix. Should the epithelium be exposed to the dry external atmosphere, keratinization occurs. The cells are all derived by differentiation from the basal cells which lie upon the basement membrane. Three main cell types are described, (1) parabasal cells, (2) intermediate cells, and (3) superficial cells. The superficial cells, and some intermediate cells, contain glycogen. The entire epithelium shows cyclic changes during the menstrual cycle, and in pregnancy, and cellular development and differentiation is controlled by the

	VAGINAL :—				
	OESTROGEN	EPITHELIUM	GLYCOGEN	pH	FLORA
NEWBORN	+		+	ACID 4 — 5	STERILE ↓ DÖDERLEIN'S BACILLI SECRETION ABUNDANT
MONTH-OLD CHILD	—		—	ALKALINE >7	SPARSE, COCCAL AND VARIED FLORA. SECRETION SCANT
PUBERTY	APPEARS		— → +	ALKALINE ↓ ACID	SPARSE, COCCAL ↓ RICH BACILLARY
MATURE	+ +		+	ACID 4 — 5	DODERLEIN'S BACILLI SECRETION ABUNDANT
POST MENOPAUSE	+ → —		—	NEUTRAL OR ALKALINE 6 — >7	VARIED DEPENDENT ON LEVEL OF CIRCULATING OESTROGEN SECRETION SCANT

Fig. 2/8 Cyclic changes in the vagina related to age

ratio of circulating oestrogens, progesterone and androgens (Fig. **2/8**). The cells do not secrete mucus, but secretions seep between the cells to moisten the vagina, and the superficial cells are constantly exfoiliated. The exfoliated cells release the contained glycogen, which is acted upon by Döderlein's bacillus, a normal inhabitant of the vagina, to produce lactic acid. This causes the normal acidity of the vagina, and explains the relative resistance of the vagina to infection. The vaginal epithelial cells can also absorb drugs, particularly oestrogens.

The epithelium rests upon a connective tissue layer containing elastic tissue, nerves, lymphatics and blood vessels, and external to this are the thick layers of interdigitating muscle fibres, which cross in a spiral manner, the main direction being oblique rather than circular. Outside the muscle is a well-developed sheath of connective tissue, which is condensed anteriorly to form the so-called pubocervical (or vesicovaginal) fascia, and posteriorly to form the rectovaginal fascia. The condensed connective tissue fuses with, and is part of, the visceral layer of the pelvic fascia.

Vascular connections

The arterial blood supply is from the vaginal and uterine arteries, which are branches of the internal iliac artery, and which form a plexus around the organ. A median artery arises from this plexus on the anterior and on the posterior walls. The arteries are called azygous vaginal arteries (Fig. **2/9**). The venous drainage, which goes to the internal iliac veins, is from a rich venous plexus situated on the muscular

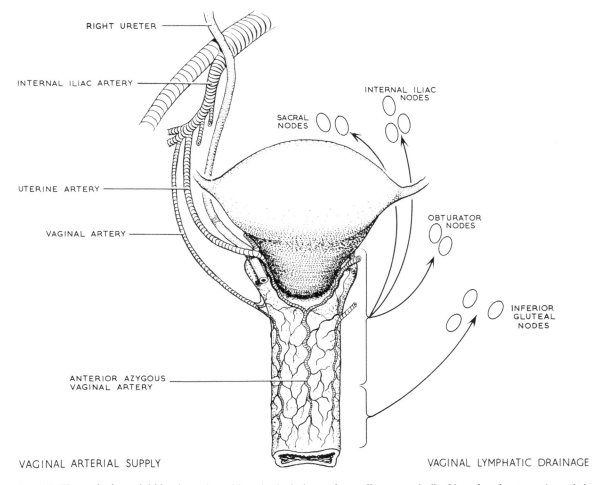

RIGHT URETER

INTERNAL ILIAC ARTERY

UTERINE ARTERY

VAGINAL ARTERY

ANTERIOR AZYGOUS VAGINAL ARTERY

INTERNAL ILIAC NODES

SACRAL NODES

OBTURATOR NODES

INFERIOR GLUTEAL NODES

VAGINAL ARTERIAL SUPPLY

VAGINAL LYMPHATIC DRAINAGE

Fig. 2/9 The vaginal arterial blood supply and lymphatic drainage shown diagrammatically. Note that the uterus is angled forward at about 90° to the vagina, and appears foreshortened

wall of the vagina, which is especially well developed at the lower end of the vagina, and which communicates with the vesical, pudendal and haemorrhoidal venous plexuses.

The lymphatic drainage of the lower third of the vagina is to the inferior gluteal nodes, near the ischial spine. Lymphatics also link with those of the upper vagina. The lymphatic drainage from the upper two-thirds of the vagina passes to the internal iliac, the obturator and the sacral nodes.

THE UTERUS

The uterus is a thick-walled, hollow, muscular organ, shaped like a pear, its apex forming the cervix which projects into the vaginal vault (Fig. **2/10**). It is located in the middle of the true pelvis, lying between the bladder and the rectum. It is flattened from before backwards, and its muscular anterior and posterior walls bulge into the cavity so that the walls are in apposition. Viewed from the front, the cavity has a triangular shape. It communicates with the peritoneal cavity via the Fallopian tubes (or oviducts) above, and with the exterior via the vaginal tube below. The uterus varies in size, being largest during the reproductive years and in women who have had children. The 'average' uterus of a nulliparous woman, measures 9cm in length, 6cm in

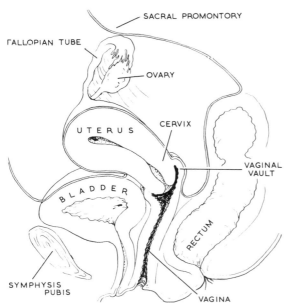

Fig. 2/10 The uterus from the side showing the anatomical relations

width at its widest part, and 4cm from before backwards, and it weighs 40 to 60g. The wall is 1 to 2cm thick, and hence the length of the cavity measures 7cm. All these dimensions are increased by about 1.5cm in women who have borne children.

Structure

Externally the uterus is covered with peritoneum on the anterior and posterior aspects, and this forms the serosal layer. Deep to the serosal layer is the muscle layer, the myometrium, which is composed of three interdigitating layers of muscle. The outer, mainly longitudinal, layer and the inner, mainly circular, layer are poorly developed, and the bulk of the myometrium is formed from the middle layer, which is composed of obliquely interdigitating strands of muscle. Deep to the myometrium is the endometrium, which is a soft layer of variable thickness made up of tubular glands, which dip into a stroma of cells held in a fine meshwork of connective tissue. A well-developed vasculature is derived from the myometrial vessels.

The uterus is made up of a *body*, or *corpus*, an *isthmus* and a *cervix* (Fig. **2/11**). The body is further divided into the area which lies above the insertion of the oviducts, and is called the *fundus*. The area where the oviducts join the uterus on each side is termed the *cornu*. The body (including the fundus) comprises the greater portion of the organ, and is formed of thick bundles of muscle. The isthmus is a constricted, annular area, 0.5cm wide, which lies between the corpus and the cervix. The proportion of muscle begins to diminish in the isthmus, and connective tissue appears in increasing amounts. The constriction at the upper end of the isthmus is called the *anatomical internal os*, and the line at the lower end of the isthmus where the endometrium changes into columnar cervical epithelium is termed the *histological internal os*. On the surface of the uterus the anatomical internal os is marked by the reflection of the peritoneum which covers the uterus, onto the superior surface of the bladder.

The *cervix* is fusiform or cylindrical in shape, and measures 3cm from above downwards, half projecting into the vagina. The proportion of muscle tissue decreases rapidly in the cervix, and in its mid portion only 10 per cent of its bulk is made of muscle, the rest being connective tissue. The supravaginal portion of the cervix is surrounded by pelvic fascia, termed the parametrium, except posteriorly where it is covered with the peritoneum of

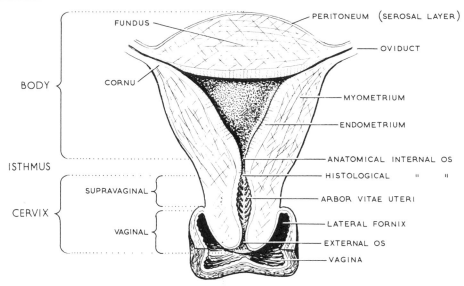

Fig. 2/11 Coronal section of the uterus showing the cavity and the cornual areas

the uterorectal pouch. The vaginal portion of the cervix is cone-shaped and projects into the vagina (Fig. **2/7**). It is covered with stratified squamous epithelium, which joins the columnar epithelium of the cervical canal at or near the external os. The cervical canal is spindle-shaped, and connects the cavity of the uterus to the vaginal cavity (Fig. **2/11**). The mucous membrane lining the canal is thrown up into anterior and posterior folds, from which circular folds radiate to give the appearance of a tree-trunk and branches. The folds are given the name *arbor vitae uteri*. The epithelium dips into the underlying stroma in a complicated system of clefts and crypts. The endocervical epithelium consists of columnar cells which secrete mucus, but the quality and quantity of this are under the control of the sex hormones.

Relations

The uterus normally lies bent forward at an angle of 90° to the direction of the vagina, but is freely mobile, rotating about a fulcrum at the level of the supravaginal cervix. Anteriorly the uterus is separated from the bladder by the vesico-uterine pouch, and posteriorly is in contact with coils of bowel and the omentum. The anterior and posterior surfaces are covered with peritoneum, but its narrow lateral surfaces are in direct contact with the broad ligament and, below, with the connective tissue, venous plexuses, arteries, nerves and the ureter, which make up the substance of the parametrium. The peritoneum which covers the anterior and posterior walls, joins at the lateral margins of the uterus to form the two leaves of the *broad ligaments*; and these two sheets of peritoneum remain in close proximity, except where they contain the ascending uterine artery, and where they diverge to accommodate the round ligament (more accurately, the round muscle) and the infundibulopelvic ligament. The broad ligament extends from the lateral uterine border to the pelvic wall. Its upper border is formed by the peritoneum covering the oviduct, and below it merges anteriorly with the peritoneum of the pelvic floor and posteriorly with the peritoneum covering the recto-uterine shelf and the uterosacral ligaments (Fig. **2/12**).

Uterine supports

These are discussed more fully in Chapter 21, but in summary are as follows: the uterus is supported from below by the muscular vagina and the fibres of the levator ani muscles which interdigitate with the middle third of the muscular vaginal sheath. An additional support of great significance is the collection of connective tissue, muscular-walled blood vessels and areolar tissue, which forms a fan-shaped sheet on each side of the supravaginal cervix, and stretches from the fascia lining the pelvic wall to join the fibromuscular cervix. This fan-shaped sheet is

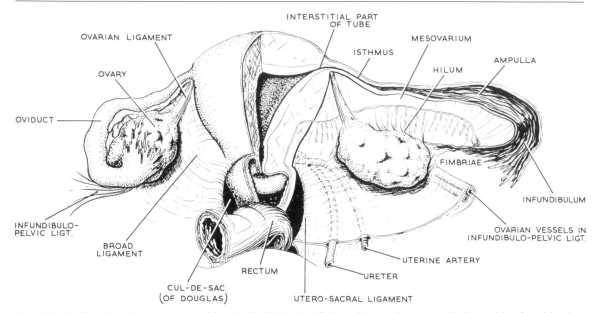

Fig. 2/12 The female pelvic organs viewed from behind. On the left the oviduct and ovary are in the position found in vivo; on the right dissection has been made

condensed posteriorly to form the *uterosacral ligaments*, and medially to form the *cardinal ligament*, or the *transverse cervical ligament* (Fig. **2/13**). Anteriorly the fascia sweeps forward down the anterior wall of the vagina beneath the bladder base. This condensation is called the pubocervical fascia. Laterally the broad ligament has a steadying effect on the uterus, whilst the round muscles play some part – although a minor one – in keeping the uterus in an anteverted position.

Vascular connections

The uterus is supplied by the uterine arteries which arise from the internal iliac artery. Each vessel runs forwards and inwards in the base of the broad ligament, and crosses the ureter above it and at right angles to it ('water *under* the bridge'), 1cm lateral to the supravaginal cervix. It gives off a descending branch which anastomoses with the ascending branches of the vaginal artery, and which supplies the lower cervix; and a circular branch to supply the upper cervix. The main trunk changes direction and passes upwards, coiled and tortuous, between the layers of the broad ligament adjacent to the lateral uterine wall, and supplies branches to the myometrium at intervals. It ends by anastomosing with the ovarian artery (Fig. **2/14**). Each branch supplying

the uterus divides, in the outer muscular layer, to send anterior and posterior branches to the myometrium, and to anastomose with those from the opposite side. These arteries give off branches at right angles, which penetrate and supply the myometrium,

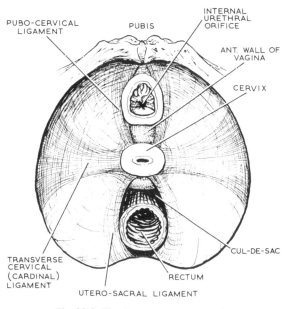

Fig. 2/13 The 'ligaments' of the cervix

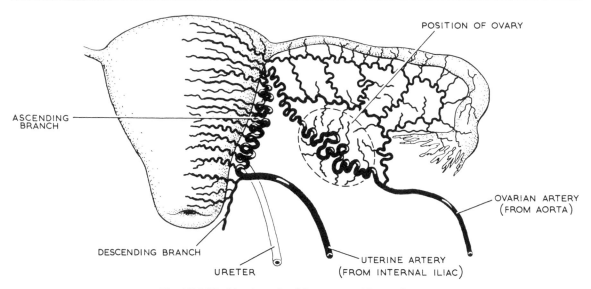

Fig. 2/14 The blood supply of the uterus, oviduct and ovary

and, entering the endometrium, form the basal arteries.

The veins of the uterus accompany the uterine artery and form pampiniform plexuses of great complexity, particularly in the parametrium where they communicate with the veins of the bladder. The pampiniform plexus drains into the uterine vein and the ovarian vein, and has communications with the vertebral plexus of veins.

Lymphatic drainage

The lymphatic drainage of the uterus consists of three communicating networks: the deepest network lies in the endometrium, the second lies in the substance of the myometrium and the superficial network is subperitoneal. The networks form collecting trunks, which pass from the corpus between the layers of the broad ligament along with the ovarian lymphatics. They then pass through the infundibulopelvic fold, and ascend on the posterior abdominal wall to join the nodes of the para-aortic group. A few channels pass along the round muscle to the superficial femoral nodes. The lowest two trunks communicate with the collecting trunks from the cervix, which pass through the base of the broad ligament to an inconstant node lateral to the parametrial node), to the nodes along the internal iliac arteries (the internal iliac or hypogastric nodes), and to the obturator nodes anteriorly. A few channels pass backwards along the uterosacral ligaments to the sacral nodes (Fig. **2/15**).

THE OVIDUCT

The oviducts, or Fallopian tubes, are two small muscular tubes, one on each side, which extend for about 10cm from the uterine cornua towards the pelvic wall, forming the upper border of the broad ligaments. The outer half of each oviduct lies in contact with the ovary, curving over its superior surface to end in the abdominal ostium. Since the tube is hollow, a direct connection exists between the peritoneal cavity and the uterus. The mucous membrane lining of the tube is thrown up into folds which almost obliterate the lumen, and which are prolonged through the abdominal ostium to form the fimbriae of the tube. The oviduct can be divided into four parts. The *infundibulum* is the outermost portion of the tube. It includes the trumpet-shaped abdominal ostium, and lies in close proximity to the ovary. The *ampulla* is the longest segment of the oviduct, is normally rather tortuous, and has a relatively thin dilatable wall. The *isthmus* is a straight, narrow, relatively thick-walled segment, and the *interstitial* portion is the short, narrow portion within the uterine wall. The size of the lumen decreases from the infundibular to the interstitial portion, where it is only 1mm in diameter; whilst the complexity of the folds in the mucous membrane increases from the interstitial to the infundibular portions (Fig. **2/16**).

The mucous membrane is lined with epithelial cells, about half of which are mucus-secreting and

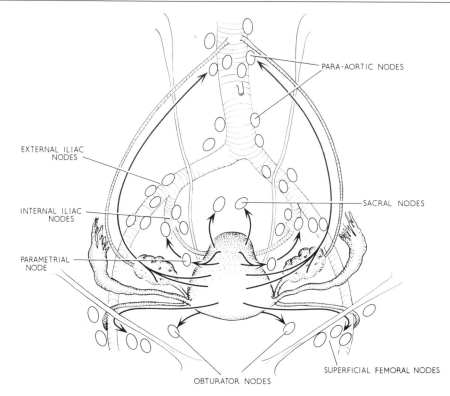

Fig. 2/15 The lymphatic drainage of the female genital organs. For clarity, the lymphatic channels have been omitted and are indicated by arrows

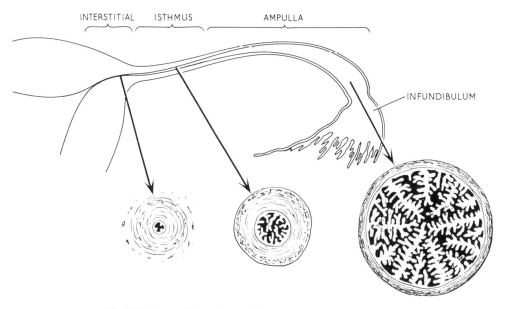

Fig. 2/16 The oviduct, showing the structure of the mucosal layer

half ciliated. The mucus secreted into the lumen is propelled towards the uterus by the action of the cilia and by peristaltic movements of the musculature of the tube. The mucus is rich in protein, and may provide nourishment for the fertilized ovum during its passage down the oviduct.

THE OVARY

The two ovaries are the homologues of the testes, and are ovoid-shaped organs. Each ovary normally lies in a shallow peritoneal fossa adjacent to the lateral pelvic wall, with its long axis in a vertical plane, but its position is influenced by movements of the uterus and broad ligament (Fig. **2/17**). The ovaries have an irregular surface, pinkish-grey in colour, and vary in size in different women, and at different times of the cycle. In the infant the ovary is a delicate, elongated structure, with a smooth, glistening surface. The ovary

of a neonate contains little stroma and mainly consists of primordial follicles. As infancy and childhood progress increasing numbers of follicles degenerate, and there is a progressive increase in stroma, up to puberty. During puberty the ovary enlarges, and in the reproductive period it averages 3.5cm in length, 2cm in breadth, 1cm in thickness, and weighs about 7g. Post-menopausally it undergoes rapid regressive changes, becoming wrinkled, white in colour and less than half the size it was in the reproductive era. Each ovary is attached to the posterior leaf of the broad ligament by a fold of peritoneum called the mesovarium, through which pass the ovarian vessels and nerves (Fig. **2/12**). The peritoneum stops where the mesovarium joins the ovary, and this part of the ovary is called the hilum. The remainder of the ovarian cortex is covered by a single layer of low columnar epithelium under which is a layer of connective tissue, called the tunica albuginea. This layer increases in density with increasing age.

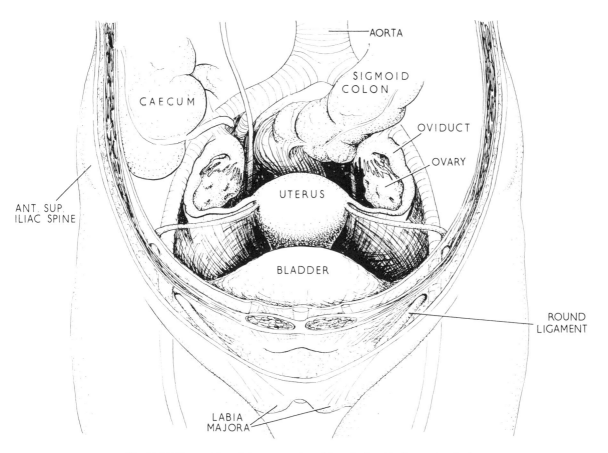

Fig. 2/17 The position of the ovary, viewed from in front in the erect patient

Vascular connections of ovary and oviduct

The arterial, venous and lymphatic connections of both ovary and oviduct are similar, and the two organs are often referred to as the *adnexae* or uterine appendages.

The *arterial* supply is from the long, slender, ovarian artery, a branch of the abdominal aorta, which arises immediately below the renal artery and crosses the inferior vena cava, the ureter and the psoas muscle on the right side, and the left psoas muscle on the left side. The vessel crosses the external iliac artery at the pelvic brim, runs between the two layers of the infundibulopelvic fold and enters the broad ligament. Within the broad ligament it runs 0.5cm below the tube, and gives off branches to the ovary via the mesovarium, and to the oviduct between the layers of the broad ligament. It ends by joining the terminal branch of the uterine artery to form an arterial arcade. The *venous drainage* is into a pampiniform plexus, and then to the ovarian veins. The right ovarian vein joins the inferior vena cava, the left ovarian vein usually enters the left renal vein.

The *lymphatics* of each adnexa drain to the para-aortic nodes, and there is some evidence of communicating trunks to the contralateral ovary via the subperitoneal lymphatic plexus of the fundus of the uterus.

The *nerve supply* of the ovary is very well developed, and arises from a sympathetic plexus which surrounds the ovarian vessels in the infundibulopelvic ligament. Its fibres derive from branches of the aortic and renal plexuses. Sensory nerves follow the arteries and are relayed in the spinal cord at the level of the tenth thoracic segment. This well-developed nerve supply accounts for the extreme sensitivity of the ovary to squeezing.

Chapter 3

Malformations of the Female Genital Tract

EMBRYOLOGICAL CONSIDERATIONS

Fertilization occurs when the male pronucleus fuses with the female pronucleus to form the zygote, which has a nucleus containing 46 chromosomes – 44 autosomes and 2 sex chromosomes – half derived from each parent. (See Appendix 1, on page 30, for further details of cell division.) At this stage the genetic sex of the new individual is established.

The formation of the gonad

By the 21st day after fertilization, the endoderm of the embryo has differentiated to form the primitive gut which is attached by a mesentery to the posterior wall of the body cavity. The body cavity is lined with mesodermal cells (the coelomic epithelium), and these cells proliferate, on either side of the root of the mesentery, to form a bulging ridge which extends the entire length of the body cavity. This is the intermediate cell mass, or the urogenital ridge (Fig. 3/1A). From it all the organs of the genito-urinary system develop, with the exception of the bladder, the urethra and the vulva.

By the 31st day, the mesodermal cells have differentiated to form mesenchyme, and this tissue further proliferates on the medial aspect of the urogenital ridge, in the cervical and thoracic regions

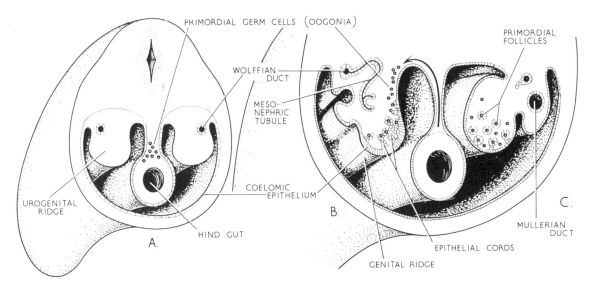

Fig. 3/1 (A) The development of the ovary. The urogenital ridge divides into a lateral portion, the tubo-ductal area and a medial portion, the genital ridge. (B) The primordial germ cells migrate into the genital ridge about 20 days after conception, and are surrounded by columns of epithelial cells from the surface of the genital ridge. (C) A later stage of development showing the primordial follicles and the Mullerian duct

of the embryo, to form the genital ridge. The genital ridge retains a covering of undifferentiated meso-dermal cells. This is the coelomic epithelium. The mesenchyme will give rise to the medulla, and the coelomic epithelium to the cortex and covering epithelium of the mature ovary. Very quickly, down-growths of cells of the covering coelomic epithelium invade the mesenchyme of the genital ridge to form epithelial cords. In the male these cords become separated from the covering epithelium, and later differentiate to form the interstitial cells, the Sertoli cells and the seminiferous tubules of the testis. In the female, a different sequence of events occurs, the columns breaking into clumps of cells which surround the primordial ova, to form the granulosa cells of the mature follicle (Fig. **3/1**B and C).

The primordial germ cells (spermatogonia and oog-onia) differentiate, at a very early stage of develop-ment, from the endoderm of the dorsal part of the hind gut (the wall of the yolk sac). They then migrate between the 20th and 30th day, passing through the mesentery of the gut to reach the genital ridge, which now forms the gonad. A theory about whether the cells become oogonia or spermatogonia suggests that this depends on their chromosomal complement. If the migrating cells contains a Y chromosome, it acts as a switch, diverting development along the male pathway and turning on a succession of male-determining genes which convert the gonads into testes. The Sertoli cells are differentiated first, followed by the Leydig cells which begin to secrete androgens. In the absence of the Y chromosome the gonad develops into an ovary. Oogonia cells are very active and multiply rapidly within the gonad, reaching a total of 7 million by the 22nd week. From this point on, cell division ceases, and there is a steady destruction of the formed cells, so that by birth only 2 million oocytes remain in each ovary, and by puberty the number has dropped to 200 000.

On entering the gonad, the oogonia become sur-rounded by the clumps of epithelial cells. These are then organized by the female evocator produced by the oogonium to form the primordial follicles. At the same time the oogonia increase in size, and nuclear maturation transforms them into oocytes. From about the 20th week, the stromal mesenchymal cells proliferate and begin to engulf and destroy any oogonia which have not acquired a protective capsule of mesodermal (epithelial) cells. They also surround the follicles to form the thecal cells. By the 28th week a number of the primordial follicles become responsive, in varying degrees, to maternal gonadotrophic hormones, and develop antra in which fluid, derived from the granulosa cells, col-lects. The primordial follicles are then called primary follicles. At the time of birth, each primary follicle contains a single germ cell (an oocyte) which begins oogenesis by initiating a reduction (meiotic) division. The first meiotic division becomes arrested in the late prophase stage until just prior to ovulation, which may occur in the case of the individual oocyte from 12 to 45 years later, or never. The second meiotic division probably occurs when the ovum is fertilized. Of the 200 000 oocytes in the ovary at puberty, 500 at most will be ovulated; the remainder will degenerate in the perimenopausal years.

It is interesting to note that the development of primordial follicles will occur if only one X chromo-some (and no Y chromosome) is present, as in Turner's syndrome (see p. 36). However, the follicles disappear during intra-uterine life unless two X chro-mosomes are present.

The male duct systems (Wolffian ducts)

In the mammalian excretory system, three successive kidneys are formed. The first, the pronephros, ap-pears in the thoracic segments of the urogenital ridge about the 24th day. The organ is made up of tubules, the medial ends of which fuse to form a duct which grows downwards to meet the cloaca (at what later becomes the prostatic urethra). This is the pronephric duct. The tubules then disappear, the duct persisting. About the 30th day, a second kidney, composed of tubules, appears in the upper abdom-inal segments, and these join with the existing pro-nephric duct to form the mesonephric (or Wolffian) duct from which the male sex duct systems are derived. Most of the mesonephric tubules disappear, but a few join the male duct system.

Meanwhile, still lower in the abdominal segments, a third and definitive kidney, the metanephros, has formed. An outgrowth from the mesonephric duct grows up to join the metanephros, forming the renal calyces, pelvis and ureter. The mesonephric (Wolf-fian) duct system develops in response to testoster-one secreted by the Leydig cells in the developing testis from about the 50th day after fertilization. In the absence of testosterone, the Wolffian duct system (the epididymis, vas deferens and seminal vesicles) fails to develop. By contrast, if the embryo is a female, only the mesonephric duct outgrowth and a few residual remnants of the mesonephric duct persist. It can be seen that a close relationship between the urinary and genital excretory system exists.

The female duct systems (Mullerian ducts)

During the period (24th to 30th day) when the pronephros is degenerating and the metanephros is forming, a fold appears in the indifferent lining of the urogenital ridge. By the 35th day a solid column of mesodermal cells (the paramesonephric duct) has formed in the fold and has grown retroperitoneally towards the cloaca.

In male embryos, development of the female duct system also begins, but is rapidly terminated, and the paramesonephric (Mullerian) ducts regress, because of an anti-Mullerian hormone (AMH) produced by the Sertoli cells in the developing testis. The effect of AMH is local, not systemic. This means that in a true intersex hermaphrodite, the excretory duct on the side of the testis will be Wolffian, the Mullerian duct having degenerated because of the local effect of AMH; whilst on the side of the ovary, the Mullerian duct is normal. Between the 35th and 40th day, in a female embryo, the Mullerian ducts have continued to grow caudally. Now the direction of growth changes and each duct grows across the midline, perhaps pulled by mesodermal fibromuscular tissue, to meet the column of cells from the other side of the body. As this occurs, the solid column becomes hollow. By the 65th day, the tubes have met in the midline and fused, the fusion beginning at the caudal end, the medial walls gradually disappearing to produce a single uterovaginal cavity. The fusion leads to a temporary overgrowth of cells at the caudal end, where the hollow tube becomes solid again, in the region of the future vagina, whilst the hollow portion forms the uterus. At the same time an ingrowth of endodermal cells from the urogenital sinus meets and fuses with the solid column of paramesonephric cells (Fig. **3/2**).

Normally at the 20th week, recanalization of the solid plugs of cells occurs. The hymen forms at the junction of the endodermal upgrowth and the paramesonephric duct downgrowth. The vagina is formed by the hollowing of the caudal portion of the paramesonephric duct, and at the upper end of this portion, recesses are hollowed out on either side of the hollow tube. These recesses, which ultimately become the vaginal fornices, mark the upper limit of the vagina. Once the hollow vagina is formed, an upgrowth of epithelium occurs from the urogenital sinus to line the vagina, the fornices and the cervix

with stratified epithelium. Thus the vaginal mucosa is formed from an ingrowth of cloacal endoderm whilst the mucosa of the tubes and uterus are formed from the canalization of coelomic mesoderm. The former becomes stratified epithelium, the latter columnar epithelium, the junction occurring in the area of the external cervical os. The cephalad portion of the fused and hollowed ducts form the uterus, and the unfused portions form the oviducts or Fallopian tubes.

The female duct system can only develop in the absence of the male duct organizer; thus in mosaics, where a Y chromosome is present, the sex is predominantly male.

The external genitalia

Up to the 45th day, the genito-urinary ducts and the gut open into a common cloacal recess. The cloaca is then divided by a septum which separates the rectal and the genito-urinary portions, the latter being surmounted by a conical protuberance, the genital tubercle. On either side of the genital tubercle, ridges develop, the genital folds; and external to them on each side swellings appear, the labioscrotal swellings. The genital tubercle forms the clitoris in the female, and the penis in the male. The genital folds form the labia minora in the female, and in the male fuse from back to front to enclose the urethral groove and to form the penile urethra. The labioscrotal swellings form the labia majora in the female and fuse to form the scrotum in the male (Fig. **3/3**). The testes only descend from the abdominal cavity into the scrotum close to the time of birth.

The indifferent primordia of the external genitalia will invariably feminize unless subjected to the influence of androgen between the 60th and 70th days of fetal life. In the normal male the androgen is derived from the interstitial cells of the fetal testes which begin to secrete hormones at the 22nd day of gestation, even before the gonad is recognizable as a testis. In the female fetus, should androgen be produced by an abnormally active fetal adrenal gland, or transferred across the placenta from the maternal circulation, before the 12th week of fetal life, the external genitalia will exhibit varying degrees of masculinization. The growth and development of the cells forming the cloaca and its conversion into male external genitalia, depends on dy-hydrotestosterone (DHT). DHT is formed in the cells of the prostate and cloaca from testosterone by the

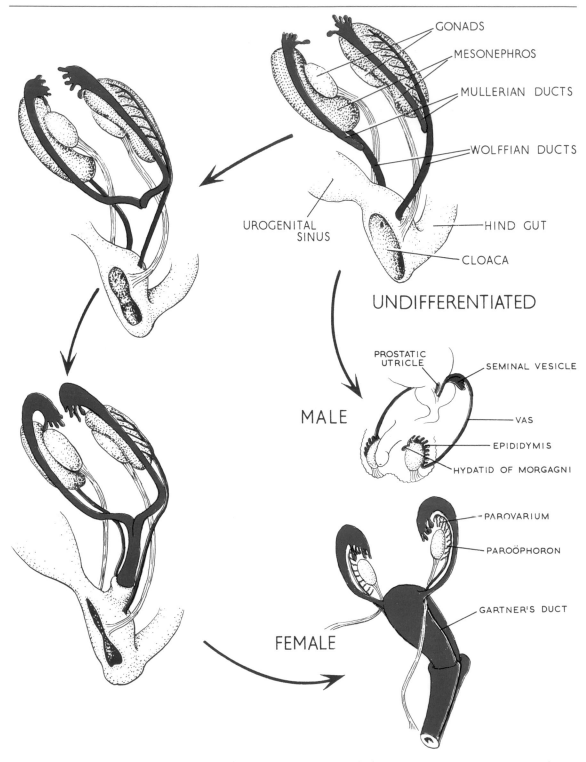

Fig. 3/2 The development of the genital organs, from the Mullerian duct in the female and the Wolffian duct in the male

7   11   40

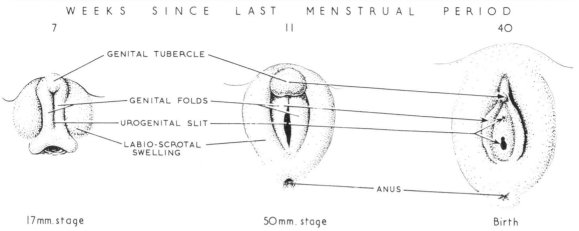

17mm. stage   50mm. stage   Birth

Fig. 3/3 Differentiation of the female external genitalia, shown diagrammatically (not to scale)

action of 5 α-reductase. In a few chromosomal males, the cells of the cloaca (and the prostate) lack 5 α-reductase, with the result that the external genitalia fail to masculinize and remain female in appearance. These men have normal Wolffian duct development (epididymis, vas deferens and seminal vesicles).

Other chromosomal males have a total tissue resistance to testosterone and to DHT, so that the Wolffian ducts fail to develop, and the external genitalia are female. The infant is brought up as a girl. The condition is called testicular feminization or androgen insensitivity (see p. 37).

The bladder and urethra

The bladder and urethra form from the anterior part of the urogenital sinus at a time when the posterior, or vaginal, part is still a solid ingrowth of cells. The cells forming the bladder proliferate and join with the downgrowths of paramesonephric duct cells which have formed the ureters.

CHROMOSOMAL SEX AND SEXUAL DIFFERENTIATION

Each cell in the body normally has a nucleus containing 46 chromosomes arranged in 23 pairs. Of these, 22 pairs are concerned with somatic characteristics (autosomes) and two are concerned with sexual characteristics. In the female the two sex chromosomes are similar, shaped like an X with shorter upper arms, and are known consequently as X chromosomes. In the male, one chromosome is an X chromo-

some, the other a much smaller Y-shaped chromosome. Just after ovulation the ovum completes the first meiotic division started so long before. This produces two daughter cells, each with a nucleus containing 22 autosomes and one X sex chromosome. There is an unequal division of cytoplasm, and the smaller cell is pressed closely to the zona pellucida and consequently is called the 'polar body'. Should fertilization occur, a second meiotic division results, and a second polar body is extruded, leaving the female pronucleus with a complement of 23 chromosomes (see p. 31). The spermatozoon, as a result of reduction division, also has 23 chromosomes, one of which is either an X or a Y chromosome. It is only by chance that an X-carrying spermatozoon, or a Y-carrying spermatozoon, penetrates the zona pellucida of the ovum and forms the male pronucleus. Once the male and female pronuclei fuse, the cells of the zygote contain 46 chromosomes once more. If there are 44 autosomes and XX sex chromosomes, the individual will be a female; if 44 autosomes and XY sex chromosomes, the individual will be a male. With each successive mitotic division, the new cells formed will normally have 46 chromosomes. In a few cases, however, the cleavage of the sex chromosomes in one of the two meiotic divisions is impaired, either failing to occur, extra pieces entering one cell, or a piece of one chromosome being displaced and translocated to join another (Fig. 3/4). These errors may involve the autosomes or the sex chromosomes, but it is the latter with which we are concerned here. For example, if cleavage fails to occur, a strain of cell line will be formed which only contains 45 chromosomes – 44 autosomes and a single sex

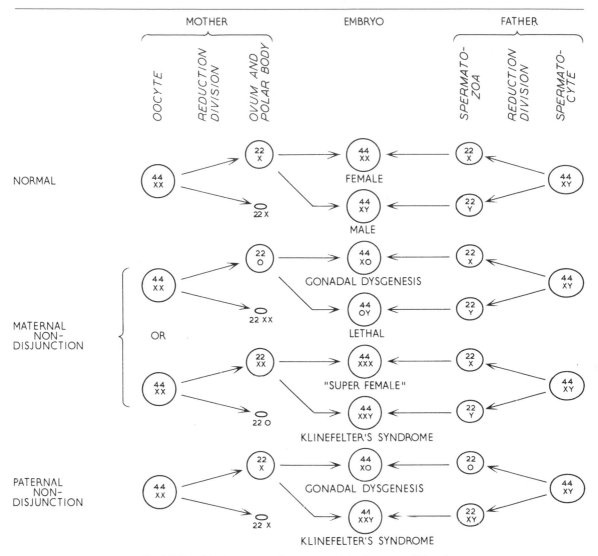

Fig. 3/4 Possible chromosomal pattern resulting from non-disjunction

chromosome. On the other hand, if the extra pieces of the X or the Y chromosomes enter one cell line, these cells will now contain 47, 48 or 49 chromosomes, made up of 44 autosomes and XXX, XXY, XXXX, XXXY or XXYY sex chromosomes.

A further chromosomal error occurs when two cell lines of different sex chromosomes content develop in the same person, forming different tissues. In the more severe forms this can produce marked errors in sexual development. The condition is called mosaicism. Although the combinations are many, most are lethal, and only a few have been encountered in clinical practice, examples being XY/XO and XY/XXY. Occasionally two spermatozoa may

fertilize a single ovum. If one spermatozoa is carrying an X chromosome and the other a Y chromosome, the individual will have tissues formed from each cell line, and will have a chromosomal mosaicism of XY/XX. Such individuals are true hermaphrodites.

These abnormalities can be investigated by examining the sex chromatin pattern of epithelial cells or leucocytes, or more completely by studying cultures of leucocytes whose development has been arrested at metaphase, when the chromosomes are most visible. A photograph of the array of chromosomes can be used to match those of similar size on the basis of length. Such a display is called a *karyotype*.

Sex chromatin pattern – the X chromosome

A much more simple, but less exact, investigation is to examine epithelial cells for the sex chromatin pattern. As has been noted, all normal female cells contain two X chromosomes. During interphase, one of these becomes tightly coiled, in contrast to the autosomes and the other X chromosome. In addition, it usually migrates to lie close to the nuclear plasma membrane, and on suitable staining is clearly visible as a dark dot 1 to 2μm in diameter. Since the dot (Barr body) represents the second X chromosome, it will not be found in the male. (Appendix 2, on page 32, gives further details of sex chromatin.) In children with ambiguous external genitalia, an examination of buccal mucosal cells gives a clear indication of the chromosomal sex. One hundred nuclei are counted. If Barr bodies are seen in more than 25 per cent of the cells, the individual is a female; if between 1 and 20 cells have Barr bodies, the individual may have mosaicism; whilst if there are no Barr bodies present, the individual is male (Fig. **3/5**).

The Y chromosome

The most powerful evocator of sex differentiation is the Y chromosome, which initially determines the nature of the gonad. The presence of the Y chromosome in the interstitial mesenchymal cells leads to the production of a male duct organizer, which stimulates the development of the male duct systems, whilst causing the female sex ducts to regress. In the absence of this substance, the genital ducts will feminize, whether an ovary is present or not. The male duct organizer has no influence on the differentiation of the external genitalia, which is primarily under the influence of androgen.

If the ovary has no germ cells, as in gonadal dysgenesis, the gonad remains asexual and is rudimentary. But since no Y chromosome is present, and consequently no male duct organizer, the direction of sexual differentiation is to the female side of neuter. As a general principle, demonstrating the pre-eminence of the Y chromosome in sexual differentiation, it can be said that 'femininity is a neuter state, and masculinity is a superimposed characteristic'. Thus if the testicles are destroyed or removed prior to puberty, the individual becomes feminine in many characteristics. If, on the other hand, the ovaries are removed, the woman does not become masculinized.

The abnormalities described may lead to ambigu-

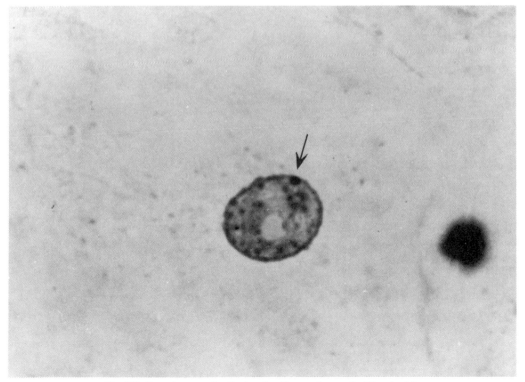

Fig. 3/5 Buccal mucosal cells showing the sex chromatin (Barr body)

ous genitalia, which should be investigated at birth, or to amenorrhoea which requires investigation in adolescence. These are discussed in Chapter 27 and in Chapter 28.

MALFORMATIONS OF THE GENITAL TRACT

From the embryological considerations just discussed, several facts can be deduced:

1. The development of the gonad is separate from that of the sex ducts, and may be normal in function even if the ducts are absent, or abnormal.
2. The close developmental connection between the genital duct system and the urinary duct system, makes it probable that a malformation of the uterus will be associated with a malformation of the ureter or kidney.
3. Abnormalities of the external genitalia may be found in association with normal internal genitalia, the error being in the response of the tissue to androgens.

Errors of sinus canalization

The main defect is that of '*imperforate hymen*'. This can always be detected if the child is examined at the time of birth, but this inspection is often omitted. In a few cases of 'imperforate hymen', mucus collects in the vagina of the young child, but generally the condition causes no disturbance until puberty, when menstruation fails to appear, although the child complains of periodic pains. With each successive menstruation, blood collects behind the obstructing membrane and, since the serum is partially absorbed, it becomes inspissated. However, with each successive menstruation there is a progressive increase in amount. This is called *cryptomenorrhoea*. Eventually over the months, or years, the vagina becomes distended with blood (*haematocolpos*) and the membrane bulges forward, tinted blue by the underlying blood. In advanced cases, blood may distend the uterus and even the tubes (Fig. **3/6**).

Examination of the girl may reveal a swelling rising from the pelvis into the abdomen, a blue bulging membrane in the vulva and a distended vagina detected on rectal examination. The treatment is to incise the membrane in a cruciate way, and to

prevent the introduction of infection into the vagina as the blood is a potent culture medium.

Less common defects encountered are complete or partial vaginal atresia, and a partial transverse membrane, which usually occurs in the upper vagina. Vaginal atresia may also be acquired, particularly in the rural areas of some Third World countries, where the vagina is packed with rock salt after childbirth to 'give it more tone' for subsequent coitus. The result is often disastrous, a narrow stenosed tube replacing the normal vagina.

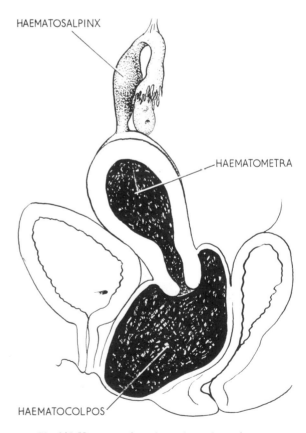

Fig. **3/6** Haematocolpos due to imperforate hymen

Failure of re-canalization of the Mullerian ducts

This will lead to atresia of the upper vagina or of the cervix.

Failure of fusion of the Mullerian ducts

In the most extreme and extremely rare form, failure of fusion of the Mullerian ducts lead to a double uterus, a double cervix and two vaginae opening into a common vulva, or into two vulvae. In most cases, however, the failure of fusion is of less marked degree, and can lead to a variety of deformities of varying significance (Fig. 3/7). Those most frequently encountered are septate vagina, uterus subseptus and uterus bicornis, unicollis. These malformations are relatively common, but often are not recognized as they are symptomless. If the uterus is bicornute, the horns may be of equal size or one may be much smaller and connected tenuously to the cervix. Should a pregnancy occur in this rudimentary horn, rupture is certain and haemorrhage will be severe. If the cavity has failed to canalize at its lower connecting end, menstruation will be dammed in the rudimentary horn, causing a haematometra and increasing dysmenorrhoea. The rudimentary horn is usually misdiagnosed as a predunculated submucous myoma, which is undergoing intermittent torsion.

The malformations do not usually reduce fertility, and should the woman become pregnant, they may cause complications which lead to their detection. Late abortion and premature labour are common because of poor implantation or because the abnormal uterus is more sensitive to stimuli. Malpresentations are frequent, especially in uterus subseptus,

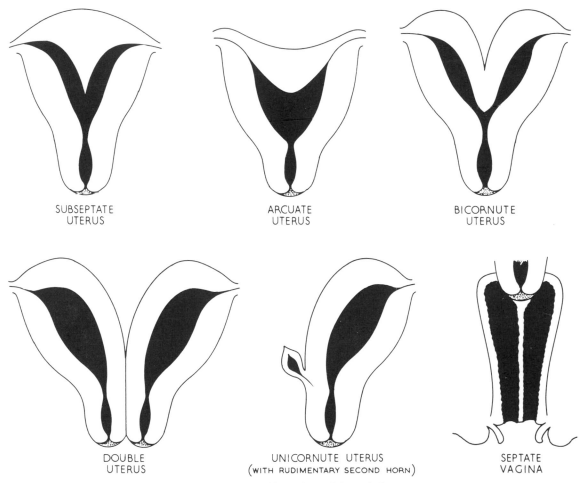

SUBSEPTATE UTERUS

ARCUATE UTERUS

BICORNUTE UTERUS

DOUBLE UTERUS

UNICORNUTE UTERUS (WITH RUDIMENTARY SECOND HORN)

SEPTATE VAGINA

Fig. 3/7 Common malformations of the genital tract

when transverse presentation is often found. If one horn of a bicornute uterus (particularly if of the bicornute, bicollis type) falls behind the horn in which the conception sac has grown, it may cause an obstructed labour. In all forms, retained placenta is usual and postpartum haemorrhage likely to occur.

Examination of the patient after delivery may show the presence of two cervices, or the uterus may appear abnormally broad in the fundal area. A hysterosalpingogram will demonstrate the deformity.

Treatment depends upon the degree of abnormality and whether it has interfered with coitus or pregnancy. Vaginal septa are best removed, as is the rudimentary horn of a uterus bicornis. When a bicornute or septate uterus has been shown to be the cause of three abortions or curtailed pregnancies, plastic surgery may be considered. An operation is performed to excise the septum or to reconstruct the two uteri into a single organ. This procedure is called utriculoplasty.

Failure of development of one or both Mullerian ducts

The absence of both ducts means that neither oviducts nor uterus is present. Amenorrhoea will be present and no treatment is available. The absence of one duct leads to a unicornute uterus, with a single oviduct attached; whilst incomplete development of one duct will give a similar uterine appearance but both oviducts will be present. Strictly speaking, there is only half of the normal vagina, but functionally it is normal. The conditions are usually symptomless, but complications may arise in pregnancy. In these cases late abortion, premature labour and breech presentation tend to occur more frequently, and the diagnosis is often only made following these events.

Persistence of male (Wolffian) duct remnants

Remnants of Wolffian ducts or tubules are fairly common, and may enlarge to form cysts of the hydatid of Morgagni in the mesovarium, or cysts between the leaves of the broad ligament. Other less common remnants may lead to cysts deep in the lateral vaginal wall (Gartner's duct cysts), in the labia minora close to the clitoris, or around the urethra.

Abnormalities of the external genitalia

The size of the labia minora varies considerably, and in some women these are large. In children, whose mothers have received androgens in pregnancy, fusion of the labia may occur. The fused labia are easily separated digitally, and should be smeared with oestrogen cream for some weeks after the separation (see Chapter 27). Androgens, either endogenous from congenital adrenal hyperplasia, or iatrogenically administered in pregnancy, can cause clitoral enlargement. The external genitals of the newborn child may be so ambiguous in appearance that it is difficult to assign it to either sex. This is discussed further in Chapter 4. Rarely the anus is found to open into the vestibule or the lower vagina, the rectal septum having failed to develop. In a few of these cases the anal orifice is constricted in the neonate, and must be enlarged to secure free egress of faeces. This can be obtained by dilatation or by surgical incision. Further plastic surgery is not required as sphincter control is excellent, vaginal contamination with faecal matter is uncommon, and the abnormality does not interfere with coitus or render it less satisfactory.

APPENDIX 1

CELL DIVISION

As is known, the nucleus of each cell which forms the organism, whether plant or animal, contains a number of chromosomes specific to that species. The chromosomes are formed of DNA linked to histones, and contain all the genetic material required to reproduce the organism. However, except for the germ cells, most of the material is masked and only that necessary to carry out the specific functions of the cell is revealed.

Cellular reproduction is not confined to the actual division, and for a specific period during the interval between cell divisions, processes are going on building up the DNA and protein content of the nucleus. But what triggers off the actual division of the cell is largely unknown. Normal somatic cellular division is a mitotic process, each daughter cell containing the normal (diploid) number of chromosomes for that species. The sex, or germ, cells undergo a different type of division, which is compensatory in character, so that the daughter cells have only half the normal chromosomal content (haploid). This is meiotic division, and during it exchange of genetic material occurs, so that the daughter cell – the ovum or the spermatozoon – expresses genetic characteristics different from its parents. Since both ovum and spermatozoon have a haploid number of chromosomes, fertilization restores the diploid complement to the new individual.

The meiotic cycle

In the first stage of meiosis the skein-like mass of chromatin separates into individual chromosomes which shorten and thicken, darker areas appearing. Soon all the chromosomes have appeared and lie very closely paired to each other, the darker areas of each member corresponding exactly in position. The paired chromosomes become even shorter and thicker, and each chromosome then splits longitudinally to form two daughter chromatids, the result being a twisted, meshed, four-strand formation, known as a tetrad. At this stage a crossing-over of genetic material occurs between the non-sister chromatids (chiasma formation). The four chromatids then join up again to form two chromosomes, which, however, have a new genetic constitution (Fig. **3/8**). The homologous pairs of chromosomes next separate towards opposite poles of the spindle, a process known as disjunction, and as a result when the first meiotic cell division occurs, two cells are produced each containing 23 chromosomes, but have different genetic constitutions. In the female germ cells, the cytoplasm divides unequally, and the cell containing only a small amount is called the first polar body.

In the second meiotic division (which occurs only after the sperm has penetrated the ovum), the chromosomes shorten and then split into two daughter chromatids, which are drawn to opposite ends of the spindle. With cell division each new cell has 23 chromosomes, but once again cytoplasmic division is unequal, and the cell with only a small amount is referred to as the second polar body. Thus the female at the end of this division has an ovum, and two polar bodies.

In the male the cytoplasm divides equally at each meiotic division and four spermatozoa are formed, each with 23 chromosomes.

Should the homologous sex chromosomes fail to separate at anaphase of either division, non-disjunction occurs. One of the cells will have an

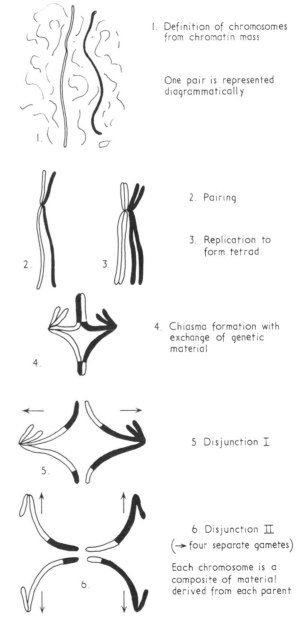

1. Definition of chromosomes from chromatin mass

One pair is represented diagrammatically

2. Pairing

3. Replication to form tetrad

4. Chiasma formation with exchange of genetic material

5 Disjunction I

6. Disjunction II
(→ four separate gametes)

Each chromosome is a composite of material derived from each parent

Fig. 3/8 Schematic representation of pairing of chromosomes and chiasma formation

extra sex chromosome, and the other will lack a sex chromosome. This is the explanation of several malformations, and the individual may have a sex chromosomal constitution of XXX, XXY or XO (YO is lethal). (See Fig. **3/4**, p. 26.)

Autosomal injury may also occur during the exchange of genetic material, fragments being deleted, translocated or fragmented. These will produce phenotypic abnormalities, one of these being 21-trisomy or Down's syndrome.

The mitotic cycle

By contrast to meiosis, mitosis, the normal way the cells of the body reproduce, is a simple process. In *prophase* the chromatin appears as a tangled skein which condenses into filaments of separate chromosomes. Soon the nuclear membrane disappears, leaving the chromosomes free in the cytoplasm as well-defined loops. A spindle then forms which grows to full size, the chromosomes lying in a median plane (the equatorial plane) where the spindle is widest. This is called *metaphase*. The chromosome then splits longitudinally, and each daughter chromatid is drawn towards its spindle pole (*anaphase*), and simultaneously the cleavage of the cell begins. This is completed and the spindle disappears, the chromosomes at the spindle pole clumping (*telophase*). The nuclear membrane reforms, the chromosomes disperse, and new nucleoli appear, which persist until the next cell division (Fig. **3/9**). Cells are not able to reproduce again at once, and the postmitotic phase may be permanent (as in ganglion cells of the central nervous system or epithelial cells), temporary as in granulocytes, or of variable length as in most cells of the body, a further mitotic division occurring when conditions are suitable. In cells which can replicate, the postmitotic phase is followed by *interphase*, when the processes leading to a further mitotic division are proceeding. During both the postmitotic phase and interphase, the other, non-reproductive, processes in the cell continue normally.

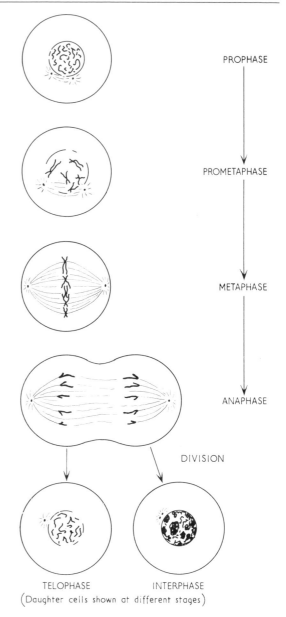

Fig. 3/9 Mitosis in animal cells

APPENDIX 2

THE FORMATION OF CHROMATIN CLUMPS – BARR BODIES

It was noted on page 25 that in the male each somatic cell has a constitution of 46 chromosomes, of which 44 are autosomes and two are sex chromosomes, one of which is termed an X chromosome, and the other a Y chromosome. In the female, each cell contains 44 autosomes and two identical sex chromosomes, which have an XX pattern. The Y chromosome is small and apparently has no function other than to contain genetic material responsible for testicular development. The female, on the other hand, has two large X chromosomes and each of the cells therefore has a 'double dose' of every gene located on the X chromosome. This genetically should produce odd results, but phenotypically the facts are otherwise, and the dilemma has been resolved by Lyon. In an hypothesis (the Lyon Hypothesis), she suggested that at a certain stage of embryonic life, probably before the 10th day, one of the X chromosomes in every somatic cell is inactivated and takes no further part in directing cellular activities. In the germ cells, however, it remains active, directing sex chromatin formation. In somatic cells the inactive X chromosome contracts, becomes tightly coiled and migrates to the nuclear membrane, where it can be seen during interphase, with suitable staining, as a dark spot – or Barr body.

Chromatin clumps are found in all body cells, but the mucosal cells from the buccal pouch or the white blood cells are the easiest to investigate. The investigation is of importance as 1 in 300 live-born children has an abnormality involving the X chromosome, and the following children should be investigated:

1. Any child with ambiguous or abnormal external genitalia.
2. Any child underdeveloped at birth which fails to thrive or is mentally retarded.
3. Female children with a lump in the inguinal canal.
4. Male children with hypospadias and an abnormally small penis.

The method is to take a smear from the inside of the cheek with a metal spatula which has a fairly sharp edge. The smear is spread thickly, and fixed in 95% ethyl alcohol at once. It is then stained with Feulgen's stain after hydrolysis with hydrochloric acid, and 100 nuclei are counted. To avoid errors, only flat, oval nuclei with well-dispersed chromatin and a well-defined nuclear membrane should be counted.

Normal unselected females from whom buccal or vaginal smears are taken have sex chromatin (Barr bodies) in 20 to 40 per cent of the cells examined. In infants with ambiguous genitals, if no Barr bodies are found, the infant is male; if more than 25 per cent of the cells have a Barr body, the infant is female; if between 1 and 20 of the cells have Barr bodies, the infant may have a mosaicism.

Chapter 4

Intersex

Intersex is a condition of imperfect sexual differentiation into either male or female. The genetic sex is the index. Thus a genetic female with male external genitalia (and perhaps male secondary sexual characteristics) is a female intersex (or female pseudo-hermaphrodite); and a genetic male with feminine external genitalia is a male intersex. The incidence of intersex is 2 to 3 per 1000. However, the intersexuality may be modified in either the male or female direction by gender sex, which is determined by the assigned sex at rearing, by appearance and social deportment, and by the direction of the sex drive. Gender sex is not an inherited characteristic, but is acquired early in life by the way the child is reared, by the way its parents and others significant to it treat it during the first three or four years of its life. The attitudes and behaviours of other people to the child enable it to behave in a way congruent to its assigned sex, in other words, enable it to develop a gender-role. It behaves as it believes a boy or girl should behave and receives praise when it behaves in the congruent way.

Shortly after establishing its gender-role the child acquires a gender-identity. It now *knows* internally that it is a boy or a girl and that this will persist to a greater or lesser degree.

Once the gender-identity has been established it is almost impossible to change it.

CLASSIFICATION OF INTERSEX

Abnormalities in sexual differentiation may derive from (1) errors in chromosomal sex, (2) errors in development of the sexual ducts due to absence of the male duct organizer, (3) anomalies in the appearance of the external genitalia or the secondary sexual characteristics, and (4) anomalies in the gender sex due to psychological influences.

Intersex may be detected at birth, or at puberty when menstruation fails to occur, or occasionally, incidentally, in later life (Table **4/1**).

Intersex detected at birth

If at the routine examination made soon after birth, the external genitalia are ambiguous; if the penis is excessively small; or if a penile urethra or hypospadias is present and no testes are palpable in the scrotum, further investigation of the child for intersex is mandatory. The investigation should include a careful history of events affecting the mother in pregnancy, and with special reference to administration of progestogens, and a history of other siblings, particularly if any died soon after birth. A rectal examination is made to identify a uterus. Buccal smears are taken to detect Barr bodies, and in special cases serum 17–OH progesterone and androgens (testosterone and precursors) are measured.

Four main types of intersex can be discerned at birth:

1. Female intersex due to congenital adrenal hyperplasia (1 in 20 000 births).
2. Female intersex due to the transfer from the mother to the fetus of certain progestogens, usually iatrogenically administered.
3. Male intersex with partially masculinized external genitalia, in which the defective development is caused by inadequacy or absence of response to the normal androgenic stimulus from the fetal testis (testicular feminization).
4. True hermaphroditism, in which both ovarian and testicular tissues are present, and which is very rare.

Most cases seen are due to congenital adrenal hyperplasia, a few are due to other causes, and are together called the 'adreno-genital syndrome'. This condition is considered further in Chapter 27.

	Chromosomal sex	Nuclear sex	Genital ducts	External genitalia	Secondary sex characteristics	Associated anomalies	When diagnosed
Female intersex							
Adreno-genital syndrome							
a. Congenital adrenal hyperplasia	XX	Positive	Mullerian	Ambiguous to male	Female if treated; otherwise male	Familial disorder 17-hydroxyprogesterone and androstendione raised	Infancy
b. Maternal ingestion of androgenic gestagens	XX	Positive	Mullerian	Ambiguous to male	Female	17-hydroxyprogesterone and androstendione levels normal History of drugs	Infancy
Turner's syndrome	XO	Negative	Mullerian	Female	Infantile	Dwarfism, webbed neck, broad chest	Childhood
Gonadal dysgenesis	XO mosaics	Doubtful	Mullerian	Usually female	Infantile	Normal height	Puberty
Male intersex							
a. Feminizing testicular syndrome	XY	Negative	Wolffian	Female	Female	Absent or sparse pubic hair. Sex-linked anomaly, i.e. other members in family will have the anomaly	Puberty or later
b. Male intersex with partially masculinized external genitalia	XY	Negative	Wolffian rarely Mullerian	Ambiguous	Infantile	None	Infancy childhood
c. Seminiferous tubular dysgenesis (Klinefelter's syndrome)	XXY or XXXY	Positive	Wolffian	Male	Eunuchoid to complete virilism	Mental deficiency common. Gynaecomastia; somatic defects	Puberty later
True hermaphroditism	XX/XY mosaic	Positive (2/3) Negative (1/3)	Wolffian and Mullerian	Ambiguous (male)	Variable	Occasionally autosomal anomalies are present	Infancy Puberty

Table 4/1 A classification of intersexual anomalies

Intersex detected at puberty

In most cases of male intersex (male pseudoherma-phrodites) and of gonadal dysgenesis the child is brought up as a girl, and the true state of affairs is only detected at puberty when menstruation fails to occur. All forms are uncommon, but gonadal dysgenesis is nearly ten times as frequent as male inter-sex with partial masculinized external genitalia, or as testicular feminization. A few cases of female intersex are detected at this time, and are mainly due to an attenuated form of congenital adrenal hyperplasia, to adrenal tumours, or virilizing ovarian tumours.

INVESTIGATIONS

The *family history* may reveal that other members of the family have either congenital adrenal hyperplasia or testicular feminization. These conditions are due to genetic defects, testicular feminization being inherited as an X-linked recessive or a male-limited autosomal dominant. Thus half the males in the family are affected.

Examination of the internal and external genitalia will define the degree of anomaly. Nuclear sex and chromosomal sex studies will further identify the condition. Laboratory investigations include the measurement of plasma androgens and 17-hydroxy-progesterone, if necessary after ACTH or HCG ad-ministration (see p. 259).

In a few cases, laparotomy is required to make a firm diagnosis.

GONADAL DYSGENESIS

In gonadal dysgenesis, primordial germ cells reach the ovary but are destroyed progressively so that by the time of puberty few remain. This means that little oestrogen is secreted, the girl is severely hypo-oestrogenic and her secondary sex characteristics fail to develop. She is also sterile, and likely to develop osteoporosis at an early age. Two forms have been described: *'pure' gonadal dysgenesis*, in which genital hypoplasia is found in an apparently normal girl who has poor breast development; and *Turner's syn-drome*, in which the genital hypoplasia is associated with short stature, shield chest, webbed neck and a variety of other deformities (Fig. **4/1**). In 'pure' gonadal dysgenesis, the sex chromosome pattern is a mosaic, usually XO/XX, whilst in Turner's syndrome

the pattern is XO. Because of the diminished oe-strogen levels, FSH levels are raised after puberty, whilst the internal genitalia remain immature and the external genitalia and the breasts remain inf-antile. If an adolescent girl presents with amenor-rhoea and is of short stature, gonadal dysgenesis should be suspected.

Most girls who have gonadal dysgenesis are short in stature because of poor growth consequent on a decreased secretion of human growth hormone (hGH). The lack of stature becomes noticeable at puberty when the expected growth spurt fails to occur. The diagnosis is made by finding raised plasma levels of FSH and LH and low levels of oestrogen. It is confirmed by a karyotype of blood cells.

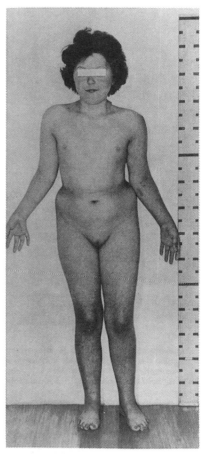

Fig. 4/1 Gonadal dysgenesis (Turner's syndrome). The patient is of short stature, has a 'webbed' neck and cubitus valgus, and is sexually infantile. Pelvic examination showed a vagina, a rudimentary uterus, but palpable gonads. (By kind permission of the Author and the Publishers of 'Triangle', *The Sandoz Journal of Medical Science*, 1967, **8**, 37.)

Treatment to increase the girl's height should begin at diagnosis: hGH, 0.2 micrograms/kg, is given three times a week. Some physicians also give an anabolic steroid (oxandrolone) which may increase the effect of hGH. An oestrogen is also given so that the breasts and genital tract develop. Usually ethinyl oestradiol at a dose of 5 micrograms is given daily for the first year, when the dose is increased to 10 or 20 micrograms. If a larger dose is required, a progestogen should also be prescribed for 14 days each month. The hormones need to be continued at least until the age of 60 to maintain bone density and prevent osteoporosis.

It is important to counsel the girl, reassuring her of the benefits of hormone medication to help her develop secondary sex characteristics, and helping her to accept her short stature and her sterility. The physician should stress that neither her height nor her sterility will diminish her enjoyment of her sexuality or her adaptation to a full and pleasurable life.

TESTICULAR FEMINIZATION
(Congenital androgenic insensitivity)

These patients are genotypic males but phenotypic females as far as their external genitalia and androgen metabolism are concerned. The gonads are morphological testes, and the anti-Mullerian hormone (AMH) has been produced by the Sertoli cells, so that Mullerian duct development is suppressed. Although the Leydig cells secrete testosterone, the cytoplasmic receptors in target tissues are unable to bind testosterone (because of an X-linked gene), so that the individual is androgen-resistant and phenotypically female. In consequence, the external genitalia are feminine, but because the Mullerian duct has failed to develop, the vagina ends as a short blind pouch. No uterus is present and the testes are found in a hernial sac or may be intra-abdominal in position. As the testes are liable to malignant change, they should be removed once puberty has occurred. Removal prior to puberty may be followed by severe climacteric symptoms. At puberty the breasts develop and there is a female distribution of body fat. Some body hair may appear, but it is usually scanty. The individual resembles a normal female (Fig. 4/2). These changes are due to the unopposed action of small quantities of oestrogen synthesized in the adrenals.

SEMINIFEROUS TUBULAR DYSGENESIS (Klinefelter's syndrome)

Klinefelter's syndrome affects approximately 1 in 1000 newborn males. The males have an extra X chromosome (47, XXY) or have a 46, XY/XXY mosaic (1 in 10 000 newborn males). Those affected tend to be taller than other children or adolescents, mainly because of longer legs, and may have a delay in speech development. After puberty, which is delayed in nearly half of the boys, they tend to have smaller testicles, and often a small penis. Thirty per cent develop gynaecomastia. During the years of growth, they tend to be shy, clumsy, lonely, to have low self-esteem and are pliant. In adult life they have a low libido. The libido may be improved by testosterone therapy. Boys with Klinefelter's syndrome need sympathetic support, counselling and encouragement to become more confident and assertive.

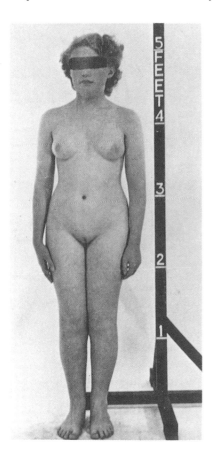

Fig. 4/2 Testicular feminization. Although apparently a female, the vagina ends in a blind pouch and the gonad is, in fact, a testis. (Reprinted from the *Brit. Med. J.*, 1955, **1**, 1174, by permission of the Author (Dr C. N. Armstrong) and Editor.)

Chapter 5

The Menstrual Cycle and Menstruation

PHYSIOLOGICAL CONCEPTS

During childhood the hypothalamus and pituitary gland are relatively quiescent, only small quantities of the trophic hormones being secreted. This quiescence comes to an end in the 2 or 3 years prior to puberty, when unknown stimuli act upon the hypothalamus causing it to produce trophic-releasing hormones. The trophic-releasing hormones, which are decapeptides, stimulate the pituitary gland to release hormones into the general circulation, and these act upon several endocrine glands to initiate the spurt of development which precedes puberty. Two of the hormones released are important in gynaecology. These are the *follicle-stimulating hormone* (FSH) and the *luteinizing (or interstitial cell-stimulating) hormone* (LH or ICSH); and it is their direct action upon the ovary which leads to the initiation of menstruation.

An important concept in this regard is to remember that the hypothalamus, the pituitary gland and the ovaries are intimately connected, and an abnormality of function in one will influence the function of the other two (Fig. **5/1**).

THE HYPOTHALAMUS–PITUITARY COMPLEX

The primary importance of the hypothalamus has been recognized in the regulation of ovulation. However, it is influenced in turn, by the emotions from higher cerebral centres and by feedback from the ovaries, so that the control of ovulation and the regulation of menstruation is complex.

The initial stimulus is due to the release of gonadotrophic releasing (or regulating) hormone, GnRH, into the hypophyseal portal vessels. GnRH reaches the anterior pituitary where it is involved in the production of FSH and LH in basophilic gonadotroph cells and in the release of the hormones from those cells. GnRH is released in a pulsatile manner in the reproductive years. The interval between pulses varies during the menstrual cycle. In the follicular phase pulses occur at 90-minute intervals, in the periovulatory period at 60-minute intervals and in the luteal phase at 200-minute intervals. The pulsatile release of GnRH stimulates the pituitary gonadotrophes to synthesize and release FSH and small quantities of LH.

Follicle-stimulating hormone is a glycoprotein. As its name implies, it stimulates the growth and maturation of between 10 and 20 primary follicles in the ovary each menstrual cycle. The number stimulated seems to be dependent upon the quantity of FSH released. (In the male, FSH stimulates the growth of the seminiferous tubules and spermatogenesis.)

The stimulated follicles mature and secrete increasing amounts of oestradiol probably because LH stimulates the theca interna cells of the developing follicles to secrete androstenedione. Androstenedione then diffuses into the granulosa cells of the follicles, where it is converted into oestradiol, under the influence of FSH. As the circulating levels of oestradiol rise, a *negative* feedback to the hypothalamus and to the pituitary occurs, which results in a reduced release of FSH. But with the further rise of oestradiol, near midcycle, a *positive* feedback results. This operates in two ways. First, by the long feedback, to the hypothalamus, oestrogen induces the release of more GnRH, which culminates in a peak release. Second, by the short feedback to the pituitary, the gonadotrophs become more sensitive to GnRH (Fig. **5/1**). These two stimuli induce a sudden surge and

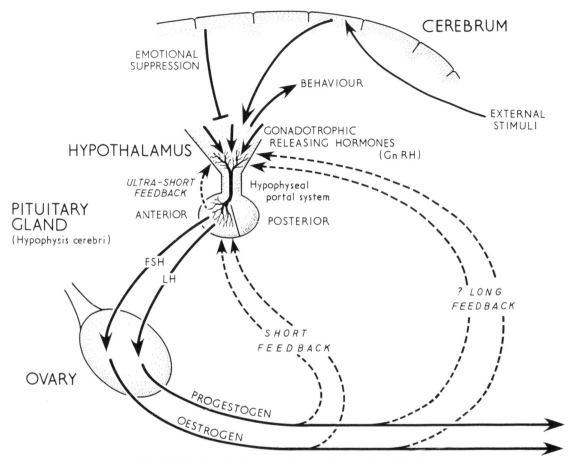

Fig. 5/1 The hypothalamus-pituitary-ovarian-uterine relationship

peak release of LH (and a smaller peak of FSH) from the gonadotrophs.

Luteinizing hormone is a glycoprotein. Acting with FSH it brings one of the stimulated follicles to full development, and within 16 to 24 hours of its surge it precipitates the release of an ovum from this follicle, which collapses.

Following ovulation, LH induces the theca-granulosa cells of the collapsed follicle to transform into lutein cells, which synthesize oestrogen and progesterone.

These two hormones feedback to affect hypothalamic and pituitary gonadotrophic function. Rising levels of oestrogen and progesterone initially inhibit FSH release, but in the absence of pregnancy, after 8 to 10 days, the levels fall, releasing the negative inhibition of FSH, and initiating a new menstrual cycle (see Fig. **5/5**).

THE OVARY

By the time of puberty, each ovary contains about 200 000 oogonia surrounded by mantles of theca-granulosa cells, and many of these have developed antra to form primary follicles (see Chapter 3). Stimulated by the pituitary gonadotrophins, each month from puberty to the menopause between 10 and 20 of the follicles mature, and in maturing synthesize and release the female sex hormones, oestrogen and progesterone. These hormones have a profound effect upon many tissues of the body, but are most active on the organs which derive from the para-mesonephric duct (the oviducts, the uterus and the vagina) and on the mammary gland. In addition, the ovarian stroma secretes small quantities of testosterone and the weaker androgen, androstenedione, indicating its bisexual attributes. The synthesis of the hormones from a common precursor, cholesterol, is

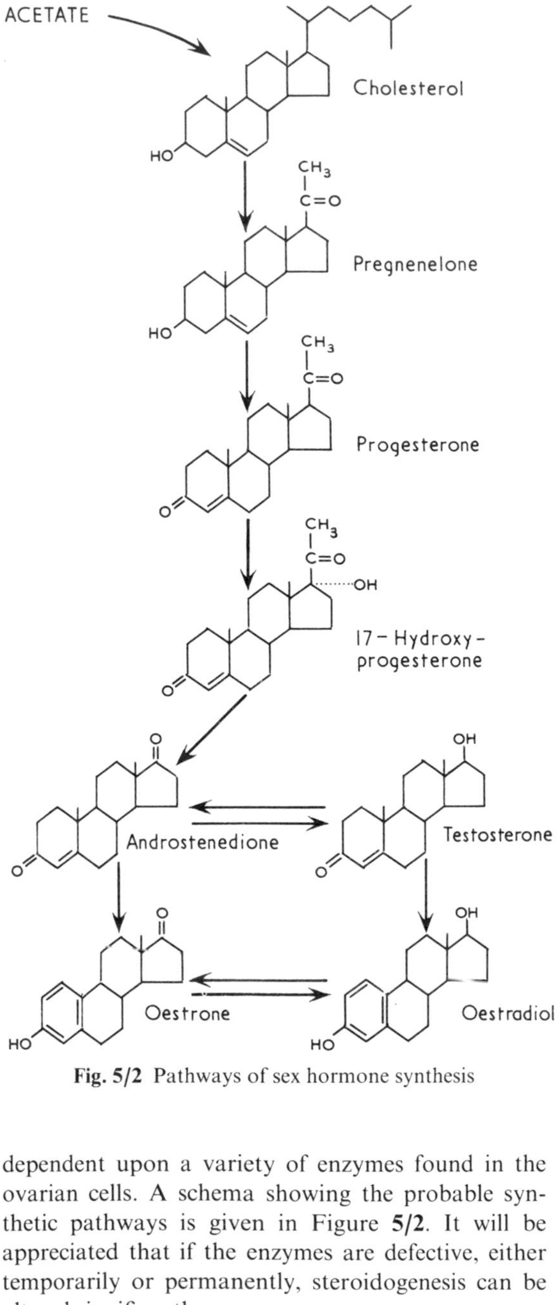

Fig. 5/2 Pathways of sex hormone synthesis

oestrone and oestriol. Oestrogens are secreted, mainly in the form of oestradiol, by the theca-granulosa cells of the ripening follicles, and are released into the blood. They are transported (bound to albumin) to tissues which contain 'target cells'. The target cells contain about 5000 molecules of a specific receptor protein which has a high affinity for oestrogens, particularly oestradiol 17 beta.

The epithelium of the genital tract and the breasts contain considerably more target cells than other tissues and consequently are particularly affected by oestrogens. The receptor protein in the target cells takes up oestradiol 17 beta from the plasma with ease. Once within the target cell, oestradiol 17 beta is transferred to the cell nucleus where it becomes bound to a new receptor, and acts on nuclear chromatin, producing a response which is determined by the nature of the receptor cells, not by oestradiol which acts as a 'switch' or 'amplifier'. Following its action, oestradiol 17 beta (and oestrone) are very rapidly metabolized (mainly to the relatively inert form, oestriol), so that the target cells may respond to the next surge of oestrogen. The oestriol (and some oestrone) is carried to the liver, where conjugation with glycuronic acid occurs, rendering the oestrogens inert. They are then excreted, partly in the faeces, and partly in the urine. Of the three 'classical oestrogens', oestradiol is the most potent, being ten times as potent as oestrone, which is ten times as potent as the weak oestrogen, oestriol.

Actions

Cellular

At the molecular level oestrogens act upon the nucleus of the target cell inducing RNA synthesis, which in turn leads to protein synthesis by the cell. Some of these proteins are enzymes which alter profoundly the activity of the cell. There is evidence that the particularly sensitive target tissues (those of the genital tract and the breast) owe their receptiveness to the presence of protein receptors in the cytoplasm and probably the nucleus, which permit the binding of a higher concentration of oestrogens (especially oestradiol) than other tissues.

Oestrogen, in the form of oestradiol 17 beta (E_2) stimulates the production of oestrogen receptors in oestrogen-dependent tissues and binds to them. The E_2-receptor complex is transferred to the nucleus where it binds to acceptor sites on the nuclear chromatin. This reaction leads to the production of messenger RNA, which directs the synthesis of

dependent upon a variety of enzymes found in the ovarian cells. A schema showing the probable synthetic pathways is given in Figure **5/2**. It will be appreciated that if the enzymes are defective, either temporarily or permanently, steroidogenesis can be altered significantly.

OESTROGENS

Metabolism

Three main oestrogens have been isolated, although many others exist. These are oestradiol 17 beta,

proteins which in turn mediate the steroid hormone response. The proteins include enzymes and other receptors. In the cell, E_2 stimulates the production of its own cytoplasmic receptor and induces the production of progesterone receptors. Progesterone regulates the process by blocking the synthesis of new oestrogen receptors and induces enzyme production which regulates oestrogen metabolism. In other words, whilst oestrogen leads to cellular proliferation in oestrogen-dependent tissues, progesterone leads to cellular differentiation. Since progesterone receptor synthesis is oestrogen dependent, pro-

gesterone indirectly antagonizes the synthesis of its own receptors and exerts control over the action of progesterone at cellular level.

The system is delicately balanced, each hormone regulating the other.

Tissues

Oestrogen has a major role in the development of female secondary sexual characteristics, and has an influence upon the psychological development of femininity, but its precise place in this is not currently defined. The principal effect of oestrogen is in the development and stimulation of the female sex organs and the breasts. This is understandable, because of the extra receptivity of these tissues to oestrogen.

The *vulva and vagina* are developed and maintained by oestrogen, the hormone influencing both the epithelial and muscular layers and stimulating the blood vessels supplying the organs. Oestrogen increases the vaginal epithelial activity, and is responsible for the deposition of glycogen in the superficial cells and consequently for the vaginal acidity. It increases the vascularity of the vagina and, together with progesterone, maintains its muscular tone and development.

The *uterus* is particularly influenced by oestrogen, which causes proliferation of the endometrium, stimulating the growth of the glands and compaction of the stroma. It increases the vascularity of the organ and causes the development of the myometrium, which at puberty changes the infantile organ into the mature uterus (Fig. **5/3**). In pregnancy, the great increase in uterine growth is largely due to the increased oestrogen secretion. After the climacteric, the atrophy of the uterus is due to oestrogen withdrawal (Fig. **5/4**). Oestrogen also affects the non-muscular tissues of the cervix, causing a softening of collagen matrix and stimulating the secretion of mucus by the cervical columnar epithelium.

The effect on the endometrium is even more marked, and in the absence of oestrogen, the endometrium becomes atrophic. If a castrated woman is given oestrogen for 2 or 3 weeks, uterine growth, and particularly endometrial growth, is stimulated, and on stopping the oestrogen an 'oestrogen withdrawal bleed' occurs. Oestrogen withdrawal bleeding usually varies in quantity from day to day and tends to persist. The stimulation of the endometrium is dose-dependent and small doses may be insufficient to stimulate development, so that bleeding is avoided. This fact is of importance if oestrogens are

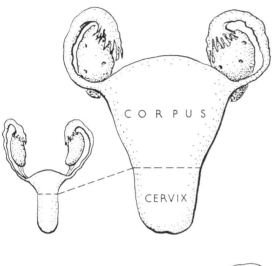

CORPUS

CERVIX

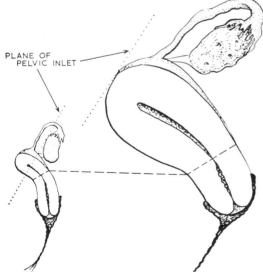

PLANE OF
PELVIC INLET

Fig. 5/3 The infantile uterus compared with the adult uterus. Note particularly the change in ratio of the corpus and cervix

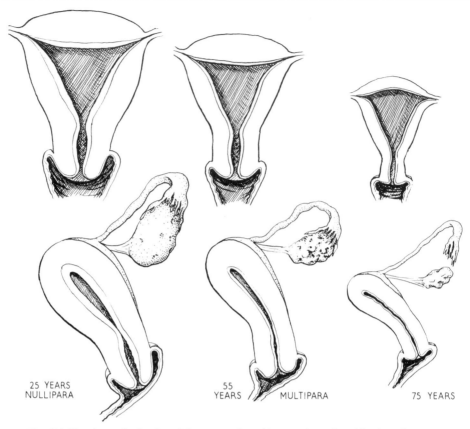

25 YEARS
NULLIPARA

55
YEARS / MULTIPARA

75 YEARS

Fig. 5/4 The change in the size of the uterus, the oviducts and ovaries with advancing age

used in the management of the vasomotor symptoms associated with the climacteric.

On the other hand, if the oestrogen-primed endometrium is further stimulated by progesterone, or if a mixture of oestrogen and progesterone is administered in place of oestrogen alone, a 'progesterone withdrawal bleed' will occur 3 to 6 days after ceasing therapy. The blood loss in this instance is much less, and of a short duration.

In certain cases, particularly in the later reproductive years, oestrogen secretion may increase, causing marked endometrial thickening. The high secretion may be constant or may fluctuate. In the latter case, when the levels are falling, the endometrial growth is not maintained and bleeding occurs. This is called 'breakthrough bleeding'. Even when the level remains high, bleeding may still occur, presumably due to disintegration of the thickened endometrium. But it should be noted that in neither of these cases is the cause of the bleeding really understood. These problems are discussed further in Chapter 7.

Hypothalamus-pituitary

The reciprocal relationship between the ovary and the hypothalamus/pituitary is mediated by oestrogen. Small quantities of circulating oestrogen produce a *negative* feedback, inhibiting FSH release and preventing follicular maturation. Larger quantities produce a *positive* feedback, stimulating an LH surge, and ovulation. Still larger doses suppress both FSH and LH release, preventing ovulation.

PROGESTERONE

Metabolism

Progesterone, which chemically has a less complex synthetic pathway than oestrogen, is secreted mainly by the luteinized theca-granulosa cells which constitute the corpus luteum, although a little is manufactured by the non-luteinized theca-granulosa cells of the follicle. In pregnancy the trophoblastic cells of the placenta also manufacture the hormone. In the tissues progesterone augments and modifies the response to oestrogen and, because of this dependency, its actions are less well understood. Progesterone is an important intermediary in the synthetic pathway from cholesterol or acetate to oestrogens, androgens and adrenal cortical steroids. As in the case of oestrogen, its biological effect is maximal on the organs formed from the Mullerian duct, and on the breasts. It disappears rapidly from the circulation due to a rapid diffusion into the target organs and fat, and to a rapid inactivation in the liver where it is conjugated. However, only about 20 per cent of secreted progesterone is conjugated and appears in the urine as pregnanediol. The fate of the remainder is not known.

Progesterone is also bound to protein receptors in 'target cells'. The number of receptors available seems to be determined by oestradiol, which explains the synergistic effect of the two hormones on many tissues. The level of progesterone (and the progesterone-like drugs, progestogens) also affects the transfer of oestrogen into the cell nucleus. The higher the level of progesterone the less the oestrogen effect and consequently the less the 'amplifier' effect. Within the cell, oestradiol is converted into the less potent oestrone by an enzyme, oestradiol 17 beta hydrogenase, and the activity of the enzyme is, in turn, induced by progesterone. It can be seen that progesterone modulates the cellular action of oestrogen in several ways.

Actions

Cellular
The action of progesterone at cellular level is regulatory, as described on page 41.

Tissues
Progesterone acts on all the organs of the genital tract, and on the breast, but only if they have simultaneously, or previously, been sensitized by oestrogen. The main action of progesterone is on the uterus, but the vagina and oviduct are also influenced. The maturation of the vaginal epithelium is hindered, and intermediate cells are desquamated increasingly, which because of their altered plasma membranes tend to form clumps. These cells contain a reduced quantity of glycogen. The cervical mucus is altered, making it more viscid and reducing its sodium content. This can be confirmed by noting the increased viscosity of a sample of cervical mucus and the absence of fern-like crystals of sodium chloride in the dried mucus. The epithelial cells of the oviduct are stimulated to secrete a clear mucus, which may aid the passage of the ovum down the Fallopian tube.

The *uterus* is the organ most affected. Progesterone increases the thickness and succulence of the endometrium by enlarging the glands and causing imbibition of fluid by the stromal cells, which become enlarged and clear, with small compressed nuclei. If the action of progesterone persists, the stroma becomes even more oedematous and is called a decidua. Progesterone also alters the enzymatic functions of the cells forming the endometrial glands, which begin to secrete mucus rich in glycogen.

Progesterone also affects other body tissues, leading to the deposition of fat. It is thermogenic, raising the basal body temperature by 0.2 to 0.5° C. It relaxes smooth muscle and ligaments, but these effects are only obvious in pregnancy. It promotes the secretion of sebum by the skin. It alters blood coagulability to some extent, although oestrogen is more implicated in this change.

THE MENSTRUAL CYCLE

The purpose of the foregoing discussion was to prepare for a description of the menstrual cycle. One further concept is essential to grasp. This is the reciprocal nature of hypothalamic/pituitary and ovarian function. Feedback mechanisms, which are essential to normal function, exist between the ovaries, the hypothalamus (the long feedback) and the pituitary (the short feedback). These feedback mechanisms are operated by the circulating levels of the sex steroids particularly oestradiol 17 beta.

ENDOCRINE RELATIONSHIPS OF THE HYPOTHALAMIC-PITUITARY-OVARIAN CYCLE

It is not known what triggers the hypothalamus to release GnRH in the years prior to puberty, but it is thought that repeated small stimuli from GnRH over the months before puberty induce the gonadotroph cells of the anterior pituitary to synthesize and to release small amounts of gonadotrophins into the

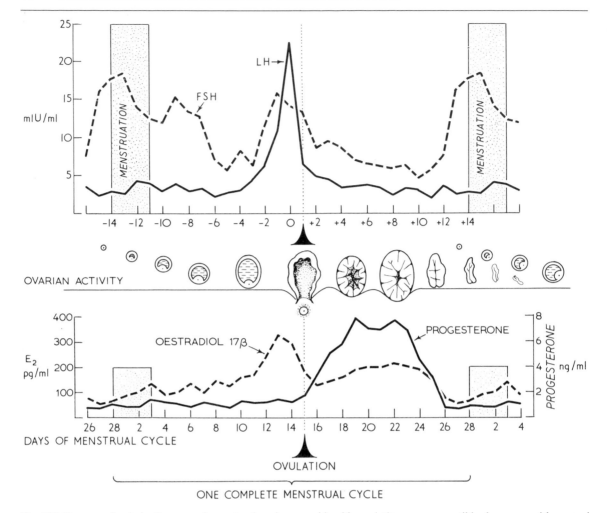

Fig. 5/5 Hormone levels in the normal menstrual cycle – considerable variations are compatible, however, with normal menstrual function. In this figure the interrelationship of ovarian steroids and hypothalamic-pituitary gonadotrophins is shown. After menstruation, rising levels of oestrogen exert a negative feedback, reducing FSH release. Towards midcycle still higher oestrogen levels exert a positive feedback causing a sudden peak release of LH which induces ovulation. An increased release in FSH also occurs. Failure of this sequence will lead to anovulation and irregular cycles. In the luteal phase, LH levels must be sufficiently high to maintain the corpus luteum until the conceptus has implanted and commenced HCG secretion, which then maintains corpus luteum function. If conception fails to occur, the corpus luteum deteriorates after about 7 days, with resulting falling levels of progesterone and oestrogen. As a consequence menstruation occurs, and FSH levels rise, initiating a new menstrual cycle

circulation until eventually sufficient amounts are released to stimulate ovarian activity. Initially follicle-stimulating hormone (FSH) is released, with only small amounts of LH.

Above a critical circulating concentration, FSH stimulates a few sensitized follicles in the ovary to mature. FSH also induces the theca cells which surround these follicles to secrete increasing amounts of oestrogen. The rising concentration of oestrogen feeds back to the pituitary and the hypothalamus in a negative way, reducing the amount of FSH released by the gonadotroph cells. Oestrogen levels continue to rise, rather more rapidly over 3 or 4 days, to reach a peak.

The LH midcycle surge: positive oestrogen feedback

Oestrogen (oestradiol) is thought to exert its negative feedback effect by inducing the release of a Gn-inhibiting factor (? LH-inhibiting factor) from

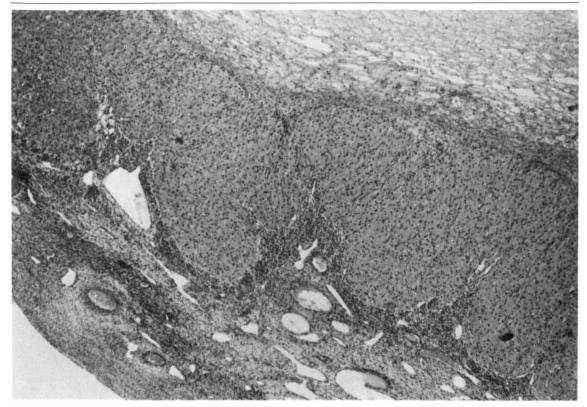

Fig. 5/6 (A) Corpus luteum. The upper part of the microphotograph shows that blood cells in the cavity are being invaded by epithelial cells. The granulosa cells show marked lutein characteristics, and superficial to this layer, the theca cells have proliferated to push cones of cells into the granulosa cell layer. Blood vessels are appearing in both cellular layers (× 40)

neurones in the pre-optic nucleus area of the anterior hypothalamus, and, at the same time, increasing cell storage of LH. The steady incremental increase of oestradiol occurs over a period of about 6 days, when it peaks. The midcycle surge of oestradiol (1) increases the sensitivity of the pituitary gonado- trophs to GnRH and (2) induces a surge release of GnRH. This is the *positive feedback*. The GnRH surge induces a small FSH and a large LH surge (which are in reality increases in the amplitude of the pulsatile surges) after a time lag, which occurs because the pre-formed Gn-inhibiting factor has to be degraded in the hypothalamus before GnRH re- lease can occur. This takes between 8 and 24 hours, so that the LH surge follows the oestradiol peak by this interval. Ovulation occurs about 30 hours (range 24–38 hours) after the LH surge.

The one follicle which, being more sensitive to FSH stimulation, has developed most quickly, now releases the ovum, and then collapses. Many of its theca-granulosa cells are luteinized and begin the secretion of progesterone. As they secrete, they proli- ferate and a corpus luteum is formed. Within 3 days of ovulation, blood vessels penetrate the luteinized cells. By the 5th day after ovulation the corpus luteum is fully functioning, and maximal quantities of progesterone are being produced (Fig. **5/6**). The circulating progesterone added to the circulating oes- trogen exerts a negative feedback on the hy- pothalamus and the pituitary, causing an altered sensitivity of the gonadotrophs to GnRH, so that LH and FSH levels fall. Unless the released ovum is fertilized and implants within 7 days of ovulation, the corpus luteum begins to degenerate, with a rapid reduction in oestrogen and progesterone secretion. This is insufficient to support the endometrium, and approximately 14 ± 2 days after ovulation, the en- dometrium breaks down and its blood vessels rup- ture, causing bleeding. Menstruation has occurred. The corpus luteum begins to degenerate with a fall in oestrogen and progesterone secretion, so that the negative feedback fails. This permits the hypo- thalamus to release increasing quantities of GnRH with the result that the pituitary gonadotrophs

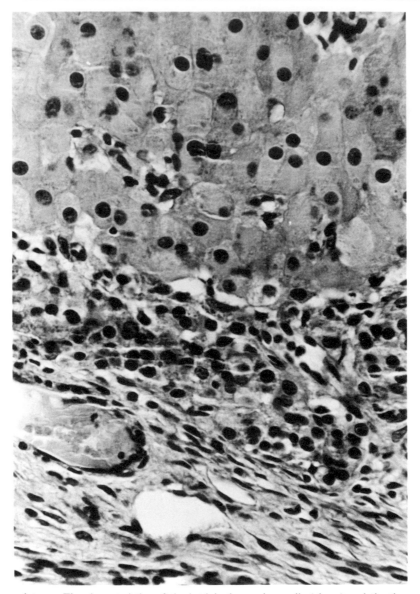

Fig. 5/6 (B) Corpus luteum. The characteristics of the luteinized granulosa cells (above) and the theca cells (below) are demonstrated (× 160)

secrete increasing quantities of FSH, which enters the circulation to initiate a new menstrual cycle by stimulating another batch of primary follicles in the ovaries. The corpus luteum degenerates further during the succeeding months, the cells undergoing colloid, fatty and finally hyaline degeneration to produce a white body, or corpus albicans (Fig. **5/7**). Should the fertilized ovum implant, its trophoblast at once secretes human chorionic gonadotrophin,

which maintains corpus luteum function and progesterone production for at least the first 40 days of pregnancy.

THE ENDOMETRIAL CYCLE

Menstruation is properly defined as the periodic cyclical shedding of a progestational endometrium,

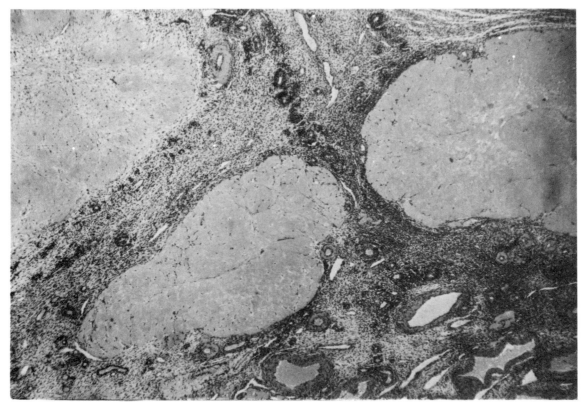

Fig. 5/7 Corpora albicantia. The cells of the corpus luteum have been replaced by an amorphous hyalinized zone surrounding a central area of scar tissue (× 40)

accompanied by blood; but the term is often used to include any periodic cyclic bleeding from the uterus. Menstruation can be considered a failure of pregnancy to occur, and the blood lost varies from 10 to 80ml, with an average of 30ml. Menstruation normally occurs at intervals of 22 to 35 days (mean 28) and the duration of the bleeding phase varies from 1 to 8 days (mean 5). This may be conveniently expressed as 5/28; indicating that the menstrual cycle (i.e. from the onset of menstruation to its next appearance) lasted 28 days, and the bleeding phase 5 days. It is also convenient, particularly since steroid therapy is available, to designate the days of the menstrual cycle. Day 1 is taken to indicate the day menstruation *starts*.

The menstrual phase

During menstruation, the superficial and middle layers of the endometrium are shed, the deep or basal layer being spared. Shedding occurs in an irregular haphazard way, so that some areas are unaffected, others are undergoing repair, whilst simultaneously other areas are being shed (Fig. **5/8**). The debris, consisting of endometrial glands and stroma, with some leucocytes and a varying quantity of blood, forms a coagulum in the uterine cavity. This is immediately acted upon by fibrinolysins and the clot dissolves. If the amount of blood within the cavity is excessive, insufficient fibrinolysins are available, and clots are passed through the cervix. Normally, however, menstrual discharge is dark red, liquid and does not clot. The discharge is expelled from the uterus by uterine contractions.

The nature of menstrual discharge

It is important to understand that menstrual discharge consists mainly of tissue fluid, (together with endometrial debris) blood only forming about 50 per cent of the total menstrual discharge. The mean quantity of menstrual discharge is 30ml with a normal range from 5 to 80ml.

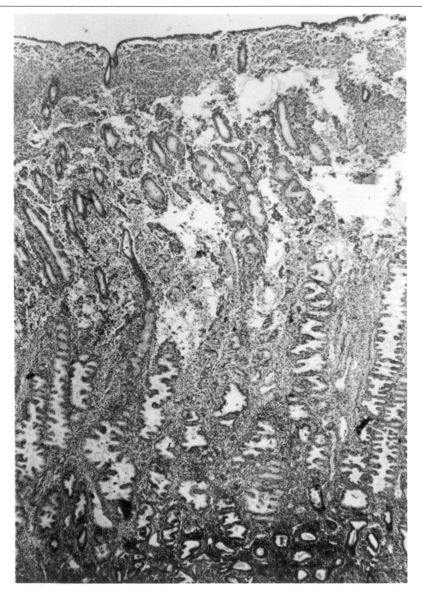

Fig. 5/8 Endometrium – early menstrual phase. The section shows beginning of focal necrosis in the superficial zone of the endometrium with small areas of haemorrhage into the stroma and infiltration with neutrophils (× 40)

The proliferative phase

At the end of menstruation, the layer of basal endometrium is covered by a necrotic zone of glandular and stromal elements, and blood clot through which the mouths of viable glands project. The remaining endometrium is infiltrated with leucocytes. Repair occurs rapidly, the epithelial surface being reformed by the metaplasia of specialized stromal cells, and by the outgrowth of the epithelial cells of the en-

dometrial glands. Within 3 days the repair is complete. This stage, the early proliferative phase, lasts from day 3 to day 7 of the normal cycle. During it, the surface epithelium is thin, the glands sparse, narrow and straight, and lined with cuboidal epithelium, and the stroma is compact. There are few mitoses in glands or stroma. Following this phase of relatively slow regeneration, proliferation speeds up, the glands increasing in size and growing perpendicular to the surface (Fig. **5/9**). The epithelial lining

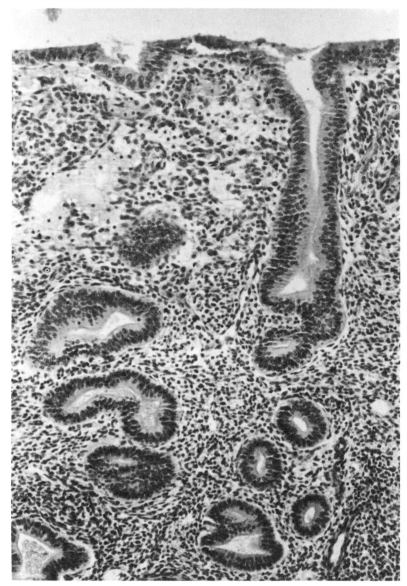

Fig. 5/9 Endometrium – early proliferative phase. Note that the glands are straight, short and narrow. The surface epithelium is thin (× 160)

becomes columnar with basal nuclei, but with no sign of secretory activity. The stromal cells proliferate but remain fairly compact, and have a spindle shape. Mitoses are common in both the glands and stroma. During the 2 days prior to ovulation, all these findings become more obvious and some of the glands become tortuous, although secretion is not seen (Fig. **5/10**). During the proliferative phase, the thickness of the endometrium increases from 1 to 3mm at the time of ovulation.

The luteal or secretory phase

The changes in this phase are due to the influence of oestrogen and progesterone on the previously oestrogen 'primed' endometrium. The luteal phase lasts from ovulation to the next menstruation, and varies in duration from 9 to 16 days. Secretory vacuoles, rich in glycogen, first appear in the glands within a day of ovulation (Fig. **5/11A**). Initially they are basal vacuoles, and displace the nuclei superficially.

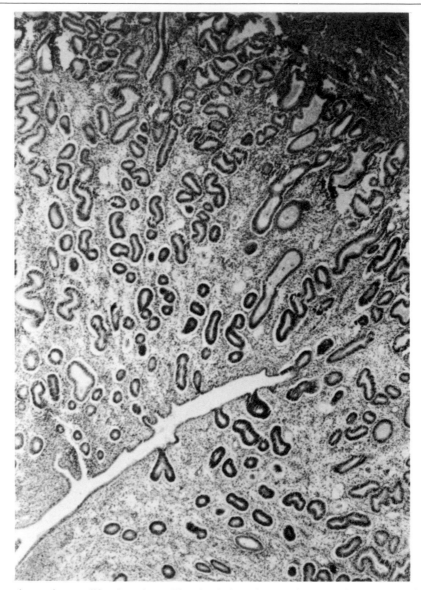

Fig. 5/10 Endometrium – late proliferative phase. The glands have become longer and tortuous, and in a few, early secretory changes may be observed. The stroma remains dense (× 40)

They rapidly increase in number and the glands become markedly tortuous (Fig. **5/11B**). By the 4th day after ovulation the secretions have streamed past the nuclei to lie in the superficial part of the cells, and the nuclei have been displaced nearer the base of the cells. By the 6th day, secretion is at its height, the glands which have discharged the mucus being low, those about to discharge the mucus being tall. The effect is a saw-toothed glandular epithelium (Fig. **5/12**).

Simultaneously the stroma undergoes changes. The cells become larger and clear as they imbibe fluid, and they are separated by tissue oedema. Near the surface there is less tissue oedema, and sheets of large clear cells can be seen, which resemble the decidual cells of early pregnancy (Fig. **5/13**).

These changes reach a maximum on the 22nd or 23rd day (of a 28-day cycle), after which growth ceases and dehydration of the stroma begins. Progesterone withdrawal has started. The endometrium

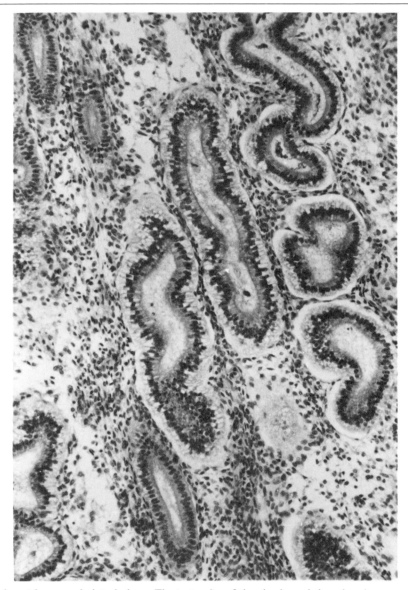

Fig. 5/11 (A) Endometrium – early luteal phase. The tortuosity of the glands, and the subnuclear vacuoles, can be seen. Note the gland in the lowest part of the picture has not been affected (× 160)

shrinks from a maximal height of 6mm, as the glands discharge their secretion, and as the tissue oedema is reduced. The stromal cells remain swollen, but the stroma becomes infiltrated with leucocytes. Two days before menstruation, these changes are marked and focal collections of extravasated blood appear beneath the surface of the endometrium. These collections increase, and the endometrium becomes necrotic in a patchy manner. Soon the surface epithelium is broken, and the necrotic endometrium and blood are shed into the uterine cavity.

THE MECHANISM OF ENDOMETRIAL BLEEDING

The basal arteries supplying the endometrium lie in the myometrium, and send off branches at right

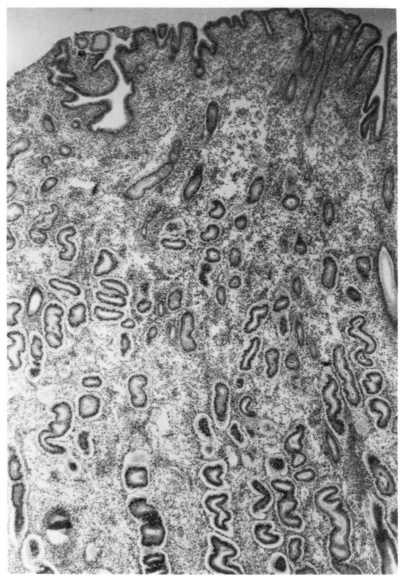

Fig. 5/11 (B) Endometrium – early luteal phase. The tortuosity of the glands and the oedema of the stroma can be seen (× 40)

angles to their course to supply the endometrium. At first, when they penetrate the basal endometrium, these arteries are straight, but as they enter the middle and superficial layers of the endometrium they become coiled. They can therefore lengthen to meet the increased thickness of the endometrium which occurs in the secretory phase of the cycle. There is little connection between each of the spiral arteries, and a single artery supplies a fairly well-defined area of endometrium. Each ends in a capil-lary network just below the epithelium, and the area is drained by a vein which runs parallel with the artery and occasionally forms arteriovenous connec-tions (Fig. **5/14**).

In the days prior to menstruation, vascular changes occur in the endometrium as the oestrogen and progesterone secretion from the dying corpus luteum diminishes. As the corpus luteum function wanes, a fall in progesterone occurs, which leads to an increase in free arachidonic acid and cyclic en-

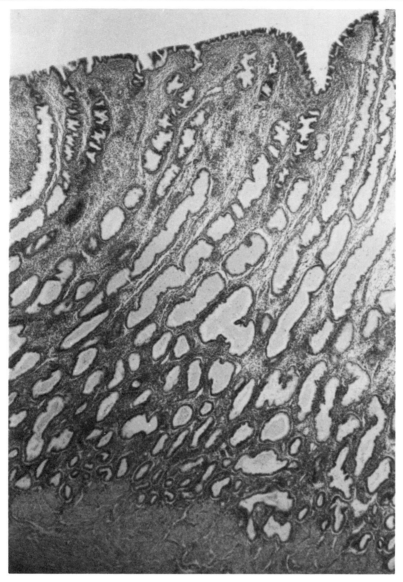

Fig. 5/12 Endometrium – 6 days after ovulation. The glands are now very tortuous with secretion in the lumen and increasing fluid separating the stromal cells. In a fertile cycle this is the day the ovum reaches the uterine cavity (× 40)

doperoxidases in the endometrium. These enzymes induce the lysosymes of the stromal cells to secrete prostaglandins, particularly $PGF_{2\alpha}$ and PGE_2; in addition PGI_2 (prostacyclin) is released in the myometrium. $PGF_{2\alpha}$ and PGE_2 are powerful vasoconstrictors and are involved in the regulation of platelet function. Prostacyclin is a vasodilator and inhibits platelet aggregation. The vasoconstrictor action of $PGF_{2\alpha}$ and PGE_2, slows the rate of blood flow through the capillaries, and a shift of fluid from the tissues to the capillaries occurs, with a resulting decrease in endometrial thickness. The stromal shrinkage leads to increased coiling of the spiral arteries, a further diminution of blood flow, and a consequent derangement of cellular function in the areas supplied. The arterial buckling increases, and the endometrium supplied becomes increasingly hypoxic, ischaemic necrosis occurring in an irregular pattern in the superficial layer (Fig. **5/8**).

Just prior to the beginning of menstrual bleeding,

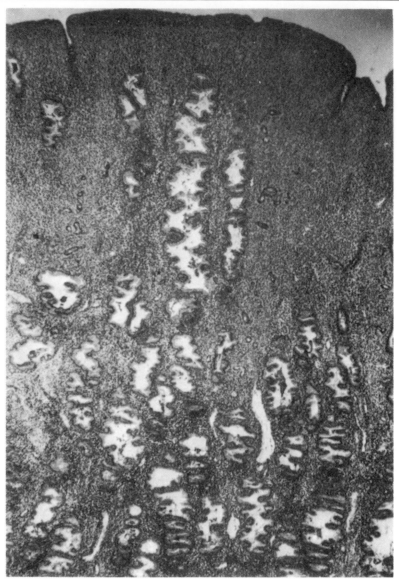

Fig. 5/13 Endometrium – 12 days after ovulation. The tortuosity of the glands is evident. The stroma beneath the surface epithelium has become predecidual with enlargement of the nuclei, and increase in the cytoplasm of the stromal cells. The basal zone of the endometrium is not affected by these changes (× 40)

a further change affects the straight part of the spiral arteries as they traverse the basal endometrium. Marked vasoconstriction occurs in individual arteries in a random fashion. The vasoconstriction persists for the next 5 or 6 days, except for short periods when relaxation occurs (probably caused by prostacyclin) and blood surges through the vessel and ruptures the already ischaemic and weakened coiled portion of the artery. In this way extravasation of blood and tissue fluid separates the necrotic endometrium, and both are shed into the uterine cavity at irregular intervals. The basal layer of endometrium is not involved, as it receives a blood supply from the main artery below the point at which vasoconstriction occurs. Regeneration of epithelial cells from the stroma and from the mouths of the glands therefore begins as soon as the overlying superficial endometrium is shed.

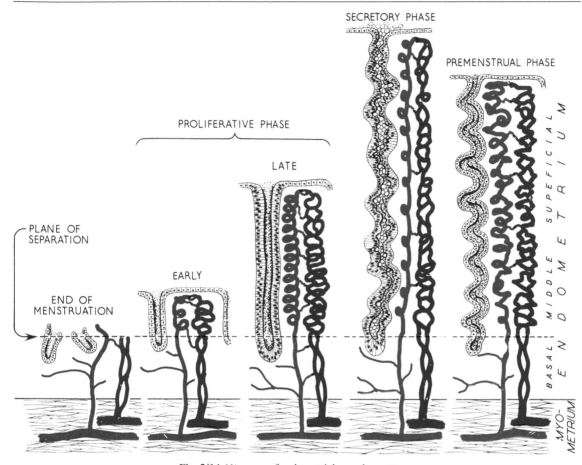

Fig. 5/14 Diagram of endometrial vascular patterns

It has been mentioned that prostaglandins released from the stroma are involved in the regulation of menstrual loss. Prostaglandins E_2 and $F_{2\alpha}$ cause vasoconstriction, whilst prostacyclin (PGI_2) causes vasodilation and inhibits platelet aggregation. The ratio between PGE_2, $PGF_{2\alpha}$ and PGI_2 may be a factor in whether the blood loss is normal or if the woman develops heavy bleeding (menorrhagia).

ANOVULATORY BLEEDING

As defined precisely, menstruation does not include anovulatory uterine bleeding. However, since the bleeding is periodic and may be cyclic, the condition may be impossible to distinguish on clinical examination, and the mechanism of bleeding is the same as that in ovulatory menstruation.

In an anovulatory cycle, the follicle ripens but because of insufficient FSH stimulation, insufficient oestrogen is secreted to provoke the positive feedback. Alternatively, the hypothalamus may be temporarily unresponsive to the positive feedback. In either event the LH surge does not occur and ovulation is inhibited. Oestrogen continues to be secreted by the theca-granulosa cells of the follicle, until it dies. The time this takes varies, and consequently the duration of an anovulatory cycle may be lengthened, although in many cases it is not. The condition can be identified by measuring plasma progesterone in the presumed luteal phase of the cycle. A plasma progesterone <15nmol/litre indicates anovulation. Another method is to examine an endometrial biopsy, which will be proliferative or hyperplastic at a time in the cycle when it might be expected to have been secretory.

Anovulatory cycles are more common at each end of reproductive life, but can occur at all ages. Before

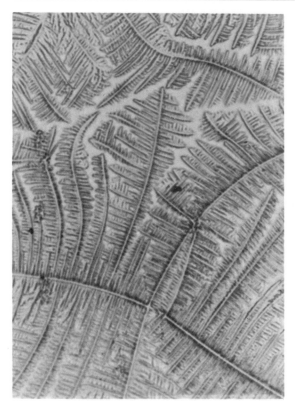

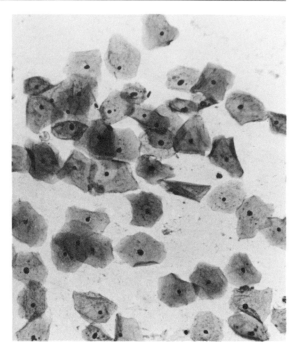

Fig. 5/16 Vaginal exfoliative cytology – late proliferative phase, note the discrete cells with small nuclei and the clear background (× 160)

Fig. 5/15 Cervical mucus – ferning

the age of 20 and after the age of 38, they may occur as frequently as one cycle in four, but between those years the incidence is probably lower than one cycle in ten, although there are considerable variations between individuals. Treatment is only required if infertility is a problem.

THE CERVICAL CYCLE

As noted earlier, the cervix uteri is influenced by the waxing and waning secretion of the female sex hormones. In the follicular phase the cells lining the clefts of the cervical canal proliferate and actively secrete a thin watery mucus. This is most marked at the time of ovulation, when a 'cascade' of mucus may be seen. The mucus contains a quantity of sodium chloride and potassium chloride, which on drying forms 'fern-like' crystals (Fig. **5/15**). The connective tissue matrix retains fluid, and this fluid retention is increased by the progesterone secreted in the luteal phase of the cycle. Progesterone also alters the quality of the cervical mucus, which becomes

viscous and poorly penetrable by spermatozoa, and no longer forms the 'fern-pattern' on drying.

THE VAGINAL CYCLE

Cyclic changes occur in the vaginal epithelium which are conveniently detected by the examination of vaginal exfoliated cells. The changes represent the ratio between oestrogen and progesterone. In the follicular phase superficial and large intermediate cells predominate, and as ovulation approaches the number of superficial cells increases. Very few leucocytes are present, so that the smear has a 'clean' appearance (Fig. **5/16**).

In the luteal phase a marked change occurs. The superficial cells are replaced by intermediate cells with folded edges. The cells tend to form clumps and leucocytes increase in number so that the smear appears 'dirty' (Fig. **5/17**).

GENERAL CHANGES IN THE MENSTRUAL CYCLE

In the follicular phase few general changes occur,

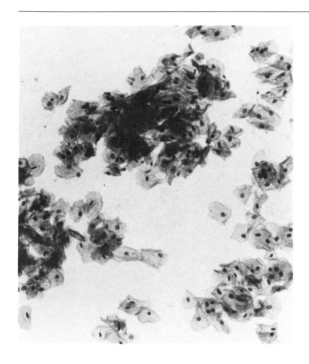

Fig. 5/17 Vaginal exfoliative cytology – luteal phase. The cells have clumped and the background infiltration of leucocytes has begun (× 160)

but ovulation may be accompanied by pain, which is lower abdominal and unilateral in type, usually not very severe and rarely lasts for more than 12 hours. If the patient complains of severe pain and is not anxious to conceive, ovulation, and hence the pain, can be suppressed by using oral contraceptives. The pain (called *mittelschmerz*) may be accompanied by a slight loss of blood per vaginam.

General symptoms occur more frequently in the luteal phase, affecting about 50 per cent of women. They are varied in character, and tend to increase as the time of menstruation approaches. They do not occur in each cycle, nor do the same symptoms occur in different cycles. The most frequently noted symptoms are irritability, lethargy, constipation, and inability to concentrate. Just prior to menstruation some women develop shadows under the eyes, and a few spots of acne on the face. Others complain of pelvic pressure. At this time, too, varicose veins of the legs tend to cause greater discomfort.

Symptoms of fluid retention occur in the luteal phase, and may manifest as abnormal weight gain, headaches and fullness of the breasts, which in a few cases become nodular and painful (mastalgia or benign mammary dysplasia). These problems are discussed further in Chapter 6.

Menstruation itself is surrounded by a veil of myth and nonsense. In the Bible it is the 'unclean time', in Ireland it is 'the curse'; in England it is 'the poorly time'. These pejorative adjectives stress the *abnormality* of menstruation, but are being replaced by a realization that menstruation is a normal function, not a manifestation of uncleanliness. There is no need to limit any activity during menstruation, and it is immaterial whether the woman uses an absorbent vulval sanitary pad, or diaper, or a tampon introduced into the vagina to absorb the menstrual flow. The latter is less obtrusive, but less efficient if the flow is heavy, and may be left in the upper vagina after menstruation, even by intelligent women. The result is an offensive vaginal discharge.

Vaginal tampons should be changed every 4 to 6 hours, and should be removed if coitus is practised during menstruation. The reason is that a few cases of severe toxic shock (due to *Staph. aureus*) have occurred amongst women using tampons, who have neglected the advice to change them often.

The few days before menstruation and the time of menstruation itself are times when an increased sexual urge is felt by many woman. Coitus during menstruation may be unaesthetic, but it is not medically dangerous, and patients who seek advice can be reassured that there is no medical reason to avoid coitus at this time.

STAPHYLOCOCCAL TOXAEMIA SYNDROME (TOXIC SHOCK)

This uncommon condition (< 1 : 25 000 cases among menstruating women per year) may be associated with menstruation but has also been reported in males and in children when it has followed infected surgical wounds, bites, furuncles and skin infections. It is characterized by the acute onset of fever > 38.9°C, sore throat, headache, aching muscles, dizziness and sometimes watery diarrhoea. A sunburn like rash develops over the skin and the conjunctiva become reddened. Three days after the onset of the fever, a dandruff-like desquamation of the skin occurs, which is followed 5 to 7 days later by epidermal sloughing on the hands and feet. Hypotension and shock develop in a proportion of these patients early in the syndrome and may be profound. The syndrome is due to infection with *Staphylococcus aureus*, which releases an endotoxin. Treatment is to restore the blood volume, and to give antibiotics which are penicillinase-resistant, such as flucloxacillin. Corticosteroids should not be prescribed.

As the condition is most often associated with menstruation, tampons have been implicated. Research has shown that tampon users are four times as likely to develop toxic shock as non-users. The risk is reduced considerably if women choose tampons made of cotton or non-enhanced rayon, and of low absorbancy. It is also recommended that tampons should be changed every 4 hours and avoided at night when a pad or minipad should be used.

Chapter 6

Disorders of the Menstrual Cycle

The 7 to 10 days prior to menstruation are a time of disadvantage to many woman. During these days, women are more likely than usual to absent themselves from work, to require hospital admission, to be involved in accidents, to commit crimes, to develop acute psychiatric symptoms and to commit suicide. Only a very small number of women exhibit these extreme features in the premenstrual period, but a much larger number of women are disadvantaged if, by chance, they have to sit for examinations, or attend interviews for jobs in the premenstruum. The disadvantage has been computed as a reduction in the total mark at an examination by between 5 and 10 per cent. During the premenstrual period, 75 per cent of healthy young women experience some degree of swelling of their bodies; 70 per cent develop one or more acneiform spots on the face; 40 per cent complain of premenstrual discomfort; and in 8 per cent of women the discomfort is sufficiently severe to be termed 'disease'. The women are suffering from premenstrual tension, or 'the premenstrual syndrome', which is a better term.

PREMENSTRUAL SYNDROME
(Premenstrual tension, PMT)

Most women notice changes in mood or develop physical symptoms at some time during the two weeks preceding menstruation. The changes are usually minor and do not disturb the women's life to any significant degree. In about 25 per cent of women the mood and physical changes are of sufficient magnitude to reduce the woman's feeling of well-being and to cause a deterioration in her interpersonal relationships, and in 3 per cent the symptoms are severely disabling. These women have the premenstrual syndrome (PMS). In the premenstrual syndrome the changes in mood and the development of physical symptoms occur between 12 and 5 days before menstruation and are relieved within 48 hours of the onset of menstruation. The symptoms may vary in character and in severity between menstrual cycles, but are always cyclic – a symptom-free period intervening between each premenstrual episode. The common symptoms are shown in Table **6/1**.

The symptoms most often reported are irritability, sadness or anxiety and the physical symptoms of abdominal and/or breast swelling, tenderness and pain.

Symptoms	
Mood (Emotional)	*Physical*
Irritability	Abdominal bloating
Anxiety	Abdominal discomfort, tenderness or pain
Nervous tension	Breast swelling, tenderness or pain
Depression (feeling sad or blue)	Feeling of weight gain
Lethargy, exhaustion, mood swings, aggression, panic	Oedema
Confusion	Headache
Craving for sweet foods	Backache
	Nausea

Table 6/1 Symptoms associated with PMS

PMS appears to be more common in women aged 30 to 45, and may become evident following childbirth or a disturbing life event.

Although PMS affects many women, the cause (or causes) of the syndrome remain unknown. A major problem in most research has been that the definition of PMS has not been clear and the methodology flawed. Many workers believe that PMS is due to an alteration in the level of the sex hormones in the premenstrual period (either an altered oestradiol: progesterone ratio, or a reduction in progesterone) but no consistent changes have been identified. A recent carefully designed study of hormonal changes across the menstrual cycle in women with PMS and in control women, showed no difference in the levels or patterns of any of the hormones measured. A recent suggestion is that the fault lies in neurotransmitter activity, particularly of endorphins, but this requires to be substantiated. Alterations in aldosterone levels have been reported by some workers but most have failed to find such changes; and this inconsistency applies to prolactin levels.

It is evident that psychological and psychosocial factors may influence a woman's perception of her premenstrual symptoms. This is demonstrated by the finding of most workers that the administration of a placebo leads to improvement or relief of symptoms in between 50 and 60 per cent of PMS sufferers, at least for several cycles. The management of a patient presenting with PMS, therefore, requires careful consideration. Initially rapport must be obtained with the patient by listening carefully to her story. Psychiatric problems should be looked for and, if detected, treated. Following this, the patient's three most severe mood and the three most severe physical symptoms should be identified, and the woman asked to make a chart, listing the severity of each symptom (on a scale of 0 to 3) each day, for at least two menstrual cycles. During this time previously taken medication should be avoided. This exercise enables the doctor to identify the problem more clearly, and helps the patient gain insight into her condition.

The exercise also emphasizes the importance of talking with the patient and offering some explanation for her symptoms. It may be especially helpful for the patient to be reassured that she is not 'just imagining her symptoms', and to have the opportunity of talking about her problems. Some women welcome the opportunity of talking with other patients in group therapy sessions. If the woman is tense or has had a 'stressful' episode, relaxation therapy may help.

Of the many drug treatments suggested for PMS, few have been studied in a properly designed trial. The medications suggested include:

* vitamin B$_6$ (pyridoxine) up to 100mg three times a day
* diuretics, including spironolactone
* progesterone (vaginal suppositories) 200–800mg daily
* dydrogesterone 10mg twice daily
* bromocriptine 2.5mg twice daily (which may help breast symptoms, but has no effect on the remainder)
* mefenamic acid 250mg 4 times a day

The drugs are usually prescribed from 2 days before symptoms are complained about (judged from the menstrual cycle diary) until menstruation starts.

Recently carefully-controlled double-blind studies have shown that pyridoxine, progesterone and dydrogesterone are no more effective than placebo in reducing the symptoms of PMS. Similar studies indicate that mefenamic acid may help some women who have severe PMS.

PERIMENSTRUAL SYNDROME

Women with this syndrome complain of symptoms occurring within 2 days of the onset of menstruation, the earlier part of the cycle being symptom free. The symptoms vary in character and severity between cycles. The most common mood symptoms are: lassitude, fatigue and lethargy. The most common physical symptoms are abdominal discomfort or bloating, a feeling of pelvic pressure; headache and menstrual cramps (dysmenorrhoea).

In some women the menstrual flow is altered, polymenorrhoea or menorrhagia being reported. It was originally thought that the symptoms were due to pelvic (broad ligament) varicosities which became congested in the perimenstrual period. This is the reason for the previously used diagnostic term 'pelvic congestion'. It is now accepted that if varicosities occur, they are secondary to the underlying vasomotor instability.

The symptoms usually cease within 24 to 48 hours of the onset of menstruation. It can be seen that the premenstrual syndrome may merge into the perimenstrual syndrome, which has been a cause of confusion.

Treatment, when required, is to prescribe analgesics for headache, and mefenamic acid (or one of the other non-steroidal anti-inflammatory drugs) for the other symptoms, particularly menstrual cramps.

DYSMENORRHOEA

Dysmenorrhoea means painful menstruation, and two types are described: (1) Spasmodic or true dysmenorrhoea, in which the pain is directly related to the onset of menstruation and is uterine in origin. (2) Secondary or congestive dysmenorrhoea, which occurs before, or during, menstruation, and may arise in the uterus or in some other organ or tissue.

Spasmodic dysmenorrhoea

This form starts 2 or 3 years after the menarche, and is maximal between the age of 15 and 25, decreasing after that time. The pain starts a few hours before menstrual bleeding begins, and ceases within 24 hours of menstruation, usually lasting less than 12 hours in total duration. The pain is cramping in character and felt in the lower abdomen, mainly in the hypogastrium. Spasmodic dysmenorrhoea is discussed at greater length in Chapter 28.

Secondary dysmenorrhoea

Secondary or acquired dysmenorrhoea is unusual before the age of 25, and uncommon before the age of 30. Two forms exist: (1) associated with endometriosis or with pelvic infection, and (2) associated with the 'perimenstrual syndrome'.

If endometriosis or pelvic infection is the cause, the pain typically starts 2 or more days prior to the menstruation, and increases in severity until late menstruation when it reaches its peak, taking 2 or more days to cease. The management is to treat the primary condition, and this is discussed in Chapters 13 and 19.

THE IRRITABLE BOWEL SYNDROME

A number of women who have the premenstrual syndrome also have the irritable bowel syndrome. The name is a compromise, indicating a lack of understanding of the disorder. There are many synonyms, such as spastic colon, nervous diarrhoea or colon neurosis. The disorder is especially common in women aged 20 to 60, who often have a background of marital stress, sexual frustration, depression or anxiety. Usually the patient complains of lower abdominal pain, often left sided, which is associated with an alteration in bowel habit. This may cause diarrhoea, constipation or alternating episodes of each. The pain is aggravated by eating or purgation and diminished by defaecation or passing flatus. In a few patients painless diarrhoea is the

only symptom and this is often limited to the early morning. Investigations must be made to exclude organic disease, including blood studies, examination of the stool for occult blood, pathogenic bacteria and parasites.

Treatment is unsatisfactory and many patients have to learn to live with their disorder, until their domestic problems are resolved. Unfortunately the condition may persist even then, and since many patients have had a variety of surgical procedures, may become fixed in the patient's personality. Recently, it has been shown that some patients with the irritable bowel syndrome have a disturbance of bowel motility leading to the alternating increased and decreased faecal transit times. A more normal colonic behaviour can be obtained if the patient eats a diet containing 15g of coarse bran daily.

If this fails to cure the complaint, mebeverine 200mg 4 times daily increases the cure rate (in the short term) to about 80 per cent. However, the disease tends to be chronic and to relapse.

IDIOPATHIC OEDEMA

Some women develop oedema which waxes and wanes periodically without any specific pattern. The oedema cannot be attributed to any disease, or to sodium-retaining drugs and has been called idiopathic, cyclical or periodic oedema. The condition affects women in their 30s and 40s, is worse in hot weather and on prolonged standing. It resembles the bloating which occurs in the premenstrual syndrome, and may occur premenstrually, but the weight gain is usually greater, often exceeding 1.5kg.

During an attack the woman's face and hands are puffy when she wakes, the oedema increases during the day, by evening her ankles and lower legs are swollen. At night the oedema diminishes but may not disappear. Eventually a marked diuresis occurs and the oedema disappears. During the attack the woman may become very irritable or depressed with resulting domestic strife.

The cause is unknown, but stress, either domestic or occupational, appears to precipitate an attack. Many of the women show considerable concern about weight and weight changes, and diet frequently. A proportion of the women are depressed (judged by psychometric testing). The essential physiological abnormality is a decrease in blood volume on standing. This leads to an increased proximal renal tubular resorption of salt and water and an increased leak of plasma into the tissues.

A few women with idiopathic oedema may have been taking diuretics for long periods, and have starved or dieted, intermittently, to lose weight. When the women start eating a normal diet or stop the diuretics, stimulation of the renin-angiotensin systems occurs, leading to oedema. The doctor should check that a woman with idiopathic oedema has not been starving intermittently or taking diuretics to 'control her weight'. If she has, she should be advised appropriately.

Treatment of idiopathic oedema is unsatisfactory. Diuretics should be avoided, and the woman should avoid tobacco, as nicotine induces antidiuretic hormone secretion. The reason for the oedema should be explained to her so that she can tell her close relatives, expecting their sympathy rather than hostility.

LOWER ABDOMINAL AND CHRONIC PELVIC PAIN

A number of women complain of a dull, nagging pain in the lower abdomen and pelvis which fluctuates in intensity and tends to be worse in the premenstruum. It may occur on either side of the lower abdomen and may be felt on different sides at different times. Many of the women also complain of deep dyspareunia and of a postcoital ache which may last for up to 24 hours. Pelvic examination usually reveals nothing abnormal.

The diagnosis is made by excluding organic causes such as chronic pelvic infection (p. 144) and endometriosis (p. 199). Laparoscopy is mandatory to exclude gross pelvic pathology. Venography via the uterus reveals that many of the women have dilated pelvic veins, but it is not yet clear if they are the cause of the pain. Recent investigations deny that previously believed causes, such as 'traumatic lacerations of the pelvic supports' and pelvic adhesions, are aetiological factors. Emotional factors, including an unhappy relationship, are often found, as is 'stress'.

Management of chronic psychosomatic lower abdominal and pelvic pain is unsatisfactory and there is no specific drug treatment. Counselling, exploring the woman's psychosexual and marital relationships, and supportive psychotherapy may help.

Chapter 7

Abnormal Uterine Bleeding

Although menstrual discharge consists of tissue fluid, (20 to 50 per cent) and blood (50 to 80 per cent), most patients perceive the loss as blood and complain of abnormal uterine bleeding.

Excessive bleeding from the uterus is a symptom not a disease, and the pattern of bleeding may be of various types. In attempting to differentiate the types of bleeding, the patient and her physician may find that they are not talking about the same condition, and time spent in elucidating the details of the amount of bleeding, the duration of the loss, the interval between episodes and associated disturbances is invaluable. When discussing menstrual disturbances, it is well to explain to the patient that when you talk about a menstrual cycle, you mean the interval from the day of onset of bleeding until the day the next episode of bleeding occurs, as many women consider the cycle to include only the interval *between* bleeding episodes.

DEFINITIONS

1. *Polymenorrhoea* (epimenorrhoea). The bleeding is cyclic, and the amount lost normal for the patient, but it occurs at too frequent intervals, the cycle being less than 22 days in duration. In the notation described in Chapter 5, 3/17 or 4/21 would indicate polymenorrhoea. Polymenorrhoea is due to a disturbance in the rhythmic release of gonadotrophins from the pituitary gland or to a relatively unresponsive ovary.

2. *Menorrhagia* (hypermenorrhoea). The cycle is of normal duration but the amount of menstrual discharge lost is excessive (>80ml). The duration of the bleeding phase may be normal or prolonged, and clots are usual. In the notation the cycle might be 5/28 or 8/28. Menorrhagia may be associated with some disturbance of the uterus, or may be due to a disturbance in the hormonal control of menstrua-

tion or to a disturbance in prostaglandin activity in the uterus. The endometrium may be hyperplastic, or normal, or the surface area of the endometrium may be increased owing to submucous myomata or adenomyosis.

3. *Polymenorrhagia*. The bleeding is excessive and the length of the cycle is reduced, the notation reading 8/20, for example. The condition is often found in chronic pelvic inflammatory disease, but both this pattern, and menorrhagia, frequently occur in anxiety states and other psychosomatic disorders.

4. *Metrorrhagia*. The term implies that the bleeding is irregular in amount, acyclical in nature and often prolonged in duration. This type of menstrual irregularity is usually due to a pathological condition of the uterus.

5. *Dysfunctional uterine bleeding* is diagnosed when investigations fail to find an organic cause for the abnormal bleeding. The dysfunction may be psychological in origin, which, acting through the hypothalamus may impair the normal reciprocal release of gonadotrophins, and consequently may impair normal ovarian steroid production or prostaglandin activity in the uterus. An increased synthesis in prostaglandins, in particular prostacyclin (PGI_2) may occur in the endometrium of some women who have menorrhagia. PGI_2 which inhibits platelet aggregation and causes vasodilatation, may be involved in the normal regulation of menstrual bleeding. The degree of hormonal disturbance varies, and consequently the endometrium may show a variety of histological patterns on curettage. The type of abnormal bleeding may be polymenorrhoea, menorrhagia or polymenorrhagia.

PHYSIOPATHOLOGICAL CONSIDERATIONS

In the discussion of normal menstruation, it was

noted that a reciprocal release of the gonadotrophins FSH and LH, and of oestrogen and progesterone would lead to menstruation if the hypothalamus, the pituitary, and the ovaries functioned normally, and if the uterine endometrium responded normally to the ovarian steroids. The influence of the emotions and illness upon the hypothalamus was also discussed, and finally the influence of other endocrine glands was mentioned.

Disturbances in these reciprocal relationships, and the effect of the emotions are involved in many cases of abnormal uterine bleeding. In other cases, organic causes such as uterine tumours, blood dyscrasias and endocrine disorders may be involved.

If the disturbance is due to a dysfunction of the reciprocal relationship between the hypothalamus-pituitary and the ovaries, caused by the effects of anxiety, depression, marital disharmony or separation, amenorrhoea or abnormal uterine bleeding may result. In the latter, the cyclic pulsatile release of

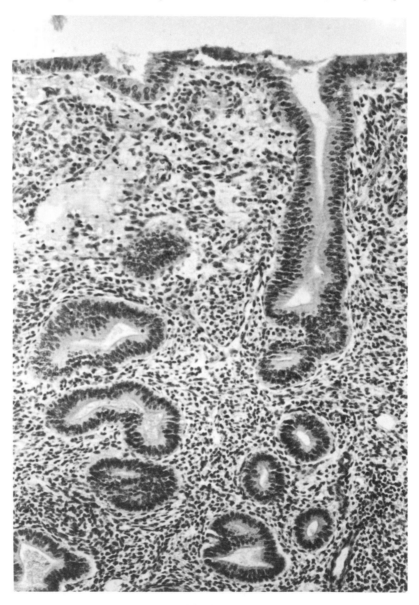

Fig. 7/1 Proliferative endometrium

gonadotrophic releasing hormone (GnRH) is disturbed. This in turn may lead to a faulty release of FSH and LH with a resulting disturbance of ovarian steroidogenesis. This may be expressed as anovulation. In many cases of abnormal uterine bleeding an endometrial biopsy in the premenstrual week will show a proliferative pattern (indicating anovulation) (Fig. **7/1**). But in many others a normal secretory pattern is found. In fact, except at the extremes of the reproductive era, when the ovary is less receptive to the effects of the gonadotrophins, a secretory pattern is more commonly found.

These observations suggest that in many cases of abnormal uterine bleeding, the cause is not directly an hormonal 'imbalance' but is due to local endometrial or myometrial dysfunction. Increased local fibrinolytic activity, which occurs in many cases of menorrhagia, may hinder the closure of gaps between epithelial cells of the endometrial capillaries. As well, high levels of plasmin may break down intra-uterine clots, increasing the likelihood of bleeding. Recently, prostaglandins have been implicated in abnormal uterine bleeding. In some patients with heavy bleeding, increased amounts of prostacyclin (PGI) and reduced amounts of PGF_2 have been found in the endometrium. Prostacyclin increases vasodilatation, inhibits platelet aggregation and relaxes the myometrium – factors which might be expected to increase blood loss.

In a few instances the disturbance operates over a longer period, and leads after an interval to uterine enlargement, particularly of the muscular layers (myohyperplasia). Myohyperplasia is due to stimulation by excessive unopposed oestrogen. Usually there is an associated increase in vascularity which is due in part to oestrogen stimulation and in part to stimulation of the sympathetic autonomic system which controls the pelvic blood vessels. The uterus is smoothly enlarged and soft, rarely exceeding the size of a 10 weeks' pregnancy (Fig. **7/2**). The bleeding pattern is one of menorrhagia, and myomata are often diagnosed erroneously.

'CAUSES' OF ABNORMAL UTERINE BLEEDING

Ovarian factors

Persistent follicular, or corpus luteum, cysts are accompanied initially by amenorrhoea but bleeding, when it occurs, tends to be abnormal, either polymenorrhoea or menorrhagia resulting until the

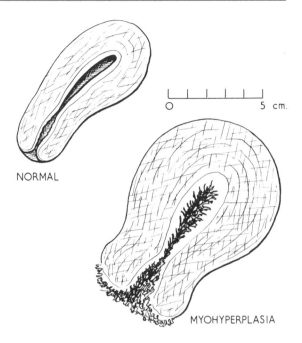

NORMAL

MYOHYPERPLASIA

Fig. 7/2 A uterus enlarged by myohyperplasia. Note the thick muscle wall when compared with a normal uterus

rhythm is restored. Functional ovarian tumours, producing oestrogen, although rare, may cause abnormal or postmenopausal uterine bleeding; but non-functional ovarian tumours do not, in general, disturb menstrual function.

Inadequate progesterone production, for whatever reason, may lead to a deficient luteal phase which is typified by an inadequate support of the endometrium, straining, 'spotting' or bleeding occurring in the few days before menstruation. An endometrial biopsy, or curettage, taken at this time will confirm the diagnosis.

In the 3 years after puberty, menstrual disturbances are fairly common: most being due to an inadequate response of the ovaries to FSH, with a consequently reduced production of oestrogen. The endometrium is inadequately stimulated and irregular bleeding tends to occur. Similarly, as the menopause approaches, ovarian sensitivity to gonadotrophins decreases, and anovulation is frequent. In these cases, bleeding from the uterus may be cyclic and normal in amount, or various abnormal bleeding patterns may result.

Uterine factors

Deep intramural and submucous myomata, which

distort and increase the endometrial surface area, are usually associated with menorrhagia, which is progressive in character and typically is worse on the 3rd or 4th days of the period. If the endometrium over a submucous myoma becomes ulcerated and thin, metrorrhagia results. Diffuse internal endometriosis (adenomyosis) and chronic pelvic infection may also cause menorrhagia. Malignancies of the uterine body and the cervix lead to metrorrhagia. The use, in recent years, of plastic intra-uterine contraceptive devices (IUD) may cause disturbances of uterine bleeding, particularly in the first few months after insertion. The bleeding may be either menorrhagic or metrorrhagic in type.

Pregnancy

A common cause of abnormal bleeding in the reproductive years is a disturbance of pregnancy, usually an abortion but occasionally an ectopic gestation. Indeed, curettage will reveal evidence of chorionic villi in a proportion of women who have abnormal uterine bleeding, and who deny the possibility of pregnancy.

Blood dyscrasias

Blood disorders characterized by disturbances in the coagulation-lysis systems or by capillary fragility, are often accompanied by menorrhagia. In many cases the symptom is the first indication that a blood dyscrasia is present.

Endocrine disorders

Pituitary disease, if it leads to an increase in gonadotrophin secretion, may cause menorrhagia. Similarly, in some cases hypothyroidism leads to menorrhagia, although hypothyroidism has been overdiagnosed and overtreated in the past.

Endometriosis

Women who have premenstrual spotting or staining may have endometriosis (see p. 199). This condition should be suspected if treatment using a progestogen does not cure the patient.

General diseases

Most chronic diseases reduce rather than increase menstrual bleeding; one exception being liver disease,

which hinders the normal degradation of oestrogen leading to hyperoestrogenaemia, and either amenorrhoea or metrorrhagia. Similarly, the administration of oestrogen by physicians for a variety of conditions, particularly in the perimenopausal age group, may cause menorrhagia or metrorrhagia, if the dose given is excessive.

Dysfunctional uterine bleeding

In over 50 per cent of cases of abnormal uterine bleeding, particularly when the pattern is that of an excessive quantity of blood (menorrhagia), no abnormal factors such as ovarian tumours, uterine myomatas, chronic pelvic infection, blood dyscrasias or endocrine disturbances are found. These cases are called 'dysfunctional uterine bleeding', although the physiopathology is unclear.

INVESTIGATION AND DIAGNOSIS

Women vary in their perception of what constitutes abnormal bleeding, and in each case the episode must be compared with the normal menstrual flow for that patient. In making a diagnosis, a carefully obtained, well-considered history is of great value. In cases where the facts are in doubt and there is no urgency for treatment, the patient may be given a placebo and instructed to keep a calendar of the duration, interval and quantity of uterine bleeding, and sometimes it is helpful to examine the patient during a bleeding episode. The patient's perception of the amount of blood lost may be inaccurate. In a study of menorrhagia in which all pads and tampons were collected and the blood loss estimated by an alkaline-haematin method, 39 of 69 patients lost less than 80ml of blood during the menstrual periods studied. The number of pads or tampons used did not correlate with the actual blood loss. However, if the pad or tampon was soaked through, if clots were prominent or if 'flooding' occurred, menorrhagia was likely to have occurred. Since the cause is psychosomatic in many cases, the patient's environment and mental attitude should be explored. The history of previous illnesses, especially those indicating a haemorrhagic tendency, must also be investigated.

The physical examination should include all systems, and not be confined to the genital tract; but the thoroughness with which this is done depends on the age of the patient and the physician's knowledge of her background. Laboratory tests include a haemoglobin and haematocrit estimation, and when necessary, tests for defects in the coagulation-lysis system and actual measurement of the blood loss.

These examinations may reveal the probable cause of the menstrual disorder, but unless the woman is a virgin or her medical history is well known to her physician, a diagnostic curettage may be required before starting therapy.

Diagnostic curettage

The purpose of the operation is (1) to exclude local lesions, such as an incomplete abortion, an endometrial polyp or malignancy, as a cause of bleeding, and (2) to obtain a representative quantity of endometrium for histological examination so that the endocrine status of the patient may be assessed, at least in so far as the sex hormones are concerned. In all women aged 35 or more, a diagnostic curettage is essential (performed preferably in the premenstrual phase following an episode of bleeding), but it may be omitted if subsequent episodes occur within 2 years, unless an abnormal endometrium has been obtained. The curettage must be performed properly and under anaesthesia, and if endometrial polyps are suspected, the cavity should be explored with a narrow sponge forceps. Diagnostic curettage should be performed *between* bleeding episodes so that an adequate sample of endometrium may be obtained, and in every case the curettings must be submitted for histological examination.

Curettage may be performed under general anaesthesia or, in selected cases, as an outpatient under local anaesthesia, or with no anaesthesia, using a Vabra suction curette.

Hysterography and ultrasonography

In obscure cases, particularly when investigations have been equivocal and treatment ineffective, hysterography, using a fluid medium and under image-intensifying screening, or hysteroscopy may reveal a myomatous polyp. The procedure can be done during a bleeding episode if a water-soluble medium is used. An alternative is to inspect the uterine cavity with a hysteroscope. Ultrasound scanning of the uterus may also be indicated.

TREATMENT

If an organic cause for the bleeding is found, treatment is directed to the primary condition, although it is well to remember that myomata, unless involving the uterine cavity, are not usually responsible for the abnormal uterine bleeding. If no organic cause is found, the condition is labelled dysfunctional uterine bleeding, and treatment depends to some extent upon the age of the patient.

During a bleeding episode

If the bleeding is heavy, bed rest and sedation are essential. If the bleeding is thought to be due to an incomplete abortion, curettage is clearly indicated, and in other cases may be used to terminate the bleeding episode by removing the endometrium. However, curettage at this time is often un-informative as regards the endometrial pattern, and if possible is best delayed until bleeding has ceased. Bleeding may also be controlled by giving an oestrogen or a progestogen by injection or orally. The oestrogen chosen is combined equine oestrogens (CEE) given intravenously in a dose of 25mg, repeated in 2 to 6 hours if severe bleeding persists. CEE acts on the coagulation system rather than on the endometrium. The progestogen usually chosen is 17-hydroxyprogesterone caproate in a dose of 125 to 250mg intramuscularly. If an oral progestogen is chosen, norethisterone 20 to 30mg in divided doses each day for 4 days is generally effective, although rather more slowly than the parenteral treatment. Bleeding stops within 24 hours, but is followed by a 'withdrawal bleeding' 3 to 6 days later. The latter stops of its own accord in a few days, but if the patient is severely anaemic, may be prevented by continuing norethisterone in a dose of 5 to 10mg daily for 20 days. Three subsequent cycles are controlled by giving oral norethisterone 5 to 10 mg daily from day 15 to day 25, or from day 20 to 25.

Patient seen when not bleeding – dysfunctional uterine bleeding

In most cases the bleeding episode, unless due to an incomplete abortion, or some other organic cause, ceases with bed rest, and the patient can be assessed in a non-bleeding phase. Treatment of dysfunctional uterine bleeding depends (1) on the type of bleeding pattern and endometrial histology, and (2) the age of the patient. In most cases, except the irregular bleeding of early adolescence, sufficient endogenous oestrogen is circulating, and the hormonal deficiency is one of progesterone. Indeed, in

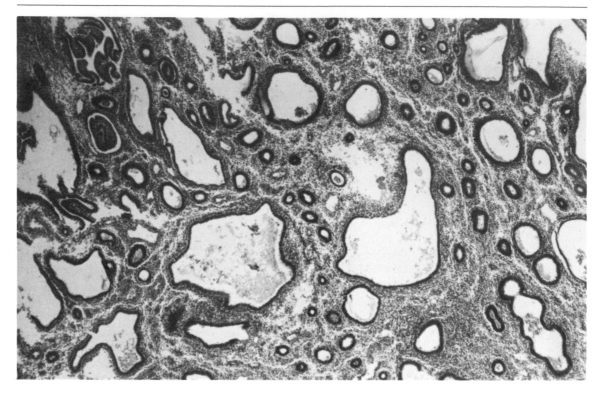

Fig. 7/3 Endometrium showing cystic hyperplasia. Note that the glands are of various sizes, but all in the proliferative phase. This is sometimes called the 'Swiss Cheese pattern' (× 40)

cystic hyperplasia excessive unopposed oestrogen is secreted. The age of the patient influences treatment, and the nearer the patient is to 40 years, the greater the place for hysterectomy, although many women over the age of 40 can be satisfactorily managed with hormone therapy.

HORMONE THERAPY

The introduction of potent oral progestogens has altered considerably the treatment of dysfunctional uterine bleeding. Since most cases are due to disturbances of hypothalamic-pituitary control, the use of progestogens to regulate the periods for a few months permits the basic disorder to undergo a spontaneous cure. Of the available progestogens, those of the 19-nortestosterone group are most suitable, as they lead to a degree of endometrial atrophy and thus aid in regulating the amount of blood lost. The particular regimen depends on the predominant type of bleeding.

1. *Polymenorrhoea*. The fault here is an inade-quate luteal phase, and the length of cycle can be increased by using an oral contraceptive from day 5, or by giving dydrogesterone 5mg from day 10 for 15 days. Since menstrual loss is normal, the 19-nortestosterones, which reduce the blood loss, are less desirable.

2. *Menorrhagia*. Heavy regular bleeding may occur from a non-secretory (proliferative) or a sec-retory (luteinized) endometrium. The latter is more commonly found in the middle reproductive years. Treatment is usually successful using a 19-nor-testosterone steroid, such as norethisterone 5mg daily from day 15 to 25, or, in milder cases from day 20 to 25. If the woman is anxious to avoid preg-nancy, she may be prescribed an oral contraceptive containing a relatively large amount of progestogen. A third choice is to give mefenamic acid 500mg three times a day with meals. The drug is started with the onset of menstruation and is given until menstruation ceases or 50 (250mg) capsules have been taken.

Women who fail to respond to these measures and who wish to avoid hysterectomy may be treated

During a severe bleeding episode

1. Curettage
2. 17-hydroxyprogesterone caproate 125 to 250mg intramuscularly or combined equine ostrogens 25mg i.v. repeated in 2–6 hours if needed
3. Norethisterone 5mg, 4- or 6-hourly for 4 days

   Note. A 'withdrawal bleeding' will occur 3 to 6 days after cessation of hormone therapy.

Management, once a diagnosis has been established

1. *Polymenorrhoea*		Oral contraceptives from day 5 to 25
	or	Dydrogestrone 5mg one to three times a day from day 10 to 25
	or	Norethisterone 5mg one to three times a day from day 10 to 25
2. *Premenstrual staining*		Dydrogesterone or norethisterone 5mg daily from day 20 to 25
3. *Menstrual pro-longation by staining*		Oral contraceptives from day 5 to 25
	or	Norethisterone 5mg one to three times a day from day 20 to 25
	or	Ethinyl oestradiol 20µg twice daily from day 3 to 7
4. *Threshold bleeding in adolescence*		Reassurance or, less commonly, norethisterone 2.5mg daily from day 20 to 25
5. *Metropathia haemorrhagica*		Norethisterone 5 to 15mg daily from day 15 to 25
	or	Oral contraceptives from day 5 to 25. In cases of failure of the above mefenamic acid 500mg three times a day may be given from day 1.

Give any of the above for 4 to 6 cycles then omit for 2 or 3 cycles, unless patients wants to continue contraception.

Table 7/1 Hormone therapy in dysfunctional uterine bleeding

with danazol. The dose is 200 to 400mg a day for a 12-week period. This regimen reduces the amount of blood lost significantly, but is associated with lassitude, muscle pains, weight gain and acne in about 30 per cent of women. The drug is expensive.

3. *Premenstrual spotting or bleeding–inadequate luteal phase.* The condition may be due to a relative deficiency of progesterone, or to endometriosis. Initially a progestogen should be prescribed. Either a 17-acetoxy progestogen (such as dydrogesterone) or a 19-nortestosterone progestogen (norethisterone) can be given from day 20 to 25 of the cycle.

4. *Prolongation of the period by intermittent scanty loss.* This is due to a disturbance of corpus luteum degeneration, and the endometrium shows a pattern of irregular shedding. Treatment is by regulating the cycle with a 19-nortestosterone from day 20 to 25, or by giving small doses of oestrogen (ethinyl oestradiol 0.02mg twice daily) from day 3.

5. *Bleeding from a poorly oestrogen-stimulated endometrium.* At each end of the reproductive period, the ovaries are relatively insensitive to stimulation by the gonadotrophins and only a small, but variable amount of oestrogen is secreted. The growth of the endometrium is reduced and bleeding can more readily occur from this poorly oestrogenized endometrium. The bleeding tends to be acyclical, and irregular in amount, varying between a scanty, dirty brown loss and a normal menstrual flow. It tends to persist, and may be indistinguishable clinically from one form of metropathia haemorrhagica. The condition has been called 'threshold bleeding'. In adolescence, reassurance is usually sufficient, as the bleeding pattern becomes normal within a few months. For the pre-climacteric woman, the treatment is that suggested for metropathia haemorrhagica.

6. *Cystic hyperplasia of the endometrium, or metropathia haemorrhagica.* This condition is also more frequently encountered at the extremes of the reproductive period, when the absence of ovulation is more common. In these cases excessive amounts of oestrogen are secreted, which cause an increased endometrial thickness. However, as no progesterone is secreted, the endometrial pattern is one of marked proliferation, or of cystic hyperplasia (Fig. 7/3). As the oestrogen levels rise, a period of amenorrhoea, usually of 6 to 10 weeks' duration, is usual; but fluctuations in the oestrogen levels then tend to occur, with the result that the thickened endometrium is no longer 'supported' and bleeding

occurs. The bleeding is acyclical and profuse. It may be prolonged in duration, but is usually painless, unless clots are expelled from the uterus. In some cases the bleeding pattern is indistinguishable from bleeding from a hypo-oestrogenic stimulated endometrium. The diagnosis can only be made by examining curettings histologically, and in older women this is mandatory to ensure that an endometrial carcinoma is not present.

The treatment of metropathia haemorrhagica depends to some extent on the age of the patient and the pathology of the curettings. Curettage itself is often curative, but if the menstrual abnormality persists, hormone treatment will usually regulate the periods. In many cases, norethisterone 5 to 10mg given from day 15 to 25 of three or four consecutive cycles suffices. Alternatively an oral contraceptive (in which the progestogen is a 19-nortestosterone) may be given from day 5 to 25 of the cycle.

SURGERY

Curettage

Although curettage is primarily performed for diagnostic purposes, it may have a therapeutic value in cases of metropathia haemorrhagica and menorrhagia. If the abnormal bleeding returns later, hormone therapy should be given or hysterectomy performed.

Hysterectomy

In the reproductive years, hysterectomy should be avoided, if possible, and reliance placed on hormone therapy. This attitude is not so important in women over the age of 40, and hysterectomy is a suitable alternative to hormone therapy in many cases. In general, it should only be performed in cases of dysfunctional uterine bleeding after failure of hormone therapy. When an organic cause for the abnormal bleeding is present in a perimenopausal woman, hormone therapy is relatively ineffective and hysterectomy is suitable treatment for most benign condi-

tions. This is discussed further in the chapters dealing with organic conditions of the uterus.

Whilst there can be no argument about the value of hysterectomy in the treatment of organic pelvic disease, the operation is used, far too often, without careful thought, to treat functional gynaecological disorders as diverse as chronic pelvic pain, dysfunctional uterine bleeding, myohyperplasia and pelvic 'infection'. The doctor suggests hysterectomy, it would appear, on the basis of 'if in doubt, cut it out', without enquiring if the origin of the disorder lies in the cerebrum rather than the pelvis, and without ascertaining if the symptoms were really only the somatic component of an underlying psychological conflict of an emotional or sexual nature. Immediately after operation an apparent cure is likely to the gratification of the patient, her husband and her surgeon alike. But within a short time other conversion symptoms appear and the patient is referred, over the years, to a variety of other surgical specialists.

The uterus, and menstruation, are to many women the core of their femininity, and the loss of the uterus has a considerable emotional response in susceptible women, particularly as it can no longer be the focus for the conversion symptoms. Depression and other psychiatric disturbances are not uncommon after hysterectomy for functional disorders, but are rare if the operation is performed for a true organic cause.

At the present time too many women are subjected to hysterectomy for insufficient reason and without pre-operative preparation for the operation. A surprisingly large number of women believe myths regarding the effect of hysterectomy on sexual function and on the development of obesity. The doctor must allow time for a careful and frank explanation to be given to the patient before hysterectomy, when incorrect ideas can be corrected and hidden fears eliminated.

Even more important, the personal physician, and particularly the gynaecologist, must realize that in psychosomatic gynaecological disorders hysterectomy should be the last rather than the first therapeutic choice.

Chapter 8

Amenorrhoea and Oligomenorrhoea

As amenorrhoea is a symptom not a disease, it may occur in many physiological and pathological conditions. In the following paragraphs the most usual of them are listed, so that the reader can see the wide range of conditions of which amenorrhoea may be a symptom. The reader may find it convenient to read this section quickly, returning to it after studying the clinical problems of investigating a case of amenorrhoea, and noting the distribution of cases amongst the various aetiologies.

Amenorrhoea may be defined as the absence of menstruation for a period which is twice that of the normal menstrual cycle of a woman who has menstruated previously (secondary amenorrhoea); or the non-appearance of menstruation in a girl who has reached the age of 16 (primary amenorrhoea).

Oligomenorrhoea means infrequent menstruation, and is usually defined as occurring when the duration of the cycle exceeds that normal for the individual by 2 weeks. Thus a patient whose normal menstrual cycle lasts 28 days, would be considered to have oligomenorrhoea if the duration of the cycle changed to exceed 42 days.

Amenorrhoea and oligomenorrhoea are therefore similar symptoms, differentiated only by a temporal factor. Hypomenorrhoea, which is defined as regular but scanty periods, also occurs. Unless found with oligomenorrhoea, it is of no clinical significance.

AETIOLOGY

Normal menstruation depends upon a normal uterus and vagina, and on the reciprocal functioning of the endocrine system which stimulates normal endometrial development. Failure of function may therefore occur at several levels, and may be physiological or pathological in nature.

Physiological causes

PREPUBERTY AND POSTMENOPAUSE

Before puberty insufficient gonadotrophins are released to stimulate ovarian function; and after the climacteric, the disappearance of the oocytes from the ovary means that it is unresponsive to gonadotrophic stimulation.

ADOLESCENCE

Irregularity of menstruation is frequent in the first 2 or 3 years after the menarche, and is due to temporary inadequate ovarian stimulation by the gonadotrophins.

PREGNANCY AND LACTATION

In pregnancy the amenorrhoea is due to FSH suppression by the large quantities of oestrogens secreted by the trophoblastic cells, and to the associated high levels of chorionic gonadotrophin. Lactation is associated with raised circulating levels of prolactin which, in turn, lead to the suppression of gonadotrophin releasing hormone (GnRH) so that neither FSH nor LH are released, the sex steroids are not synthesized in the ovaries and amenorrhoea is usual.

PRIMARY OVARIAN FAILURE (PREMATURE MENOPAUSE)

In about 5 per cent of cases, primary ovarian failure (premature menopause) is the cause of secondary amenorrhoea. Some of these women have a familial tendency to a premature menopause (that is the ovarian follicles disappear and the woman reaches the menopause before the age of 40). In other women, follicles are present but auto-antibodies may 'block' gonadotrophin receptors in them, so that the woman 'reaches' the menopause. The diagnosis is made by finding that the FSH level is greater than 20–40IU per litre and the oestradiol level is less than 100pmol/litre on at least two occasions.

One woman in three, diagnosed as having ovarian failure, unexpectedly ovulates and menstruates some years after the diagnosis. This change is assumed to be due to reversal of the 'block' to gonadotrophin stimulation. These cases have been called the 'resistant ovarian syndrome'.

The two types of ovarian failure cannot be differentiated, even by laparoscopic biopsy of the ovaries, as the tissue sample may not reflect the state of the rest of the ovary.

Treatment is unsatisfactory, but hormone replacement should be started to prevent bone loss (see p. 275). Hormone replacement may also be followed by spontaneous ovulation. Gonadotrophin-releasing hormone analogue has been used to permit the remaining follicles to develop instead of remaining atretic because of the high FSH levels, but there is no evidence that the drug induces the change, and GnRH analogue treatment usually fails. If a woman with primary ovarian failure desires a pregnancy, IVF using donated ova, is the preferred treatment.

Pathological causes

CHROMOSOMAL CAUSES

Male intersex, and other chromosomal abnormalities such as ovarian agenesis, are obvious causes of amenorrhoea, and should be considered in all cases of primary amenorrhoea as about one-fifth of cases are due to this cause (Chapter 4).

MALFORMATIONS OF THE GENITAL TRACT

Absence of the uterus is clearly incompatible with menstruation, whilst if vaginal atresia or imperforate hymen is the defect, menstruation will occur (cryptomenorrhoea), but no blood will escape per vaginam. This is sometimes called false amenorrhoea (Chapter 3).

UTERINE CAUSES

Surgical removal of the uterus or radiation damage will result in amenorrhoea, and the symptoms may be found in cases of tuberculous endometritis. Trau-

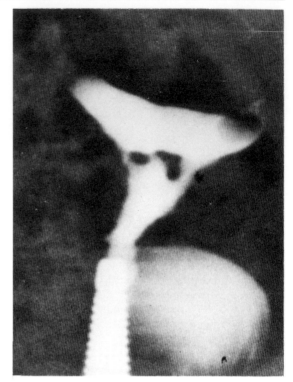

Fig. 8/1 Asherman's syndrome. The patient had amenorrhoea of two years' duration following an induced abortion. The hysterogram shows the filling defects caused by the intra-uterine adhesions. The diagnosis was confirmed by the passage of a sound under anaesthesia

matic uterine amenorrhoea, due to the formation of intra-uterine adhesions from over-enthusiastic curettage, for late puerperal bleeding, is another cause. This is referred to as *Asherman's syndrome* (Fig. 8/1). The diagnosis is made by curettage and hysterogram, and by the failure of bleeding to occur following progesterone therapy. Treatment is rather unsatisfactory but some success has been obtained by (1) careful curettage or the use of a hysteroscope to break the adhesions, (2) the insertion of an intra-uterine device, or a Foley catheter for a short period of time, (3) dexamethasone 20mg intramuscularly every 4 hours for 36 hours to prevent adhesion reformation and (4) cyclic oestrogen and progesterone for 2 cycles to aid regeneration of the endometrium. Recently the adhesions have been vapourized using an Nd-YAG laser directed through a hysteroscope. This method may supersede the older methods.

In some countries such as India, *endometrial tuberculosis* is an important cause of amenorrhoea, but these cases are becoming less frequent as tuberculosis

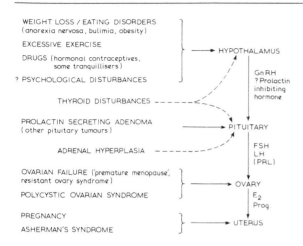

WEIGHT LOSS / EATING DISORDERS
(anorexia nervosa, bulimia, obesity)

EXCESSIVE EXERCISE

DRUGS (hormonal contraceptives,
        some tranquillisers)

? PSYCHOLOGICAL DISTURBANCES

THYROID DISTURBANCES

PROLACTIN SECRETING ADENOMA
(other pituitary tumours)

ADRENAL HYPERPLASIA

OVARIAN FAILURE ('premature menopause',
resistant ovary syndrome)

POLYCYSTIC OVARIAN SYNDROME

PREGNANCY

ASHERMAN'S SYNDROME

HYPOTHALAMUS
GnRH
? Prolactin
inhibiting
hormone

PITUITARY
FSH
LH
(PRL)

OVARY
E₂
Prog

UTERUS

Table 8/1 The aetiology of secondary amenorrhoea

control measures are implemented. In the developed countries of the world endometrial tuberculosis is a rare cause of amenorrhoea.

OVARIAN CAUSES

1. *Agenesis and dysgenesis.* If gonadotrophins are released rhythmically, the growth of a number of follicles will occur in the normal ovary, with the cyclic release of oestrogen and progesterone. In cases of ovarian agenesis and dysgenesis (Chapter 4), no, or few, follicles are present, and no, or inadequate, oestrogen is synthesized. This results in amenorrhoea.

2. *Ablation or radiation*, will eliminate ovarian responsiveness to gonadotrophins.

3. *Persistent follicle cysts.* So long as the oestrogen level remains high and does not fluctuate, the endometrium will be supported and the changes presaging menstruation will not occur. Amenorrhoea may therefore be present.

4. *Granulosa-theca cell tumours*, which synthesize large amounts of oestrogens, may lead to amenorrhoea during the reproductive period of life for similar reasons.

5. *Polycystic ovarian syndrome.* A syndrome of oligomenorrhoea or amenorrhoea (or, occasionally dysfunctional uterine bleeding), hirsutes and sometimes obesity, together with infertility, was first described by Stein and Leventhal. The cyst may be single or there may be multiple small follicles. Both can be detected by ultrasound. The multifollicular ovaries tend to occur in women who have amenorrhoea associated with severe weight loss. When a

single follicular cyst is present, the level of oestradiol in the plasma is high; with multilocular cysts the level is normal. In these cases the amenorrhoea is probably the consequence of a derangement in oestrogen metabolism. The syndrome has excited much interest because of the obscurity of its aetiology and the dramatic response to treatment. The current explanation is that the condition is due to inappropriate stimulation of the ovaries by gonadotrophins. The basal concentration of LH is raised, whilst that of FSH is relatively lower than in a normal menstrual cycle. The increased basal level of LH leads to a hypertrophied theca interna and to the increased secretion of androstendione and to a lesser extent testosterone from the ovary. At the same time the reduced level of FSH results in inadequate development of the granulosa cells.

Oestradiol secretion from the ovaries is comparable to that found in normal women in the early mid-follicular phase. Oestrone levels are raised, most being derived from the conversion of androstendione. These changes provide an inappropriate feedback to the pituitary with resulting anovulation and amenorrhoea. The hirsutism is due to the effects of the excess circulating free testosterone.

Oestrogens, mainly oestrone, are produced in peripheral sites by the conversion of the androgens, but this secretion is constant, and the cyclic release of gonadotrophins ceases. However, LH continues to be released in excess.

The condition is self-perpetuating until it is treated.

The diagnosis is suggested by the symptom complex. It can be confirmed by the detection of polycystic ovaries by ultrasound and a raised LH:FSH ratio. Free testosterone levels (in saliva or plasma) are also raised.

Four problems may require treatment. First, the endocrine disturbance. Second, the obesity. Third, the hirsutism. Fourth, the infertility.

The endocrine disturbance may be corrected by suppressing gonadotrophin release by prescribing a combined oral contraceptive containing 50 micrograms of oestrogen. Obesity responds to some degree

Weight loss	20–40
Polycystic ovaries	15–30
Pituitary insensitivity (post pill)	10–20
Hyperprolactinaemia	10–20
Primary ovarian failure	5–10
Ashermann's syndrome	1–2
Hypothyroidism	1–2

Table 8/2 The causes of secondary amenorrhoea (per cent).

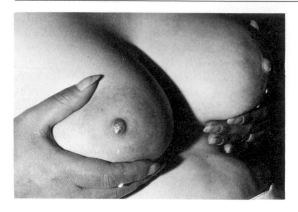

Fig. 8/2 Galactorrhoea. The patient had delivered 18 months previously. Lactation has persisted since that time with amenorrhoea. Examination showed a 'superinvoluted' uterus and lactating breasts

to diet and exercise. Hirsutism, which may be most distressing to the patient, can be reduced or eliminated (see p. 91).

When the main problem is infertility, the doctor must first establish that the only apparent barrier to conception is anovulation associated with the polycystic ovarian syndrome. In a few women the anovulation is due to hyperprolactinaemia, and if raised prolactin levels are found, treatment with bromocriptine is indicated. If the prolactin levels are within the normal range, therapy is started using clomiphene. This may be supplemented by a single injection of HCG, 5000 units, given at the time of the oestrogen peak. If pregnancy does not occur after 4 to 6 courses of clomiphene, pure FSH in daily doses adjusted to the level of serum oestradiol will usually achieve the development of a follicle. Ovulation is induced by an injection of HCG (5000U). Using these regimens, ovulation occurs in 90 per cent of cases, but the pregnancy rate is only 50 per cent. These methods supersede ovarian wedge resuction as tubal adhesions occur in at least 10 per cent of cases and, if pregnancy occurs, the ectopic gestation rate is eight times that found in a 'normal' population.

The full-blown syndrome is uncommon, but recent investigations using ultrasound of healthy women show that about 20 per cent had polycystic ovaries at the time of the studies.

PITUITARY CAUSES

1. *Pituitary tumours.* Amenorrhoea may be caused by pituitary tumours. In many cases there is other evidence of disturbed pituitary function.

2. *Hyperprolactinaemia and prolactin-secreting tumours.* Prolactin secretion by the pituitary gland is inhibited, under normal conditions, by the prolactin-inhibiting factor (PIF) released by the hypothalamus. PIF is composed mainly of dopamine.

In certain circumstances, prolactin release is permitted. Dopamine receptor blocking agents (for example, phenothiazines) or dopamine depleting agents (e.g. reserpine or methyldopa) may lead to raised plasma prolactin levels. Hypothyroidism with raised TRH levels may also produce hyperprolactinaemia, by the direct action of TRH on the galactophore cells in the pituitary. Hyperprolactinaemia may also occur in some women using oral contraceptives, or after ceasing to take the drugs, presumably due to a raised sensitivity of the galactophores to oestrogen, which stimulates prolactin release. However, the most common cause of hyperprolactinaemia is a microadenoma of the pituitary.

Raised prolactin levels suppress the oestrogen mediated release of GnRH from the hypothalamus which in turn blocks the LH surge needed for ovulation. Hyperprolactinaemia may also interfere with the actions of the gonadotrophins in the ovary itself.

In most cases of hyperprolactinaemia, amenorrhoea is the only finding, although, in about one-third, galactorrhoea is also present (Fig. **8/2**).

Hyperprolactinaemia accounts for about 20 per cent of cases of secondary amenorrhoea. The diagnosis is by finding raised prolactin levels in the blood plasma. Unfortunately, no consensus exists on the upper limit of normal. A recent suggestion is that a level < 700mU/litre is 'abnormal'. This finding must be followed by estimation of the visual fields, and CAT scan, or coned radiography to detect a prolactin secreting tumour, which may be a macro- or a micro-adenoma. A macro-adenoma requires treatment as do some micro-adenomas. This is discussed on page 78.

Hyperprolactinaemia is usually associated with amenorrhoea, but other patterns of disturbed hypothalamic-pituitary-ovarian function may occur such as oligomenorrhoea, hypomenorrhoea, irregular menstrual bleeding and, possibly, infertility.

Hyperprolactinaemia produces the menstrual disturbances by interfering with normal pulsatile GnRH secretion and release.

Treatment is needed if a macro-adenoma is detected, or if the woman desires to become pregnant, but in *all* cases prolonged follow-up is important as a proportion of women with hyperprolactinaemia eventually develop a tumour or a micro-adenoma. Many of the women have signs of oestrogen deficiency, such as poor vaginal lubrication and vaginal atrophy. In some women the sexual response is reduced.

2. *Hypopanpituitarism.* During severe antepartum haemorrhage, or more commonly postpartum haemorrhage with shock, arrest of the blood supply to the anterior lobe of the pituitary may occur, and be followed by complete or partial ischaemic necrosis of the lobe. The degree of necrosis is directly related to the severity and duration of the haemorrhage and shock. All the hormone-producing cells of the pituitary are affected, and absence of these trophic hormones profoundly alters body endocrine functions. The deficiency of growth hormones and prolactin lead to an absence of lactation and to the atrophy of the viscera, but fat and muscle deposition is normal and the patients do not become cachexic. The absence of the melanotrophic hormone leads to pallor and depigmentation of the nipples and areolae. The absence of adrenocorticotrophin leads to a marked reduction in circulating hydrocortisone, aldosterone and androgen, with consequent reduced insulin tolerance, a poor water diuresis, diminished sweating, increased sensitivity to cold, the falling out of hair from the pubic, the axillary and the eyebrow areas, and a loss of libido. The absence of thyrotrophic hormone leads to apathy. The absence of gonadotrophins leads to amenorrhoea and uterine atrophy. The danger of the disease is that hypothermic episodes or hypoglycaemic coma occur frequently. Treatment is effective in preserving life, and consists of giving daily doses of prednisone 5mg, thyroxine 0.2mg, and, possibly, testosterone. The condition is also known as Sheehan's syndrome.

HYPOTHALAMIC CAUSES

The predominance of the hypothalamus in regulating the menstrual cycle is shown in the finding that once chromosomal and congenital anomalies are excluded as causes of amenorrhoea, over 60 per cent of cases are due to hypothalamic malfunction. These are mainly due to environmental and psychosomatic (emotional) factors which inhibit the release of the gonadotrophin-releasing hormone (GnRH) or affect dopamine metabolism. Amenorrhoea is frequently found in *severe depression* (melancholia), and may occur after a change of work, separation or severe marital disharmony. In a few cases, organic lesions of the hypothalamus cause amenorrhoea. In such cases, the endocrine disturbance is marked, and the amenorrhoea only one symptom of a complex. Acute and chronic illness, acting upon the hypothalamus may cause amenorrhoea. Amenorrhoea may be caused by acute starvation, resulting from famine, or because of strict dieting, or excessive exercise which a woman adopts to achieve and to maintain a fashionably slim figure. A few young women develop *eating disorders, particularly bulimia and anorexia nervosa.* Not all women with bulimia become amenorrhoeic, but most develop menstrual disturbances, either irregular menstruation or oligomenorrhoea. In all patients with anorexia nervosa there is evidence of hypothalamic dysfunction, which is thought to be due to weight loss but may be associated with a psychological disturbance. The factors result in amenorrhoea. The endocrine abnormality is one of low circulating levels of oestrogen and of LH, but FSH levels are not always low. Treatment is to restore the woman's weight by persuading her to eat more. Once her weight is regained, (but often after some delay) the endocrine dysfunction is restored to normal and menstruation resumes. Ovulation-inducing drugs are contraindicated unless anovulation persists when the woman's weight is normal. The prescription of oral contraceptives to restore menstruation is also contraindicated.

OTHER ENDOCRINE CAUSES

Hypo- and hyperthyroidism may cause oligomenorrhoea or amenorrhoea, but in the latter other signs of excessive thyroid activity are usual. If any doubt exists the TSH level should be measured. If TSH is high or undetectable, free T_4 should be measured.

ADRENAL CAUSES

A few women who are infertile, with oligomenorrhoea, hirsutes, acne, and sometimes obesity are found to have no ovarian enlargement. Estimation of plasma 17 oxosteroids shows raised levels. These women are thought to have mild post-pubertal adrenal hyperplasia. Treatment with prednisone 2.5 to 10mg a day usually restores regular ovulatory cycles in less than 4 months' treatment, with a high chance of pregnancy occurring. The hirsutes is reduced to some extent. If no improvement occurs within 6 months, the diagnosis may be polycystic ovarian syndrome. Adrenal hyperplasia, as part of the adrenogenital syndrome and of Cushing's disease, is another cause, as androgens oppose the effect of oestrogen on the endometrium.

OVARIAN CAUSES

These have been discussed on page 73.

IATROGENIC CAUSES

During the use of oral contraceptives or after ceasing to use them, amenorrhoea may develop. Oral (and 'injectable') hormonal contraceptives suppress GnRH release by a negative feedback. In certain women complete suppression occurs with resulting amenorrhoea, presumably because of a greater hypothalamic sensitivity to the sex steroids. Post-pill amenorrhoea occurs because the suppressive effect persists for some months after contraception has been discontinued. Amenorrhoea, after ceasing to take 'the Pill', of short duration is not unusual and responds without treatment. Should the amenorrhoea persist for longer than 12 months, as it does in about 7 women in every 1000 who have ceased to use 'the Pill', investigations should be started to exclude an organic cause. Post-hormonal contraceptive amenorrhoea, of rather long duration, is more common if the woman has chosen 'injectable' contraception, particularly if medroxy-progesterone has been administered. If the latter has been used, the amenorrhoea may last up to 1 year. Similarly, large doses of the phenothiazines and certain hypotensive agents cause amenorrhoea, which in view of the diseases for which the drugs were required, is probably beneficial to the patient.

INVESTIGATION OF AMENORRHOEA

Study of large series of cases of secondary amenorrhoea (not due to pregnancy), suggests that most result from a failure in the pathway between the hypothalamus and the pituitary.

Most cases of secondary amenorrhoea are due to (1) hyperprolactinaemia, (2) weight loss, as in anorexia nervosa or following severe dieting or from psychological disturbances or (3) hypothalamic 'insensitivity' following exogenous oestrogen (e.g. oral contraceptives) or progestogen (e.g. injections of medroxy-progesterone acetate).

It follows from the above that a careful history and clinical examination (during which weight changes, hirsutism and galactorrhoea must be sought) will reveal obvious endocrine disturbances and will eliminate congenital anomalies of the genital tract, such as imperforate hymen, absent uterus or ambiguous genitalia, as causes. If the latter are present, special laboratory investigations are required, including examination of the buccal mucosal cells for nuclear chromatin (Barr bodies) (see p. 27), and karyotyping. If the physical examination, including the pelvic examination, reveals no abnormalities, laboratory tests should be started.

Of the many tests proposed, most are only required for research purposes, and a relatively simple sequence of tests will elucidate the cause of most cases of amenorrhoea.

The following tests are currently considered essential in the proper investigation of amenorrhoea. In certain situations additional investigations are needed.

1. *X-ray pituitary fossa*. Although a pituitary tumour is unusual if the prolactin level is normal and the amenorrhoea of less than 2 years' duration, about 1 per cent of normo-prolactinaemic amenorrhoeic women have been found to have a small pituitary tumour. It is for this reason that the procedure is considered essential.

2. *Hormone assays*.
   (a) FSH (and LH if polycystic ovarian syndrome is suspected, as its diagnosis is supported by a raised LH level). An FSH level $> 170 \mu g/l$ indicates ovarian failure.
   (b) Prolactin (hPr). A raised prolactin level on two or more occasions makes cone radiography or CAT scanning of the pituitary fossa essential.
   (c) TSH (and serum T_4 (ETR)). Although hypothyroidism is unusual in women whose prolactin level is normal, it occurs in 1 to 2 per cent of amenorrhoeic women.
   (d) Oestradiol 17 beta (E_2). Some authorities routinely measure plasma oestradiol, but there is evidence that more information is obtained from the 'progestogen stimulation test'.

3. *Progestogen stimulation test*. The test depends on the fact that progesterone is unable to provoke uterine bleeding in the absence of sufficient circulating oestrogen ($E_2 > 150 pmol/l$). Medroxy-progesterone acetate 5mg is given each day for 5 days. If this provokes normal menstrual bleeding within 7 days it can be assumed that the woman

Investigation of secondary amenorrhoea

1. History (duration, illness, drugs, eating behaviour, hormonal contraceptives).
2. Clinical examination (including weight).
3. X-ray pituitary fossa.
4. Measure or test, the following:

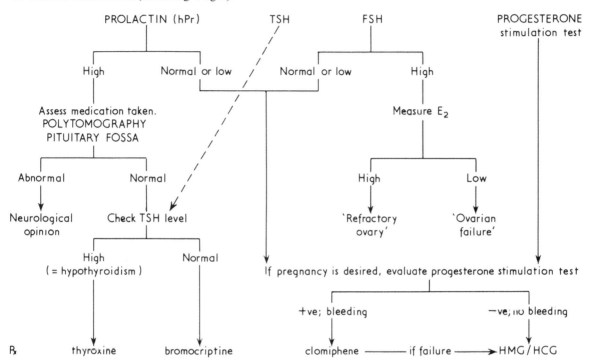

Fig. 8/3 The investigation and treatment of secondary amenorrhoea

has normal circulating levels of oestradiol and that a response to clomiphene may be anticipated, provided that hPr levels are normal. If the bleeding is scanty or absent, it is unlikely that ovulation can be initiated using clomiphene.

4. *Diagnostic curettage.* In countries where tuberculosis is common, diagnostic curettage may be indicated, but in most situations it is not necessary.

THE EXTENT OF THE INVESTIGATIONS

The purpose of the investigations is to exclude organic disease (especially a prolactin-secreting microadenoma of the pituitary gland); and to help the woman become pregnant. Unless organic disease is suspected, amenorrhoea of less than one year's duration does not need investigation, as most women start menstruating in this time.

After this period, the investigations outlined should be undertaken, although in certain circumstances they may be instituted earlier.

In the absence of an organic lesion, amenorrhoea represents no danger to the woman, and treatment should only be offered if she desires to become pregnant. In every case, the woman is entitled to a full explanation of the presumed cause of the amenorrhoea.

The sequence of the investigations and the outcome is shown in Fig. 8/3. The distribution of cases of amenorrhoea amongst various aetiologies depends on the population examined. A common distribution would be:

Primary amenorrhoea	5%
Secondary amenorrhoea	
due to:	
Hyperprolactinaemia	30%
Weight loss, excessive exercise	30%
Post-pill	25%

Ovarian failure	5%
Systemic disease	3%
Hypothyroidism	1%
Polycystic ovary	1%

TREATMENT

Treatment depends on the identified cause of amenorrhoea. If ovarian failure (premature menopause) is diagnosed by the finding of a raised FSH level and a low plasma oestrogen level (on 2 or more occasions), it is impossible to induce ovulation, although treatment may be needed to control menopausal symptoms.

In other cases of secondary amenorrhoea, treatment is only indicated if the woman desires to become pregnant. In this event, the other factors involved in infertility should have been excluded before specific treatment for anovulation and amenorrhoea is adopted.

Weight loss (including anorexia nervosa)

Until the woman regains her normal weight, drug treatment to restore ovulation and menstruation is of no value. Treatment should be directed to encouraging the woman to begin eating again. This may require psychiatric consultations and psychotherapy. About 75 per cent of the women will regain their body-weight, but not all will menstruate; ovulation-inducing drugs may help these women.

Hyperprolactinaemia

Three groups of women who have hyperprolactinaemia can be identified. The largest group is made up of those women who have raised serum prolactin levels but no evidence of a prolactinoma (functional hyperprolactinaemia). The second group consists of women who have a microadenoma (<10mm in diameter); and the smallest group of those women who have a tumour which extends out of the pituitary fossa (a macro-adenoma).

Women who have functional hyperprolactinaemia require assessment at 1–3-year intervals, including a CAT scan, but do not require treatment unless they desire to become pregnant, when bromocriptine is usually effective in inducing ovulation.

Women who have a micro adenoma do not need treatment unless they are infertile or oestrogen deficient (for example, have a dry vagina) but they need to be assessed each year.

Women who have a macro adenoma require treatment. Until recently, the choices were treatment with dopamine agonists, trans-sphenoidal partial hypophysectomy or radiotherapy to the pituitary gland. Most physicians have now accepted that the primary treatment is a dopamine agonist, such as bromocriptine. Bromocriptine supresses the secretion of prolactin and causes the tumour to shrink in over 90 per cent of cases. This effect persists if medication is stopped after several years treatment. Surgery and radiotherapy are less successful, may cause hypopituitarism and are followed by a recurrence of hyperprolactinaemia in at least 20 per cent of cases.

Bromocriptine is given initially in a dose which reduces serum prolactin levels to the normal range, and then treatment is continued with a smaller maintenance dose (2.5 to 7.5mg/day). Surgery is only advised if treatment with bromocriptine fails.

Follow-up, during treatment with bromocriptine and after ceasing to use the drug, is important: regular measurements of serum prolactin and an annual CAT scan are essential.

It is known that the increased oestrogen secretion which occurs in pregnancy may induce the prolactinoma to grow. If it is a micro-adenoma this rarely occurs, but if the patient has a macro-adenoma, growth is more likely. A patient who has a macro-adenoma should avoid becoming pregnant until the tumour has shrunk to lie completely within the pituitary fossa, as shown by a CAT scan. If shrinkage has failed to occur in spite of adequate treatment with bromocriptine, surgery should be considered. When the patient becomes pregnant, bromocriptine should be stopped. The pregnancy should be monitored by enquiring about clinical symptoms of persistent headache or impaired vision, but visual fields need not be assessed, nor are serial measurements of prolactin of any benefit. Clinical symptoms should lead to a CAT scan and treatment with bromocriptine.

Hypothyroidism

Treatment with thyroxine is indicated.

Hypothalamic-pituitary dysfunction

In these cases, which form a large group of women with secondary amenorrhoea, the body-weight is normal, FSH, LH, hPr, TSH (or T_3 T_4) levels are normal, and there may be a history of taking contraceptives. If the amenorrhoea has persisted for more than 12 months, ovulation can be induced in over 80 per cent of women using clomiphene initially, and gonadotrophins, if clomiphene fails to induce ovulation. The progesterone stimulation test helps, in these cases, to determine the best initial approach to treatment. If a withdrawal bleed has not occurred following the test, clomiphene alone is unlikely to be successful.

Clomiphene is an 'anti-oestrogen' in effect (although it is actually a weak oestrogen). It binds to oestrogen receptors in the cytoplasm of 'target' cells, as does oestradiol. But when the clomiphene-receptor complex is transferred to the nucleus it induces very little synthesis of new receptor and the cell becomes relatively insensitive to the effects of endogenous oestradiol. This inhibits the negative feedback mechanism with the resulting release of GnRH and subsequently of FSH and LH. Clomiphene may also act directly upon the hypothalamus, causing the release of FSH. Since each patient's response to the drug varies, the smallest possible dose should be given to avoid overstimulation of the ovaries. In subsequent months the dose is increased if ovulation fails to occur. After 4 months of unsuccessful treatment a period without treatment should be offered as it has been found that spontaneous ovulation and pregnancy may occur in this interval (Table 8/3).

If the progestogen stimulation test is negative the regimen is often unsuccessful, but is worth trying for 2 or 3 months. Should anovulation persist after the regimen outlined, the patient should receive either human menopausal gonadotrophin (HMG) and human chorionic gonadotrophin (HCG) or gonadotrophin releasing hormone (GnRH) in pulsed doses subcutaneously. Human pituitary gonadotrophin (HPG) may be used in place of GnRH but is in short supply and is expensive.

HMG and HCG: In this regimen 3 ampoules of HMG (Pergonal) are given on days 1, 3, 5, followed by HCG 10 000U on the day the main follicle has reached 20–25mm in diameter (as determined by ultrasound). The dose of HCG must be individualized, for example, if more than one follicle is >20mm in diameter the ovulating dose of HCG is omitted, and unprotected intercourse is avoided in that cycle. In spite of these precautions the multiple pregnancy rate exceeds 20 per cent.

The use of the gonadotrophins, HMG and HPG, is not without hazard to the patient, as the dose which induces ovulation varies considerably between patients, and indeed between treatment cycles in the same patient, and is very close to that causing super-ovulation and pathological ovarian enlargement. It must be stressed that the drugs should only be used after the patients have undergone meticulous investigations, both by clinical and laboratory methods, and the patient must be cared for in a special centre which has an efficient laboratory facility

GnRH: In this development, pulsed injections of GnRH in a dose of 5 to 20μg are given, intravenously or subcutaneously, every 90 minutes via a battery-operated auto-infusion pump. Ovulation is detected using ultrasound and the pulsed injections are continued until pregnancy is confirmed to ensure good decidual development. The injections may have

Stage	Month	Dose
1	1	Clomiphene 50mg daily for 5 days
2	2	Clomiphene 100mg daily for 5 days
3	3	Clomiphene 150mg daily for 5 days
4	4	Clomiphene 200mg daily for 5 days
5	6–8	No treatment
6	9	Clomiphene 100mg daily for 5 days + HCG 5000 IU 7 days later
7	10	Clomiphene 150mg daily for 5 days + HCG 5000 IU 7 days later

If ovulation occurs at any stage, maintain the regimen which produced it for 3 months. If ovulation fails to occur move to the next stage. Ovulation is determined 9 to 16 days after starting the course, by observing a rise in the daily basal body temperature, or by finding significant quantities of progesterone in the plasma. Clomiphene is given from day 1 to 5 of the cycle.

Table 8/3 Therapeutic regimen using clomiphene to induce ovulation

to be given for 20 days or more. The patient continues her normal life during this time. The advantage of pulsed injections of GnRH is that the careful monitoring required for the other two regimens is not needed, the cost of treatment is less and the pregnancy rate higher. To maintain corpus luteum function following ovulation GnRH may be continued or HCG 1500IU given every fourth day for three injections.

THE RESULTS

With increasing discrimination of the various causes of anovulatory amenorrhoea, and with more precise therapy, higher rates of ovulation and conception have occurred. Ovulation may be expected to occur in 85 per cent of women investigated and treated appropriately; and between 65 and 75 per cent will become pregnant. However, pregnancy wastage is high. Over 20 per cent of the pregnancies abort spontaneously. The rate of multiple pregnancy is also high, if clomiphene or HMG is required to induce ovulation. Most of the multiple pregnancies are twin pregnancies. Clomiphene use is associated with a rate of about 10 per cent, and that of the gonadotrophins of more than 25 per cent. Multiple pregnancy, in turn, may lead to pre-term labour and a raised perinatal mortality.

The proportion of women who ovulate and conceive following treatment of oligomenorrhoea is lower (as is the proportion of regularly menstruating anovulatory women), in spite of treatment similar to that given to anovulating amenorrhoeic women. Only about 30 to 40 per cent of this group ovulate.

It is interesting to note that the regularity of menstruation and the occurrence of ovulation in patients with secondary amenorrhoea (particularly if this follows oral contraceptives), oligomenorrhoea and regularly occurring anovulatory cycles who have been treated with clomiphene or gonadotrophins, improves after ceasing therapy. Over the next year, or longer, 60 per cent of women will continue to have regular menstruation and spontaneous conceptions will occur in about half of them. It appears that the 'fertility drugs' initiate the regular release of GnRH from the hypothalamus in many women.

FOLLOW-UP

Women who have hyperprolactinaemia (usually associated with amenorrhoea and often galactorrhoea), and in whom no tumour is detected should be followed up by annual estimations of hPr, and skull X-ray, as a number of them will eventually show evidence of a pituitary tumour. This is more likely if the hyperprolactinaemia occurred spontaneously rather than following pregnancy or the use of oestrogenic hormonal contraceptives.

TREATMENT SUMMARY

Assuming pregnancy desired:
1. *FSH raised = ovarian failure*
   (do karyotype, with banding to exclude Y-line of cells).
2. *Weight loss or obesity*
   Help woman regain normal weight before giving any ovulating inducing drugs.
3. *hPr raised (repeat), TSH normal, pituitary fossa normal*
   Rx bromocriptine.
   (Also give if woman has symptoms, but does not desire pregnancy.)
4. *hPr raised and TSH raised*
   Rx thyroxine.
5. *LH raised, FSH normal = PCO*
   Confirm by ultrasound or laparoscopy: then clomiphene.
6. *FSH normal, hPr normal, progesterone stimulation test, positive or oestradiol normal*
   Clomiphene initially. If failure, give HMG + HCG. If that fails, either GnRH pulsed injections or HPG + HCG.

Chapter 9

Human Sexuality and Psychosexual Problems

Alone of the mammals, man does not mate instinctively in response to a special group of visual and nasal stimuli produced by the female, but must learn techniques. Alone of the female mammals, the female human engages in copulation at times other than when ovulation is imminent. The primacy of sex as a basic human instinct has produced patterns of sexual behaviour in tribal societies, from the most primitive to the most sophisticated, which are a product of the environment and culture pertaining to that society. In primitive tribes what appears at first sight to be sexual freedom, is often sex hedged in with a variety of complex taboos which proscribe certain activities and encourage others. In the New Guinea Highlands, young men and women are encouraged to engage in 'leg carrying' in which physical contact usually just short of, but often including, coitus is permitted and promiscuity accepted; but once the couple have paired off and have married, strict prohibitions on the female are enforced. Amongst Eskimos a guest is normally offered the services of one of the host's wives for copulation, and if she fails to provide sexual satisfaction, the husband is shamed. In certain Indian (and other) societies, homosexuality in youth is not condemned but considered natural, being replaced, as the youth grows older, by a heterosexual attachment to a bride chosen by the family he had not seen prior to the marriage ceremony. Islam permits polygamy, but enjoins that each wife is treated equally in every respect, whilst Judeo-Christian societies consider polygamy evil but tacitly accept the presence of prostitutes. To a large extent the Christian belief that sex is evil, and even within marriage is permissible solely for reproductive purposes, stems from the writings of Augustine; whilst the concept that woman is inferior to man comes from an earlier ecclesiastic, Pope Gregory. The pronouncements of the two early Christian theologians were further codified during the turbulence of the Reformation, when male authoritarianism and female subjugation were confirmed. This led to the 'double standard' of sexual behaviour – the male was permitted to seek sexual satisfaction with women, but the female was expected to remain a virgin until marriage and then submit to male dominance.

Rescue from the rigid pattern in Western society only came with the writings of Freud who suggested that sex was a basic instinct to be enjoyed by both partners, and that coitus not only formed the centre of physical expression but extended beyond the mere physical act of copulation. In Western societies today a much more open approach to sexual behaviour is apparent in both sexes, and a much freer atmosphere has arisen in which sexual matters may be discussed. Despite this, the majority of adolescents continue to obtain their knowledge, or lack of knowledge, of sexual behaviour from inhibition-bound parents who still believe that sex is dirty; from the collected myths of their peer-group; from a small amount of biological information obtained at school or church; and from experimentation with adolescents of the other or the same sex. In most modern Western societies, the myth of male supremacy and of female submission and the concept of a 'double standard' regrettably persist. A more rational cultural pattern would be to accept, as normal, the urgency of the sexual drive, providing that in obtaining an outlet for this drive neither partner suffers exploitation.

THE SEXUAL DRIVE

Five criteria serve to identify the sex of an individual, (1) gonadal sex, (2) nuclear sex, (3) hormonal sex, (4) external genital morphological sex, and (5) gender identity or psychological sex. Because of an error in determining the sex at birth, or in early childhood, following a cursory examination of the external genitalia, a child may be raised in the opposite psychological sex. Gender identity, particularly if imprinted in the first two years of life, is extremely difficult to change should the error not be discovered until puberty. This implies that sexual behaviour is learned, and the psychological and cultural influences which fashion it are not easily reversed.

The relative influences of genetic and environmental factors on the sexual drive have not been fully elucidated. It is possible that individuals differ in their inherent sexual drive (or libido), but this factor has little influence compared with psychological and social influences in childhood and adolescence. These play the major part in determining a person's sexual drive. Because of the 'double standard' still prevalent in society, women are more affected by psychosocial influences than men. This has led to the erroneous belief that women have fewer sexual needs and a lower sexual drive than men. The basis of this observation is that many women seem slower to respond sexually, reach orgasm less frequently and appear to 'demand' sex less than men.

These attributes are not innate; they are due to the faulty conditioning of girls in childhood in regard to their sexuality. For example, a mother who brings up her daughter to believe that sex is 'dirty', that pre-marital sexual intercourse is sinful, that it is a wife's duty to submit passively rather than to enjoy coitus, that men are sexually expert, sexually aggressive and have no thought for the needs of women, is likely to produce a woman with impaired sexuality.

Because of this negative conditioning, a woman may accept her role as a sexual puppet to be manipulated for the man's pleasure, and believe that her sexual function is only to be a receptacle for semen and for a growing fetus. She has been 'taught' not to expect to enjoy sex as much as a man.

A further reinforcement of the conditioning that sex is unpleasant can result from a traumatic sexual experience in childhood or adolescence (for example, incest or an early sexual assault). Such an experience may markedly reduce a woman's sexual drive. (In the case of a man, it can also cause sexual problems and may contribute to premature ejaculation or impotence, which is more correctly termed erectile failure.)

The importance of intelligent sexual upbringing by informed parents or by teachers, is obvious. Childhood conditioning that sexuality is disgusting and dirty, to be hidden beneath bedclothes and not mentioned, that the naked body is indecent and that the genitalia do not exist, can lay the foundations for a deficient sex drive in adult life.

During adult life, sexual drive varies considerably in different people and at different times of their lives. In general, the sex drive is strongest in both sexes from adolescence until late in the third decade, after which it declines slowly. This information is a generalization, as many individuals and couples continue to have a high sexual drive until old age.

The drive is altered by outside interests. Men may have a reduced drive, because of pressures of work, or excessive alcoholic consumption; whilst the demands of childrearing and the effect of endogenous depression may reduce the drive in women. By contrast, many women find a resurgence of their sexual drive during and after the climacteric.

During periods when the sexual drive of one partner is low, the couple may find pleasure and often sexual excitement if they cuddle each other and enjoy the tactile stimulus of two bodies close together.

Although humans, both male and female, differ in the intensity of their sexual drives, conflict generally only occurs in a relationship if one partner has a high sexual drive and the other has a low drive. In other words, the relative sexual drive between partners is more significant than the absolute sexual drive of each.

As I have mentioned, women have the same sexual drive as men, although they may have been culturally conditioned to suppress it. Only recently, and only in certain strata of society, has this belief been acknowledged and women have been able to obtain sexual equality with men.

In an equal sexual relationship, sex is not something done to someone, but something mutually pleasurable which is done together, *with* each other rather than *for* the other. Unfortunately, this ideal situation is rare. Most adults enter a sexual relationship with a collection of acquired inhibitions and 'hang-ups' towards sexuality. Yet equality in a sexual relationship demands that each partner has some knowledge of human sexuality, is comfortable in his or her own sexuality, and is able to communicate openly with the other partner so that both can choose what is right for them.

Considerable evidence is now available that the problems of disparate sexual drive in a relationship are aggravated if the partners are unable to talk openly to each other about their sexual desires. The lack of communication is mainly due to inhibitions about human sexuality induced during childhood and adolescence. Often a vicious circle occurs during which the sexual relationship becomes distorted and frustrations mount. Much disharmony in a sexual relationship can be reduced, or eliminated, if the couple are able to talk openly with each other about their sexual and other needs, and, during sexual intercourse, pleasure each other.

Unfortunately, because of ignorance about sex, because of an upbringing in which sex was either not mentioned, or treated as somewhat shameful, an individual's ability to be comfortable about sex, to communicate about sex and to have a shared responsibility for sexual pleasure is often muted. In such a relationship (by which I mean an agreed commitment to another person, whether legalized or not) sexual problems may occur.

As each partner is unable to communicate openly and freely about his or her sexual needs or desires, frustrations increase.

These frustrations can lead to a variety of psychosomatic symptoms and help is required. But a doctor can only help to resolve the problems resulting from sexual inadequacy if he or she has the basic knowledge and understanding of human sexuality, is comfortable in his or her own sexuality, and is able to communicate to the person in a clear, nonjudgmental way.

THE HUMAN SEXUAL RESPONSE

The human sexual response in women and in men can be divided into five phases although the distinction between each phase is often blurred and one tends to merge into the next, provided the appropriate stimulation occurs. The phases are: (1) the desire phase, (2) the excitement (or arousal) phase, (3) the plateau phase, (4) the orgastic (orgasm) phase, and (5) the resolution phase.

Sexual desire is stimulated by the sight, touch, or smell of another person or by seeing erotic material. It may merge imperceptibly into the excitement phase or be suppressed by inhibiting stimuli.

In the *excitement phase* the breasts respond by erection of the nipples, tumescence of the areolae and increase in mammary size due to congestion of the capillary plexus. Simultaneously, the clitoris increases in width, and the labia minora become softer and thicker from passive venous congestion, reaching a peak in the short plateau phase. The degree of clitoral and labial response varies from woman to woman. During the excitement phase the pelvic

tissues, including the vaginal submucosa, become congested and fluid transudes between the vaginal epithelial cells to cause what Masters and Johnson term 'the sweating phenomenon'. The vasocongestion surrounding the lower third of the vagina produces swellings or 'cushions' around the introitus, which caress the entering penis.

The pleasure of the excitement phase is intensified in both sexes if the couple pleasure each other sexually. This is also called foreplay, but mutual pleasuring is a more descriptive term. Mutual pleasuring involves cuddling and body contact. It involves stroking and body exploration with fingers, tongue, lips and thighs. It involves specific stimulation of each partner's erotic zones by fingers, lips or tongue – in a woman her breasts and clitoral area, sometimes her anal area; in a man, his penis, scrotum and anal area. Mutual pleasuring is a learning experience and has no set formula. Each partner's needs and desires are unique, and each has to discover what turns on the other partner to the greatest extent.

In the *plateau phase*, the physiological changes which occurred in the excitement phase increase and the woman may wish to be helped to reach orgasm by digital or oral stimulation of her clitoral area, or she may be ready for and desirous of feeling her partner's penis contained in her vagina. The movement of the man's penis as he thrusts and withdraws indirectly stimulates the clitoris so that the woman may reach orgasm. However, orgasm during penile thrusting occurs in fewer than half of sexually stimulated women. This may be because of the rapidity of the man's passage from the plateau to the orgastic phase. If the woman does not reach orgasm during penile thrusting she may wish her partner help her reach orgasm by oral or digital stimulation.

Orgasm

It was believed that a woman can have two types of orgasm, a 'clitoral orgasm' and a 'vaginal orgasm'. An error of observation and of deduction by Freud is responsible for this. He maintained that the clitoral orgasm was an immature form, which was obtained by masturbation, and that vaginal orgasm only developed with sexual and psychological maturity, when the centre of sexual sensitivity was transferred from the clitoral area to the vagina. The deduction from this was that masturbation is immature, and a woman who can only reach an orgasm by masturbation is immature and psychosexually impaired, whilst a woman who develops a vaginal orgasm is sexually and psychologically mature. This Freudian view is erroneous. Most sexually responsive women are able to reach orgasm by direct or indirect clitorial stimulation. Many women can reach orgasm by stimulation of the anterior vaginal wall. There appears to be a clitoral-anterior vaginal wall sensory arm of the orgasmic reflex.

Thus orgasm in women differs little from that in men, with the exception that in the male ejaculation occurs. Stimulation of the clitoral area by manipulation, or by the movement of the penis as it is thrust in and out of the vagina (which may cause clitoral stimulation indirectly) brings the woman to orgasm. In addition, many women obtain additional pleasurable sensations from the vagina, so that an orgasm is neither clitoral nor vaginal but both. It is triggered by clitoral stimulatory impulses being relayed to the lumbar spine where a reflex mechanism occurs. Efferent fibres carry impulses which cause clonic rhythmic pelvic muscular contractions. The reflex is under the control of psychic influences which can be facilitatory or inhibitory, the latter leading to a failure of orgasm.

During orgasm, the perineal muscles, the medial fibres of the levator ani and the sphincter ani muscles contract rhythmically and involuntarily, as do the muscles of the vaginal barrel and the uterus (to a lesser extent). The orgasm is said to be more intense if the erect penis in inserted deeply into the vagina at the time, and is gripped and released rhythmically by the contracting muscles. Many other muscle groups, particularly of the lower abdomen and back, contract at the height of the orgasm, and a deep feeling of relaxation, ecstasy (in the original sense), relief and lethargy follows. The woman has entered the phase of *resolution*. In the initial moments of resolution, the clitoral area is exquisitely sensitive (which is analogous to the exquisite penile sensitivity immediately after ejaculation), but this rapidly passes and decongestion of the vagina, the labia minora and the clitoral area occurs over a period of 5 to 10 minutes. The phase of resolution may last minutes or may merge into sleep lasting hours, depending on the circumstances. A few women (15 per cent according to Kinsey) are able and desirous of obtaining multiple orgasms during coitus, the same sequence of phases following more rapidly with each orgasm (Fig. **9/1**). If the woman is stimulated to the plateau phase but fails to achieve an orgasm, the resolution phase may be prolonged, the decongestion of the pelvic tissues only occurring slowly and imperfectly. Repeated stimulation and failure to achieve orgasm may lead to physical and mental frustration, and is a possible underlying cause of many psychosomatic gynaecological complaints. It may also lead, protectively, to a reduction in libido, or the woman may seek to obtain satisfaction with other sexual partners, or to sublimate her frustrations in other forms of activity.

THE TWO PARTS OF SEXUAL AROUSAL

It will be realized that the sequence of the phases of sexual arousal merge into each other and that the separation was made for descriptive purposes.

In both women and men the sequence of sexual arousal has two distinct parts. Both are mediated by psychic or physical sexual stimulation (and usually, but not necessarily, by both). Both can be inhibited to a greater or lesser degree by subconscious influences.

The first phase is controlled physiologically by the parasympathetic nerves. During it, vasodilatation and vasocongestion of the pelvic organs occurs. In a man, this causes penile erection as blood fills the cavernous spaces in the penile cylinders. In a woman, it leads to vaginal lubrication and to the congestive cushions which form around the lower part of the vagina. Failure of the stimulation to produce these changes causes impotence in a man and general sexual dysfunction, so-called 'frigidity', in a woman.

The second part of sexual arousal is controlled physiologically by the sympathetic nerve supply. During it, clonic muscle contractions of the pelvic muscles occur; in other words, the person has an orgasm. Initially the contractions are limited to the perineal muscles but later many other muscle groups

10 % NO ORGASM	50% ORGASM WHEN CLITORIS STIMULATED	25% ORGASM DURING COITUS	15% MULTIPLE ORGASMS

Fig. 9/1 The orgastic response in women

are involved. The sequence is the same in both sexes, and the pleasurable effect spreads through the whole body. But in a man orgasm is usually accompanied by the emission of seminal fluid from the prostatic area along the urethra and then its periodic, spasmodic ejaculation.

Failure of this sequence to proceed in an orderly way leads to premature or retarded ejaculation in a man and lack of orgasm in a woman.

Whilst penile erection and vaginal lubrication can occur with adequate stimulation in a person who has a spinal transsection, indicating that it is a reflex, there is a controlling centre for sexuality in the brain. The sexual centre is in the thalamic and limbic areas of the old cortex and is closely related to the 'pleasure centres' of the paleocortex. Sex and pleasure are related anatomically as well as psychologically!

The spinal reflexes which control erection and ejaculation in a man and vaginal lubrication and swelling in a woman are normally subservient to the cerebral sex centres (which control the pleasure of orgasm). They in turn receive and transmit impulses from most neural areas and circuits in the brain. Thus the human sexual response is influenced by multiple influences acquired from infancy onwards. These influences derive from experiences, memories, emotions, associations and thoughts. Because our culture treats sexuality as taboo, to some extent the influences are more likely to be inhibitory than facilitative and to induce, in the susceptible person, fear or anxiety about their sexuality. But equally the inhibitions can be overcome and sexual response facilitated by the positive emotions of love, or by fantasy.

Only if people can escape from the negative conditioning of their culture and the couple can abandon themselves to the erotic experience, will their sexual response be maximal, and full sexual pleasure achieved.

MASTURBATION

Tactile stimulation of the external genitalia is universal in childhood, and in adolescence masturbation is general both in males and females. Masturbation (either auto-masturbation or mutual masturbation) is a normal sexual developmental occurrence which diminishes in frequency, or is omitted, once heterosexual relations begin. During sexual development it plays an important role in enabling the individual to realize his or her response to sexual stimuli. It is obvious from this that masturbation causes no physical or mental damage and should give rise to no feeling of guilt. In fact the only problems associated with masturbation result from anxiety induced by the erroneous cultural beliefs which have developed over the centuries in Judeo-Christian societies. In these cultures masturbation was associated with guilt, with shame and with evil. It was considered to lead to mental defectiveness on the one hand, and impotence in marriage and premature senility on the other. Only in recent years has it been recognized that these statements are nonsense; but even today some gynaecological textbooks state that clitoral hypertrophy, pelvic congestion, menorrhagia and leucorrhoea are caused by excessive masturbation.

The cure for all this mythology is to educate adolescents that masturbation causes no harmful physical effects, that it is a normal appropriate method of sexual expression, and that as heterosexual relationships develop, the frequency of masturbation diminishes.

In certain circumstances, such as bereavement or prolonged separation from a lover, women (and men) may return to masturbation as a means of sexual release rather than seeking a new sexual partner. Because of our cultural attitudes, this may occasion guilt, and the medical counsellor should make every effort to reassure the woman that masturbation is beneficial to her physical and mental health rather than the reverse.

COITUS

It should be clear from what I have written that many of the myths regarding sexual behaviour, masturbation and coital technique, are indeed myths, and what the couple do in privacy by mutual consent is normal and natural. There are no abnormal coital positions, and whether copulation occurs with the man above and the woman recumbent, or the woman above and the man recumbent, or the couple lying side by side, or the penis entering the vagina from the rear, is a matter which is individual and dependent upon the circumstances at the time. It is also normal for couples to prefer orogenital or digital sexual stimulation occasionally or usually. Many women experience orgasm only after digital stimulation of the clitoral area, or from cunnilingus, or prefer one of these methods as a change from penile-vaginal contact. Similarly, a man may enjoy fellatio in preference to coitus from time to time.

Coitus takes place frequently in the early years of sexual activity, often occurring once every 24 hours. The frequency falls after 1 or 2 years to the 'mean' of two to three times a week, and as middle age supervenes, to once a week or less. But as has been noted, there is a marked individual variation and there is no standard norm from which deviations can occur. What is suitable for that couple is normal. 'Excessive' coitus has no harmful effects, and 'infrequent' coitus, if this pattern is acceptable and not frustrating to both partners, is equally innocuous. It is only when the sexual drive of one partner fails to be satisfied or sublimated, that problems arise.

PROBLEMS ASSOCIATED WITH COITUS

First coitus

Attempts at a first coitus can be distressing to a woman, particularly if she has had a sexually repressed upbringing and has acquired little, or inaccurate, knowledge about sex. The discomfort is aggravated if the man lacks knowledge, is clumsy and is unwilling to arouse the woman sexually before attempting penetration of her vagina. Failure to enjoy the experience can lead to sexual problems (in either or both partners).

These problems can be reduced if a woman, who has not previously had sexual intercourse, seeks a medical examination from a sympathetic knowledgeable doctor or marriage counsellor. He or she is able to explain basic sexual matters to the woman, or better to the couple, and can recommend contraceptives should the couple desire them.

Coitus during menstruation and pregnancy

There is no medical reason why coitus should not take place during menstruation if the couple desire it. The belief that coitus at this time is dangerous as the tissues are fragile and that infection may occur is nonsense and the only objection is an aesthetic one.

Coitus during pregnancy is also surrounded by taboos. In one Pacific Island Group coitus is interdicted, but a substitute wife is provided for the male. In fact, coitus in early pregnancy is safe provided the man is gentle, and need only be banned when a patient has threatened to abort, or is a recurrent aborter. During pregnancy the woman's libido often changes. Some women have a greatly increased sexual drive, in others the drive diminishes.

Coitus becomes more complicated technically in later pregnancy, especially if the man-superior position is chosen. Other coital positions, especially rearentry, offer solutions and coitus can continue as long as both partners mutually wish to continue. Alternatively, sexual tension can be relieved by genital manipulation, either digitally or by cunnilingus. These varieties of sexual expression are satisfying and safe, except that the man should avoid blowing into the woman's vagina during cunnilingus because of the potential hazard of the air entering a blood vessel and causing a fatal air embolism.

There is no truth in the myth that sexual activity, including orgasm, in a healthy pregnant woman can induce abortion or induce premature labour, nor will it lead to fetal infection if continued up to the time of confinement.

In the puerperium, coitus can be resumed as soon as the woman wishes and finds it enjoyable.

SEXUAL COUNSELLING

In the past few years it has been evident that many problems brought to the attention of doctors have a basis in disturbed relations between the partners. Frequently the problem is a sexual one, and is the result of childhood inhibitions about human sexuality leading to an inability to communicate on sexual matters.

All too often in the past the doctor, lacking the perception and embarrassed because of his own sexual 'hang-ups', has failed to detect the underlying problem and has treated the symptoms with tranquillizers or mood elevators, with little success. This approach has been aggravated by the absence in medical curricula of any discussion of, or education about, human sexuality. Luckily for patients and doctors this is changing.

Two main problems exist which prevent many doctors from counselling patients with sexual problems. The first is a lack of knowledge about human sexuality. The second is the doctor's inability to discuss such problems without embarrassment, in common language (avoiding the solace of jargon) and without the doctor imposing his value judgments on the problem. Medical students and doctors, like most people in society, have attitudes to sexuality and its expression which may cause them anxiety and discomfort. They become defensive, judgmental and may lose the concerned objectivity necessary for counselling.

Counselling skills can only be obtained by the student becoming aware of his own sexual inhibitions, confronting and overcoming them, and learning to communicate in a compassionate, factual manner with his patient. This type of experience is best obtained in experiental sessions in which role playing is used.

A further problem may arise in discussing disturbed sexual relations. In the majority of them, it is essential to involve the other sexual partner if therapy is to be successful. The aphorism, used by Masters and Johnson, that 'in human sexual problems there is no uninvolved partner' is valid.

Counselling about sexual problems, which includes problems of infertility, contraception, abortion, is an important part of gynaecology, and it is one which is acquiring increasing importance as the more gross gynaecological conditions requiring surgery become less frequent.

SEXUAL DYSFUNCTIONS IN WOMEN

The biphasic nature of the sexual response and the fact that sexuality is usually a mutual experience can, in the absence of appropriate responses, or because of subconscious inhibition of those responses lead to several forms of sexual dysfunction.

All forms of sexual inadequacy may lead to marital disharmony, to depression or to a variety of psychosomatic disorders. Of course, if the woman does not perceive that she is sexually inadequate, or accepts her inadequacy, the problem is minimized. In such cases she may 'fake' sexual enjoyment, including orgasm, to please her partner. Recent evidence suggests that, over a period, this leads to more, rather than less, marital discontent, and open discussion between partners is to be encouraged.

Such discussion is often impossible, even when the woman feels that she is missing sexual pleasure, without skilled, sympathetic counselling. With skilled sympathetic counselling, most of the problems will be resolved and the couple will reach a better, more pleasurable sexual relationship.

Women have three forms of sexual dysfunction:
1. Inhibited sexual desire.
2. Dyspareunia (including vaginismus).
3. Orgastic dysfunction.

The causes of all forms of sexual dysfunction are complex and multiple, and to some extent overlap. Although ill-health, depression and fatigue may be a cause, and must be excluded, psychosexual factors are more frequent and significant.

A significant factor in producing sexual dysfunction (with the exception of the organic causes of dyspareunia and apareunia) is a negative attitude towards sexuality as a means of mutual pleasuring. This often occurs from faulty upbringing by parents whose view of sex is that it is something shameful to be endured, not enjoyed, and to be suppressed rather than treated as a normal, integral part of living. In this environment a woman, by erroneous 'imprinting', by negative conditioning and by suppression of the limited information available to her, perceives sex as 'dirty'. This attitude may have been reinforced by a traumatic first sexual experience in which the man sought relief without attempting to give the woman any pleasure, or having any real feeling for her needs. It may also be enhanced by a religious orthodoxy in which negative attitudes to the joy of sex are rigorously encouraged.

Additional factors may be a lack of communication with the male sexual partner about sexual matters, so that he is never told what stimulates her sexually, and has never tried to find out for himself. To this may be added the problem that the man fails to provide sufficient 'foreplay' to arouse the woman to the plateau stage and once his penis is in her vagina reaches orgasm and ejaculates rapidly.

This complicates the problem, for the same psychosocial factors which lead to a reduced libido and failure to reach orgasm in a woman, are involved in premature ejaculation and erectile failure – the two most common male sexual problems. Of the three forms of sexual dysfunction in women, inhibited sexual desire is the most severe and the woman who has it is usually sexually up-tight. The woman who has orgastic dysfunction may enjoy sexuality but knows that she is missing out on greater enjoyment.

The management of sexual dysfunction begins by the doctor obtaining a comprehensive sexual history including the woman's attitudes to her body and to menstruation. A general history should be obtained with particular reference to physical illness and psychiatric problems, such as depression. When this information has been obtained and evaluated, the doctor is better able to attend to the psychosexual problem. In this regard an acronym is helpful. The acronym is LEPERS:

Listen   for hidden signals
Explore   the patient's attitude to sexuality
Provide   information
Examine   relationships
Reduce   anxiety
Suggest   strategies

	Clinical Syndrome	
	Male	Female
1. *Inhibited sexual desire*	——— No arousal ———	
2. *Fear of sexual (genital) activity*	Primary erectile failure (impotence)	Vaginismus
3. *Impairment of sexual arousal.* Absence or inadequate vaso-congestion* due to failure to respond to erotic stimulation from anxiety, guilt or fear of injury.	Reduced libido and secondary erectile failure (impotence)	Reduced libido
4. *Impairment or failure of orgasm.* Extremely rapid, or absence of clonic rhythmic contractions of pelvic musculature due to inhibition of genital tactile or psychic erotic stimulation.	Premature ejaculation	Orgastic dysfunction
	Retarded ejaculation	

* In the male, penile erection; in the female, vaginal lubrication and perivaginal swelling.

Table 9/1 Sexual dysfunctions

– permission giving
– specific treatment

In the treatment of a woman's orgastic dysfunction, particularly, her partner usually should be involved. If his inhibitions prevent him from co-operating, or if the woman believes his inhibitions prevent her from communicating her needs to him, the treatment will fail. The medical counsellor should talk with the man separately, after talking with the woman, so that he may assess and discuss each partner's sexual beliefs and anxieties.

The objectives of therapy are to alter an existing destructive attitude to sexuality; to reduce or resolve any underlying interpersonal sexual conflict, anxiety or fear; and to enable the couple to create an environment in which sexuality is perceived as a joyous, mutually pleasurable experience.

To achieve these objectives the counsellor, through discussion with the woman, seeks to help her examine her attitudes to sexuality and discover what stimulates her sexually. It also enables her to find out what diminishes her sexuality. When she has found what turns her on she can make her partner aware of her sexual desires. In other words, the counsellor seeks to help the couple express their sexual needs to each other. With the knowledge of each other's sexual desires and needs, the couple are given sexual 'tasks' to enable them to overcome hidden conflicts, anxieties and fears.

The sexual tasks have been described by Masters and Johnson, by Kaplan and by others (see bibliography). They start with 'sensate focus' exercises, go on to erotic zone stimulation (breasts and genitalia) and then to 'non-demanding coitus'. These tasks are reinforced by sessions with the therapist who explains problems revealed during the tasks. As each task involves an increasing awareness of the 'pleasuring' nature of sexuality and as each is completed successfully, the couple move on to the next task. But should either partner fail to find pleasure in the task (or refuse to complete the task), the counsellor discusses the possible causes, so that alternative routes to sexual pleasure can be found. Not all of the tasks are needed in each case, but a selection helps most couples with a sexual problem.

Inhibited sexual desire

Women with *inhibited sexual desire* (previously called generalized sexual dysfunction) are not sexually aroused even when sexually teased by their partner and may find such teasing distasteful. The condition may have been present since puberty or may be acquired after some months or years of marriage. If both partners have inhibited sexual desire, problems are not perceived, but if one sexual partner has an inhibited sexual desire and the other has a normal or a raised desire and is easily sexually aroused, problems become manifest. These problems are perhaps less marked in women because of a woman's genital morphology. A woman who has an inhibited sexual desire may accommodate her man's sexual needs by accepting, although obtaining no enjoyment from sexual intercourse; but a man who has inhibited sexual desire will make his partner sexually frustrated. Some women who have *inhibited sexual desire* are able to enjoy caring for their partner in other ways but seek to avoid the sexual advances he may make. In the more resistant cases, the woman not only has an inhibited sexual desire, but finds all sexual advances unpleasant, threatening and revolting.

A few doctors believe that inhibited sexual desire and orgastic dysfunction can be treated by giving the patient injections or tablets of testosterone or one of its salts. Recent carefully controlled trials have shown that testosterone provides no benefit (compared with placebo) in the treatment of these conditions. It should not be prescribed.

Sexual exercises may help to resolve inhibited sexual desire but the results are poor; nor is any other therapy more successful. However, the doctor may be able to help the woman (and her partner) to adjust to, and cope with, their sexual problems.

Dyspareunia, apareunia, vaginismus

Apareunia and dyspareunia are symptoms. The former implies that the penis has not been permitted, or has not been able, to penetrate the vestibule and enter the vagina; and the latter that coitus is painful. The pain and discomfort may be introital or may only occur on deep penetration.

As with many problems of sexual behaviour, the fault may lie with the male or with the female. Apareunia may be due to impotence or to gross malformation of the penis on the part of the male; or to local diseases of the pelvic organs, or to psychosomatic disturbances, on the part of the female. The last two factors are also the causes of dyspareunia. As well, ignorance or inexperience may prevent normal coition.

The local causes of dyspareunia must be sought and eliminated before deciding that the condition is psychosomatic in origin. Local causes include malformations of the lower female genital tract; scarring and contraction following inexpertly performed pelvic floor repair and operations for uterovaginal prolapse; the use of rock salt to 'tighten' the vagina after childbirth; infections (particularly trichomoniasis and vaginal candidiasis); or tumours of the vagina and rectum. In most of the cases the woman complains of pain during attempted insertion of the penis into the vagina. This is introital dyspareunia. Deep dyspareunia is felt when the erect penis is fully inserted, or in the hours following

coitus. The deep dyspareunia occurring during coitus may be caused by chronic pelvic infection, endometriosis or by a prolapsed ovary, but pain occurring in the hours following coitus is always psychosomatic in origin.

If examination confirms that the fault does not lie with the male, and that no organic causes of dyspareunia are present in the female, the condition is of psychosomatic origin, and often presents as *vaginismus*. This condition is due to an involuntary tightening of the muscles which surround the vaginal introitus and lower third of the vagina. The muscle spasm may be so marked that coitus is impossible, and even vaginal examination using a single finger provokes an intense spasm. The spasm may involve not only the pelvic floor muscles, but the adductor muscles of the thighs (which have been called graphically 'the pillars of virginity'). Occasionally partial penetration is possible before pain is felt, so that the patient may complain of either introital or deep dyspareunia.

The cause of vaginismus lies in inadequate or faulty sex education, particularly if a belief has been acquired that sex is 'dirty', or a fear that the introduction of the penis will damage the woman. Occasionally vaginismus can be traced to a sexual assault occurring during childhood or adolescence, or to the initial forcible, clumsy, coital attempts by an ignorant or inhibited man. In all these instances, fear is the root cause.

Treatment of dyspareunia depends on the cause. Local conditions may be readily remedied, but vaginismus often requires longer management, and the patient must be involved in her own therapy. It must be stressed to her that she is anatomically normal and not 'small made', and that cure is certain, provided she is able to insert a finger or an object into her vagina.

As many women are ignorant of the appearance and anatomy of the vulva, the counsellor describes this with diagrams and/or photographs. The woman is then induced to look at her vulva using a mirror whilst the therapist identifies and discusses its anatomy.

The woman is next induced to try and insert a finger into her vagina, and is given instructions to continue the exercise at home. In many cases both sexual partners are seen together and the woman is induced to let the man insert his finger. The alternative is for the doctor to try to insert a small Cusco's vaginal speculum. Once a finger is accepted, two fingers (or a larger speculum is inserted) until three or four fingers are accepted. If a speculum is used it should be shown to the woman after being inserted into her vagina.

When the woman is able to accept three fingers or a moderately large speculum into her vagina without contracting her levator muscles, she is ready to try sexual intercourse. Both she and her partner should be seen together so that the therapist can stress the need for slow non-demanding foreplay so that she obtains good vaginal lubrication. As well, a coital technique may be suggested in which the patient flexes and abducts her thighs during coition. This leads reflexly to pelvic muscles relaxation.

Occasionally the vagina requires dilatation under anaesthesia, until at least three fingers can be introduced, the perineal muscles being stretched or 'ironed out'. Following dilatation, some patients obtain help by using vaginal dilators, not to keep the vagina dilated, but as psychological props until coitus is attempted again. But it is to be remembered that the best vaginal dilator is the erect penis. In postmenopausal women, who have early vulvo-vaginal atrophy, oestrogen cream helps to make the tissues more supple, but if the patient menstruates normally, she is producing adequate amounts of endogenous oestrogen, and exogenous oestrogen is of no value. Occasionally plastic surgery is required to enlarge the vaginal orifice which has been narrowed by scarring, but the operation is not required for vaginismus and indeed may aggravate the problem by producing a sensitive scar in the introitus.

The management of dyspareunia, especially when due to vaginismus, requires that the patient has confidence in the physician who has the time, sympathy and patience to persuade her that her childhood conditioning was wrong, so that she may be persuaded to adopt a more open attitude towards sex.

Orgastic dysfunction

As I noted earlier in this chapter, the sexual drive is influenced by childhood conditioning and cultural taboos. The term 'frigidity' has been used (mostly by men) to describe women who have a low sexual drive (or libido), women who fail consistently to reach orgasm, and women who do not regularly reach orgasm. Frigidity is an inexact, pejorative term and should be avoided as it implies a permanent sexual maladjustment.

The problem is not frigidity but one of two differ-

ent sexual dysfunctions: first, inhibited sexual desire and second, orgastic dysfunction (anorgasmia and infrequent orgasm). Inhibited sexual desire has been discussed earlier in this chapter. Orgastic dysfunction will now be considered.

A few women with orgastic dysfunction may never have reached orgasm although they are able to respond sexually to a greater or lesser degree. Most women with orgastic dysfunction have a 'situational' orgastic dysfunction: they can reach orgasm in one situation but not in another. For example, a woman may fail to reach orgasm during coitus, but may regularly reach orgasm by masturbation or in dreams; or she may reach orgasm sometimes but not always during coitus.

A woman who has orgastic dysfunction needs to learn to enjoy her body and particularly her genital area. She may achieve this by learning to stimulate her clitotral area herself, or permitting her partner to do it. If she chooses to masturbate, she may have to be taught how to. Many women who are unable to reach orgasm during love play, by cunnilingus or during coitus, may learn to reach orgasm by masturbation. In fact masturbation is of considerable help in resolving anorgasmia. Many women prefer not to have their partner present when they masturbate, at least until they are accustomed to the practice. Many women also have to be taught how to masturbate, by the sexual counsellor. In this situation the axiom that the partner should be involved does not apply.

A woman who is anorgasmic may find that she has to masturbate for a prolonged period, often

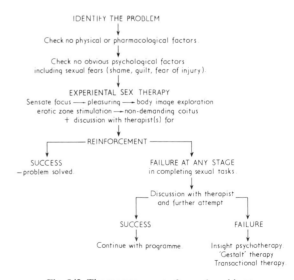

Fig. 9/2 The management of sexual problems

exceeding an hour in her early attempts, before she reaches orgasm. Masturbation can be tiring and the use of a vibrator is often helpful. The stimulation of the clitoral area by a vibrator helps many women reach orgasm more quickly and enjoyably than digital masturbation.

If she chooses to involve her partner she must be sure that he has the sensitivity to stimulate her vulval and clitorial area at her suggestion and under her direction, so that she is in control. With patience most women reach orgasm in one of these two ways.

When the woman has reached orgasm by clitoral stimulation, the couple proceed to 'non-demand' coital techniques, which seek to enhance the woman's sexual arousal. These techniques include longer periods of foreplay, and coitus with the woman in the superior position, the man's penis contained in her vagina whilst he (or she) continues to stimulate her clitoris.

The latter technique is termed 'non-demand' because the partners are instructed to relax and to refrain from feeling the need to 'perform' but, instead, to concentrate on pleasuring.

The importance of fantasy in sexual arousal has not been explored fully, but the evidence indicates that fantasy can enhance sexuality, enabling the couple to have a more intense sexual relationship. A problem which may arise and need explanation is the guilt felt by one partner during sexual exchanges when he or she fantasizes about some other experience or memory. This guilt is unnecessary as many people in close sexual relationships use fantasy from time to time.

If the counsellor finds that there is a barrier to progress in joint sexual exercises, he should suggest masturbation and fantasy as an alternative. He (or she) should also stress that an orgasm reached by masturbation is not 'less feminine', nor 'inferior', nor is it less 'normal' than an orgasm achieved by orogenital or digital clitoral stimulation or one obtained during coitus.

It will be clear that these strategies are aimed at altering the individual's and the couple's destructive attitudes to sexuality in several ways. First, they shift the couple's objective away from sexual performance and achievement: ('He expects me to have an orgasm, so I fake one' or 'I don't really want sex but to show I'm normal I pretend to enjoy it'), to giving and receiving pleasure. Secondly, they modify the tendency of the dysfunctional partner to stand aside and observe herself, what Masters and Johnson call 'spectatoring'. Instead they teach her to abandon herself and focus exclusively on the pleasurable erotic experience which envelops her. Thirdly, by communication, they help to resolve any interpersonal sexual conflicts. In short, they aim to make sex a joyous experience.

Whilst most women (and men) with sexual dysfunction respond to these techniques, a few fail to obtain the attitudinal changes. The arrest of response may occur at any stage of the programme and generally indicates that the individual has a major underlying intrapsychic or inter-personal problem. In such an event further psychiatric intervention is needed which may be by using psychoanalysis, transactional analysis or any other modality favoured.

The techniques outlined were introduced initially by Masters and Johnson and have many variants. All have produced better results than the earlier method of an authoritarian approach by a psychiatrist using 'traditional' methods and the administration of androgens. The latter were supposed to improve libido, either by enlarging the clitoris or by some neuropharmacological effect. There is no unequivocal evidence of the latter, and it is known that orgastic capacity is not related to clitoral size.

OTHER SEXUAL PROBLEMS

HIRSUTISM

The development of body hair is to some extent genetic. Certain races, for example, Chinese, are relatively free of body hair. Other ethnic groups, for example, Southern Europeans, appear to have much more body hair. The difference can be explained by a lack of hair follicle sensitivity to androgens amongst the Chinese.

Some women have increased, or excessive, hair growth in abnormal places, compared with the others of their ethnic group. These women are hirsute, and are often disturbed about their hair distribution as they perceive it to diminish their femininity.

Hirsutism is not the same as virilism, although women with virilism are usually hirsute. Virilism may be due to virilising ovarian or adrenal tumours, which are both rare; or to a delayed appearance of congenital adrenal hyperplasia, which is even more rare. The signs of virilism, in addition to hirsutes, are clitoral enlargement, amenorrhoea, voice deepening, a receding hairline, breast atrophy and an increased muscle mass.

In most cases of hirsutism, the condition is due to the 'benign androgen excess syndrome'; but hirsutism may occur as a part of the polycystic ovarian syndrome. In both instances signs of virilism are absent, but in the latter oligo- or amenorrhoea and obesity are usual.

The hirsutism is due to increased circulating levels of testosterone, mainly free (unconjugated) testosterone, due to increased production rates. The free testosterone level in the plasma is raised in over 90 per cent of hirsute women (although the total testosterone levels may be within normal limits when it is postulated that the hair follicles are hypersensitive to androgenic stimulation).

Unless signs of virilism are present there is no need to start intensive investigations, and a diagnosis of hirsutism due to the 'benign androgen excess syndrome' can be made on clinical evidence and confirmed by measuring the free plasma testosterone level.

A few gynaecologists also order a single measurement of androstenedione, serum hormone-binding globulin (SHBG), cortisol, FSH, LH, and 17-α hydroxyprogesterone to exclude rarer causes of hirsutism such as Cushing's syndrome, congenital adrenal hyperplasia and polycystic ovaries.

The management of the problem is broad. The physician enquires about any associated psychosexual problems, perceived as due to the hirsutism. He offers information about cosmetic aids, such as bleaching, shaving (which, contrary to popular belief, does not accelerate hair growth), waxing, the use of depilatory creams and electrolysis. Electrolysis is expensive and painful and should be undertaken by an expert, but only if the excessive hair is sparse and coarse.

Drugs should be prescribed with care. Some improvement is likely if a contraceptive pill is used. A more effective drug, cyproterone acetate, is now available. It is a competitive inhibitor of androgens at peripheral receptors and may also reduce androgen synthesis. Cyproterone acetate, 100mg is given from day 5 to 14 of a menstrual cycle, and ethinyl oestradiol 30μg is given from day 5 to 25 to maintain cycle control and prevent conception. The oestrogen is given to regulate the menstrual cycle, as it tends to be irregular, with dysfunctional bleeding, if cyproterone alone is used.

Any response in reducing hirsutism is uncommon in less than 3 months, and usually the drug needs to be continued for 9 months to achieve maximal effect. Cyproterone can then be withdrawn, but further courses may be needed if hirsutism recurs. About 20 per cent of women fail to respond.

Side-effects occur in between 10 and 20 per cent of women. These include lassitude (20 per cent), increase in body-weight (18 per cent), loss of libido (10 per cent) and breast discomfort (9 per cent).

Other studies suggest that the diuretic, spironolactone, which inhibits androgenic action by occupying binding sites on target tissues, and has direct anti-androgenic properties is to be preferred. Spironolactone 200mg a day, in divided doses, has been effective in reducing hirsutism, over a period of 3 months and if continued maintains the improvement. About half of the women taking spironolactone develop polymenorrhoea, but oral contraceptives will regulate the menstrual cycle.

In fact, oral contraceptives should be prescribed routinely if the woman is sexually active and does not use a contraceptive method. This is because if she becomes pregnant and the fetus is male, he may be feminized by the androgenic effect of spironolactone. If the woman is obese in addition to being hirsute, advice should be given for her to reduce her weight, if possible, as spironolactone is more effective if the woman's weight is in normal range.

FEMALE HOMOSEXUALITY (LESBIANISM)

In Judeo-Christian societies homosexuality is considered an evil, male homosexuality being a greater evil than female homosexuality, or lesbianism. Lesbianism has been condoned, if disapproved of, for years, but only recently has homosexuality between consenting adult males been accepted as legal in Britain. In other English-speaking countries, homosexual contacts between adult males remain a crime. To the average person in these countries the homosexual is a pervert, an object of ridicule, an emotionally sick person; judgments which reflect the society's emotional attitudes to sexual behaviour more than a scientific appraisal of the homosexuals' problems.

Between 2 and 5 per cent of women are homosexual, that is the woman prefers the continuing company, the emotional and physical contact of a person of her own sex and preferentially responds erotically to another woman. Why women are homosexual is unknown, but it is thought that homosexuality is due to conditioning during childhood, rather than being due to an inherited trait or an hormonal disturbance.

A homosexual's identification of her gender role is confused by parental attitudes during the most active period of her physical and psychological development, and this later inhibits her from developing a heterosexual eroticism. The responsibility falls mainly upon the parents or guardians, and homosexuality may result from an excessive dependence upon or poor relationship with one parent. However, there is no reason why lesbians should not live a full and happy life if society will let them; and in fact the gynaecological problems of the female homosexual are no different from those of her heterosexual sister.

HYSTERECTOMY, PROBLEMS FOLLOWING

If hysterectomy is performed expertly and for an adequate reason, such as dysfunctional uterine bleeding which cannot be controlled by hormones; large symptomatic myomata; endometriosis or chronic pelvic inflammatory disease, the result is usually most successful. The patient is relieved of her symptoms and is grateful. Unfortunately, in many countries, hysterectomy is resorted to far too frequently and with too little reason, the physician being unable, or unwilling, to devote sufficient time to determine that the underlying disorder might be better treated by non-operative means. This surgical approach is not without danger and psychosomatic problems may be considerable.

The frequency of hysterectomy is higher in countries where surgeons are paid a fee for service rather than a salary. Thus the rate of hysterectomy per 1000 women of various age groups in Australia, Canada and the USA is twice that of the rate in Scandinavia and in Britain. In England and Wales in 1977 one woman in every 250 aged 20 or more had the operation. Many of these operations were performed for apparently trivial reasons, at least in

so far as no pathology was found in the uterus in half the cases.

Following operation, about one-third of women are mildly or moderately incapacitated for 3 months, and one-fifth for longer. Some studies show that women who have had a hysterectomy are twice as likely to become depressed compared with women who have had a cholecystectomy. A careful, recent study, however, showed that there was no increase in psychiatric morbidity after hysterectomy and that three times as many of the women compared with controls, had a Present State Examination Score $\geqslant 5$ when assessed pre-operatively.

About one quarter of women who have had a hysterectomy with ovarian conservation performed when they were aged 40 or less will develop menopausal symptoms within four years and a similar proportion reach menopause before the age of 45.

These data suggest that if hysterectomy is suggested for conditions other than uterine cancer, the doctor has the obligation to talk with the woman and her partner to explain the need for the operation, other choices available and to discuss psychological and psychosexual matters when appropriate. If the gynaecologist feels unable or uncomfortable about this, the woman should be referred to a psychiatrist or a psychologist for assessment.

Hysterectomy should be avoided except for very cogent reasons, and especially if the woman has pre-operative depression or is under the age of 40 at the time of operation. This opinion is strengthened by recent evidence that women who have had a hysterectomy in the premenopausal years have an increased risk of developing cardiovascular disease.

When the operation is performed for an adequate reason most women adjust rapidly, particularly if the ovaries have not been removed, but to some the idea of the mutilation causes considerable anxiety. This anxiety must be resolved before operation, if the best results of hysterectomy are to be obtained. The anxiety stems from several widespread misconceptions. These are (1) that after hysterectomy the patient is no longer sexually desirable, and becomes an 'old woman', (2) that coital capacity is impaired, and (3) that hysterectomy is followed by obesity. The basis of these misconceptions is that, in the past, the ovaries were often removed at hysterectomy and severe climacteric symptoms resulted. Each patient who is to undergo hysterectomy must receive a full explanation of the reason for the operation and of its extent. She should be reassured that hysterectomy does not render her less desirable sexually or induce premature senility; and that coital capacity is in no way impaired, the vagina in fact being lengthened, rather than shortened, after total hysterectomy. It should also be pointed out that obesity is not a consequence of the operation, but of overeating, and a reluctance to resume normal physical activity. Finally, it must be stressed that apart from amenorrhoea and the inability to conceive, the patient who has undergone hysterectomy should have no disability interfering with her habitual way of life.

SEXUAL ASSAULT (RAPE)

In Britain and Australia rape is defined as 'the unlawful carnal knowledge of a woman without her consent by force, fear or fraud'. In the USA many States specify more particularly what constitutes rape, but essentially the laws imply the same definition. It should be noted that if the woman is less than 16 years of age, or is mentally defective, it is no defence that her consent was obtained; nor is it necessary for the penis to penetrate the vestibule, or ejaculation of semen to occur, before the crime of rape can be sustained.

A woman who has been raped needs to be treated with great care, and the usual hospital routines should be minimized. This has been recognized in many areas, where 'rape crisis centres' have been established. The woman is seen in a non-institutional environment which is staffed by a trained social worker and empathetic nurses. The doctor who is called in to examine the woman has also received training in dealing with the psychological and social problems associated with rape, as well as being able to determine whether rape has occurred. Often rape can be confirmed, but in many cases the doctor can only give an opinion.

The examination should take place in the presence of a third person, and the consent of the woman obtained in writing. The history of the alleged assault should be obtained and recorded, the emotional state of the woman should be assessed, the presence of bruises or scratches on her arms or body should be sought and the vulva should be carefully examined to detect blood, bruising or the presence of seminal staining. Laboratory investigations include the examination of a vaginal smear for spermatozoa, and later a serological test should be obtained to exclude a sexually transmitted disease.

In over 60 per cent of rapes, the assailant is a relative or friend or an acquaintance of the woman, and frequently the rape takes place in the home of the victim or the assailant.

As pregnancy is a possibility if the rape has taken place during the ovulatory period, the question of curettage should be discussed with the woman. Obviously removal of the endometrium will prevent nidation if the ovum happened to have been fertilized. The operation should at least be suggested to the woman for her consideration.

SEXUALITY AFTER THE CLIMACTERIC

Sexual desire and the sexual drive are unaltered after the climacteric in 60 per cent of women, are increased in 20 per cent, and diminished in 20 per cent of women. The most important influence is the pattern established in the woman's reproductive years: if she had an active, pleasurable sexual life then, she is likely to have a similarly enjoyable sexuality in her older years. Studies in the USA have shown that 70 per cent of couples questioned said that their sexuality was not diminished at least to the age of 65, and many are sexually active into their late seventies.

A woman's sexual potential persists for longer than a man's and any decline in sexual activity is likely to be due to his failing capacity to respond. However, with encouragement his sexuality can be aroused.

It is important for the counsellor to know that certain changes may occur in men. With increasing age it may take longer for a man to have an erection, the erection may go and return more frequently during sexual pleasuring, ejaculation may take rather longer to occur in response to penile thrusting and the refractory period before further coitus is desired may be longer. Some women observe these changes in their partner and erroneously believe that the apparent reduction of sexual interest by the man is because she is growing older and her body is 'less desirable to him' than previously. This may be the case in some instances but in others it is due to the changing nature of male sexuality with increasing age. Reassurance by the sexual counsellor can do much to reduce a woman's anxiety about this.

A problem which arises is that women live longer than men. Because, by convention, many women believe that a man should initiate sexual advances, older women, either single or widowed, have a reduced chance of finding a suitable partner than do older men. This may cause psychosomatic problems because a woman's libido may be high. She should not feel guilty or embarrassed about this, and in the event of failing to find a suitable sexually active partner, may masturbate to relieve her sexual tension. If she consults a doctor, she should be told that this is normal, healthy and beneficial to her.

SEXUAL EDUCATION IN ADOLESCENCE

The child's attitudes towards sexuality reflect largely those of his parents. If the parents consider sex to be 'dirty', nudity to be 'indecent' and bodily excretory functions 'unmentionable', the child is likely to believe that sex is something to be concealed or sniggered about in the peer-group.

Today there is great ferment and confusion in people's minds regarding sex, and the prevalent increasingly permissive attitude by society to sexuality imposes a considerable conflict in the young adolescent. Despite this, conventional Western society is still largely puritanical in cultural attitudes towards sex, and this has occasioned a dissemination of pornography. The word of mouth, and the pulp magazines which purvey pornography are readily available to the adolescent so that his original confusion is compounded, and he is increasingly concerned about concepts of sexual behaviour. What is right? Should he follow group attitudes, or should he think for himself? Unfortunately, all too often, he has no facts on which to base his concepts, and his only information about sex is derived from misinformation and myths secretively learned from his peers, or from the mass media.

The need for the adolescent to obtain factual information about the physical and psychological manifestations of sex and human reproduction is even greater in today's permissive atmosphere than it was in the past. And this need is even more urgent for an adolescent girl than it is for an adolescent boy, because of the accepted 'double standard' of sexual behaviour.

Most psychologists would agree that sex education is best given by the child's parents, mainly by their observed attitudes to sex, by their sexual behaviour to each other, and by answering the child's questions about sex factually and correctly. However, it is clear that many parents are either too ignorant to explain sexual matters, or are unwilling to discuss sexuality with their children. Education authorities have attempted to meet the problem by introducing 'hygiene' or 'personal development' instruction into the school curriculum, and parent-teachers associations have attempted to supplement this by lectures. Unfortunately the instruction in both leaves much to be desired, partly because the instructors are not always the most suitable persons to convey factual information on sexual matters.

It would seem that the individual whose background, ethos and training are most suited to undertake the task of sex education may be a physician.

Chapter 10

Infertility or Childlessness

It is a pertinent comment on human behaviour that whilst one large group of women are seeking to have unwanted pregnancies aborted, another large group is as earnestly seeking to achieve a pregnancy. In times past the woman was always blamed; but in recent years it has been shown that the male partner is at fault in about 30 per cent, the female partner in 30 per cent and factors affecting both account for the remaining 40 per cent of cases.

About 10 per cent of married couples fail to achieve a pregnancy between puberty and the menopause, and infertility causes so much distress that they require sympathy, understanding and help. But our limitations in helping must be realized, and the couple should be deterred from embarking on the harrowing and expensive path of a multiplicity of visits to gynaecologists, hormonologists, acupuncture specialists, and the sorry crowd of quacks and pseudoquacks that lie in wait. Despite this warning, investigations to seek the causes of infertility are worth while. A number of women become pregnant during the investigation, and more become pregnant after treatment (including artificial insemination with donor's semen, when the man is sterile). A number of women become pregnant following investigation and treatment, but neither can be claimed to be the reason for the pregnancy. Taken together about 55 per cent of couples will achieve a pregnancy. The older the female the less is her chance. The investigations should be carried out in a systematic manner; the couple should be told at the outset that about three visits at approximately monthly intervals will be required; and the steps adopted should be explained in detail so that their full co-operation can be obtained.

DEFINITION

Infertility can be diagnosed when the couple have not achieved a pregnancy after a year of normal coitus. Although a woman may visit her physician prior to this time to make sure that her genital tract is clinically normal, further investigations are unnecessary except in special circumstances, as 90 per cent of women desiring to become pregnant do so within 12 months of trying. Although a further 4 per cent become pregnant in the next 12 months, the advantage of investigation after one year of normal coitus is that minor defects may be corrected early, the sexual drive in the early years of marriage is maximal, and psychosomatic factors contributing to infertility increase as the months and years pass.

THE SCOPE OF THE INVESTIGATIONS

In the past three decades a great deal has been written regarding the investigations considered essential. During the years the investigations have multiplied, but the number of women becoming pregnant after the multiplicity of investigations has remained relatively unchanged. At the present time too much is being done, with too little thought for the underlying derangements of reproductive physiology and for the very important psychosomatic factors involved in ovulation, fertilization and implantation. In general, the physician is approached initially by the female partner, but after the initial discussion and clinical examination to ensure that the patient has no general disease which would render pregnancy hazardous to her, and that her genital organs are clinically normal, he should insist that the male partner be examined. It is clear that a time-consuming, possibly expensive investigation of the female is pointless if, for example, the male has azoospermia.

FACTORS IN INFERTILITY

In analysing the multiple causes of infertility, it is helpful to classify the main cause. Several clinics have reported their analyses in the past two decades. The proportions of infertile couples placed in each category varies, depending on the population investigated and the referral procedures. In Table **10/1** factors affecting fertility are shown.

It will be observed that in 10 to 20 per cent of couples investigated no cause to account for the infertility is found. Despite newer investigatory techniques in recent years, this proportion has not altered significantly. It is also important to know that when this group of 'cause unknown' is followed up for 5 or more years, about 4 women in every 10 become pregnant without further treatment.

One speculation is that psychosomatic factors may play an important part in these cases acting via neurohormones to alter ovulatory or oviductal function.

Table **10/1** gives some indication of the areas of investigation made to determine (1) that adequate numbers of spermatozoa are deposited around the cervix, (2) that ovulation occurs, (3) that the oviduct is patent and so permits the ascending spermatozoon to fertilize the descending ovum, (4) that the endometrium is 'prepared' hormonally to receive the fertilized egg, and (5) that the patient is psychologically 'prepared' for pregnancy.

Male factor	25–40 per cent
(defective spermatozoon production, insemination difficulties)	
Gross pelvic pathology in the female	5–12 per cent
Cervical factor	1–5 per cent
Uterine factor	<4 per cent
Tubal factor	30–50 per cent
Ovarian factor	3–10 per cent
Unexplained, after investigation	10–20 per cent

Table **10/1** Factors influencing fertility in several large studies

THE MALE PARTNER

Ideally the husband should be interviewed on one occasion separately from his wife. The history of past or present illness, of occupation (excessive heat may reduce spermatogenesis), of sexual habits (infrequent coitus or impotence) and of social habits (smoking particularly) should be noted. If he is healthy, the physical examination need not consist of more than inspection and palpation of the genitalia, attention being paid to the size and consistency of the testicles and the presence or absence of varicocele of the spermatic cord. However, many a man, although prepared to go to the initial interview with his wife, is reluctant to be examined. Provided he is prepared to submit a specimen of seminal fluid for examination and it is normal, the physical examination can be omitted.

Seminal analysis

The specimen should be obtained by coitus interruptus, or by masturbation, collected in a dry, clean glass jar and brought to the laboratory within 2 hours of production. Coitus should be avoided for 2 days prior to the test, and then take place on the morning of the test. Alternatively, a masturbation specimen may be produced in the laboratory. If the couple have a religious or moral objection to the methods outlined, normal coitus should take place and the wife present herself 6 to 12 hours later for a *postcoital test* made at the presumed time of ovulation. The test will confirm or deny the presence of semen in the vagina, but cannot replace a properly performed semen analysis in evaluating the man's contribution to the infertility problem.

The postcoital test is also used to determine if the sperms are able to penetrate cervical mucus, and may give an indication of immunological problems as a cause of infertility (see p. 100).

In some clinics a sample of the man's semen (and the woman's serum when appropriate) is examined for antisperm antibodies.

The range of results in normal fertile men is wide, and for this reason only the lower limits of normal are given. The rule 2, 2, 6, 6 may help as a memory aid. The volume should be more than 2ml; the count more than 20 000 000 spermatozoa per ml; the motility more than 60 per cent, 2 hours after production; and more than 60 per cent of spermatozoa should be normal in shape. When the count is less than 20 000 000 per ml, the *quality* of the semen becomes increasingly important; but the count is the most important factor in dividing 'good' from 'poor' semen, since as the count falls so do the values of all the other measurements. A single report of a 'poor' semen has no prognostic value, and no opinion must be made *until three seminal appraisals* at 2 to 3 week intervals have shown the semen to be subnormal.

Azoospermia (the absence of spermatozoa) may be due either to defective spermatogenesis or to damage to the ducts along which the spermatozoa pass. Defective spermatogenesis follows abnormal development of the testes, late or non-descent of the testes, or damage to the testicular blood supply. Mumps, contracted after the age of 12, is complicated by orchitis in one-third of cases, and in one-third of these azoospermia results. Damage of the spermatic ducts is usually due to infection, particularly gonococcal, which causes epididymitis and occludes the vas deferens.

Oligozoospermia, which may be severe, may be caused by deficient spermatogenesis or by alterations in the ambient testicular temperature, a raised temperature reducing spermatogenesis. Work in a hot, humid climate; the wearing of tight underpants which approximate the testicles to the crutch; inguinal testicles and varicocele, may produce oligozoospermia.

The initial investigation of the man is to obtain a semen specimen and make a seminal analysis. If this shows a 'normal' semen (Table 10/2), and his partner confirms that he ejaculates in her vagina, no further investigations are needed.

If the test shows oligospermia, and this is confirmed on two further seminal analyses, the man should be examined to exclude a varicocele of his spermatic cord. If this is found, it should be treated surgically. At the same time, a stained slide of the semen is examined for pus cells. The presence of pus cells suggests prostatic infection, which is investigated by the two-glass urine test and by prostatic massage, so that a further sample can be examined bacteriologically. If infection is diagnosed, treatment with appropriate antibiotics is indicated.

If the seminal analyses show azoospermia or oligospermia, in the absence of varicocele of the spermatic cord, or prostatic infection, the plasma FSH level should be estimated on two or more occasions. Raised FSH levels indicated severe testicular damage and no treatment is available.

Normal or low FSH levels associated with the azoospermia or severe oligozoospermia (< 5 million spermatozoa), suggests damage by infection of the epididymis or the vas deferens. Currently no effective surgical anastomosis has proved effective, but vaso-epididymal anastomosis using microsurgical techniques may offer some hope in the future.

Moderately severe oligospermia (> 5 million but < 20 million spermatozoa) associated with normal or low FSH levels, suggest inadequate stimulation of spermatogenesis, and treatment may help, provided there is not also testicular damage. This can be excluded by a testicular biopsy. If the biopsy shows nothing more severe than focal tubular atrophy, treatment with clomiphene 50mg daily for 80 days may improve the quantity and quality of the semen sufficiently to permit fertilization.

Serum antibodies (in either partner) against spermatozoal surface antigens may be a cause of infertility but their presence seems of limited significance in evaluating infertility. If a negative postcoital test, taken in the pre-ovulatory 2 days, is found on three or more occasions sperm antibodies may be sought in bromelin-treated cervical mucus or by a radio-labelled antiglobulin test. If such antibodies are found, treatment is rather unsatisfactory. Corticosteroid therapy, methylprednisolone 96mg daily for 7 days (given to the male in the second half of his partner's menstrual cycle) for 2 or 3 cycles has been suggested; as has AIH. In the latter the husband's semen is introduced into the uterine cavity via a polyethylene catheter. The pregnancy rate of these methods in uncontrolled trials is about 20 per cent.

Until properly controlled double blind trials of this medication have been made, the treatment cannot be validated, and should only be used in a research programme.

Some authorities recommend that the fructose, zinc and acid phosphatase levels of the seminal fluid are also measured in cases of azoospermia and oligospermia. The seminal fluid makes up 90 per cent of the ejaculate. Two-thirds of it derives from secretions of the seminal vesicles, which are rich in fructose. One-third comes from prostatic secretions which contains zinc and acid phosphatase. Low levels of fructose and zinc, or high levels of acid phosphatase, suggest that the man has low grade vesiculoprostatitis. Treatment of this condition with antibiotics may improve the sperm count and increase sperm motility.

In addition, an infertile man should reduce his

Volume	2ml
Count	20 000 000 per ml
Motility	more than 60 per cent motile within 2 hours of ejaculation
Normal forms	more than 60 per cent

Table 10/2 Normal semen (lower limits)

consumption of alcohol and cigarettes as these affect the quality of the spermatozoa.

However, there is no evidence that abstention from coitus improves sperm quality, indeed there is evidence of the opposite, that excessive congestion of spermatozoa in the epididymis decreases sperm motility.

Surgical correction of a varicocele improves seminal quality in about 50 per cent of cases, although the wives achieve a pregnancy much less frequently. The administration of vitamins, steroids, thyroxine and gonadotrophins, whether animal or human, have proved of no value in improving the quality of the seminal fluid, and azoospermia is at this time untreatable.

Infertility may also be caused by impotence; by consistent ejaculation of semen into the bladder. Some urologists recommend artificial insemination of the husband's semen (AIH) in these cases, with varying success. Semen is collected and introduced into the upper vagina at ovulation time to bathe the cervical os. Artificial insemination of a donor's semen (AID) is being increasingly used when the male has azoospermia or severe oligozoospermia, as societal and demographic changes have reduced the 'supply' of babies available for adoption.

The donor should be of the same ethnic group as the male partner. He should be healthy and have been tested serologically to exclude syphilis and AIDS and by smear (and culture) to exclude gonorrhoea, during the week before he donates his semen. If the woman is Rhesus negative, a Rh negative donor should be selected.

The express consent of the donor of the sperm, the woman and her husband (if she is married) should be obtained before proceeding to insemination, and the donor must remain anonymous.

Insemination can be made with fresh or with frozen semen. The insemination is made at ovulation time, judged by observing the basal body temperature rise, the oestradiol peak, the LH peak, or the quality of the cervical mucus. A quantity of fresh semen (usually about 1ml) is injected gently into the cervix, and, in the case of fresh semen, the remainder is placed in the upper vagina to bathe the cervix. Two or three inseminations are made each month over a 2- to 4-day period, and are repeated, unless pregnancy occurs, for 3 to 6 cycles.

The organization of an AID service using frozen semen is rather more complicated but, once established, is easier to run. Specimens are obtained from healthy donors and placed in plastic 'straws' each containing 0.5ml. The straws are frozen in liquid nitrogen. The pregnancy rate is said to be increased if a cervical cap is used following insemination.

The pregnancy rate using fresh semen over a 6-month period, is 60 to 70 per cent. That using frozen semen is less than 55 per cent. This may be increased if AID is performed for each month for 12 months.

THE WOMAN

The woman should be examined either at the initial interview, or at the visit following. At the interview the history of past illnesses and operations should be elicited, and the patient's sexual behaviour, including coital technique, should be discussed. It should be noted that orgasm is not necessary for conception, and the loss of semen from the vaginal orifice post-coitally is normal. Nor is there any evidence that the normal methods of contraception ultimately lead to a reduction in fertility, or that vaginal tampons for control of menstrual blood flow reduce fertility. A detailed analysis of menstrual patterns should be obtained, and the patient's social habits (tobacco, alcohol) assessed. Finally, an assessment of the patient's underlying psychology, particularly relating to sex, should be obtained.

A physical examination and laboratory tests should establish that disease is absent. The laboratory tests should include: urine examination and blood examination (a test for syphilis and a haemoglobin estimation are minimal). The examination is made to detect abnormalities which might interfere with childbearing and child-rearing, and is preventive medicine in the true sense. The pelvic examination is made to detect any gross abnormalities of the genital tract (for example, an 'unruptured' hymen, vaginismus, partial or complete absence of the vagina or uterus, uterine myomata, tubal or ovarian swelling). At this time the opportunity should be taken to make a cervical smear, which is examined for suspicious or malignant cells.

Abnormalities found at the general and pelvic examination require correction, and the method adopted will depend, to some extent, on the seminal appraisal of the male partner. It is surprising that in about 1 per cent of infertile couples, apareunia or dyspareunia is the cause. The cause of this is vaginismus, which is caused by marked spasm

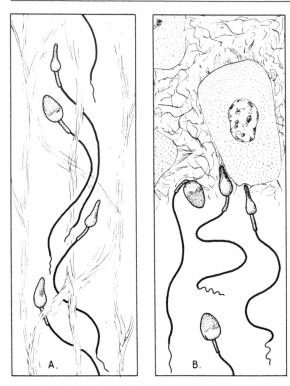

Fig. 10/1 Model of cervical mucus showing the helical 'tunnels' which form in the ovulatory phase; and the impenetrable meshwork occurring in the progestational phase. (From Odeblad, E. *Acta Obstet. Gynec. Scand.*, 1968, **47**, supp. 1, p. 57.)

of the levator ani muscles, and is psychological in origin.

'Cervical factor'

Since the spermatozoa must penetrate the cervical canal and avoid being trapped in its clefts and tunnels, the cervix has long been considered a major factor in infertility. The alterations in the cervical mucus caused by the cyclic release of oestrogens and progesterone have been described (see p. 56), and the rising tide of oestrogen prior to ovulation induces a flow of clear, watery, stretchable, elastic mucus from the cervical columnar cells. Progesterone produced by the corpus luteum alters the mucus, which becomes scanty, thick and viscous (Fig. **10/1**).

Deep cervical cautery or conization would reduce cervical secretions and are a rare 'cause' of infertility. Most cases in which the cervical factor has been incriminated as the cause of a couple's infertility are due to the failure of the sperm to reach and to fertilize the ovum. In most cases the inability of the sperm to penetrate the cervical mucus at ovulation time is due to defective sperm function (probably immunological) rather than to a 'hostile' cervix. As the sperm has first to penetrate the cervical mucus, this is an obvious place where the dysfunction may be observed. Currently the postcoital test (PCT) is used to evaluate this problem.

Several problems arise which limit the prognostic value of the postcoital test. The first is the need to perform the test on one of the two days before, or on the assumed day of, ovulation. The second is that the criteria for a 'positive' test vary between clinics. The third is that in a proportion of negative tests sperm can be aspirated from the cul-de-sac. The fourth is that pregnancies follow cycles in which the PCT is negative.

With these limitations, a positive PCT, that is one in which at least 5 sperms/per HPF are seen to be moving progressively forward 12 hours after the intercourse, excludes a 'cervical' cause for the infertility. If three successive PCTs are negative, some gynaecologists arrange for a Sperm Cervical Mucus Contact Test (SCMC test). In this test samples of the husband's sperm and a known fertile donor's sperm are mixed with cervical mucus (taken at ovulation time) from the wife and from a fertile female. The results are shown in Table **10/3**. The treatment of the 'cervical factor' is unsatisfactory. As many cases are thought to have an immunological basis, the use of condoms for 6 months, and the use of corticosteroids have been used with limited success. Occasionally cervical ectropion associated with marked mucorrhoea may hinder spermatozoon penetration, and if detected may be treated with cauterization. Again the scientific value of the procedure remains to be proved, although some pregnancies follow its use.

Uterine factors

The uterus may be a cause of infertility because of malformation; infection, especially tuberculosis; damage, especially Ashermann's syndrome; or because the endometrium is not sufficiently developed to receive the fertilized egg. In reality, in the last condition, it is not the uterus which is at fault, but the endocrine control of endometrial development. The main problem seems to be defective corpus luteum function, which may in turn follow defective follicular function.

Penetration of wife's cervical mucus with donor's semen	+	−	+	−
Penetration of donor's cervical mucus with husband's sperm	+	+	−	−
Diagnosis	Specific immunological problem in couple	Cervical mucus of wife abnormal	Specific immunological problem in male	Problem in husband *and* wife
Treatment	AID Intra-uterine AIH or ?IVF	?Ethinyl oestradiol 0.01mg b.d. day 5–12	AID or corticosteroids to male	?

Table 10/3 Sperm-cervical mucus crossed hostility test

The belief that a retroverted uterus (in the absence of pelvic infection) is a cause of infertility has no basis and cannot be sustained.

Tuberculosis as a factor

In certain countries, genital tract tuberculosis may manifest itself only in a complaint of infertility. In the USA and Australia, for example, the incidence is less than 0.5 per cent of all infertile patients investigated, but in Israel it is 5 per cent and in the developing countries, e.g. India, over 15 per cent.

In such countries, infertility investigations must include a diagnostic curettage with investigation by histopathology and guinea-pig inoculation for the presence of endometrial tuberculosis (see p. 147).

Tubal (oviduct) factor

The spermatozoon fertilizes the ovum in the outer third of the oviduct, and the fertilized egg is propelled gently along the tube, taking 3 days in the journey to reach the prepared endometrium. For this to occur, the oviducts must be patent and functional. This led Rubin, and later others, to develop instruments for determining the patency and, to some extent, the function of the oviducts. The instruments release a supply of CO_2 gas (carbogen), which flows at a regulated pressure and quantity through a cannula placed firmly in the cervical canal. Rubin's test has been replaced by hysterosalpingography, in which an oily or water-soluble radio-opaque contrast medium is injected through the cervix. Its passage through the uterus and oviducts is monitored by image-intensified television. The procedure is best performed just prior to mid-cycle. The patient may be given an analgesic injection of pethidine 100mg prior to the procedure but this is not usually needed.

A uterine cannula is introduced into the cervix, the contrast medium is injected slowly under television screening, and permanent radiographs are taken at appropriate intervals (Figs. **10/2** and **10/3**). If hystero-salpingography shows apparently occluded oviducts, the procedure is repeated 1 month later. Tubal occlusion, especially in the outer portion of the oviduct, should be further investigated by inspecting the oviducts at laparoscopy and by injecting a dye (usually methylene blue) transcervically. This investigation enables the gynaecologist to give a better evaluation of the prognosis if surgery is contemplated.

The laparoscope may be used in place of hysterosalpingography to inspect the pelvis and to determine tubal function, although there is no evidence that a higher pregnancy rate follows its use. Some gynaecologists use the method in preference to hysterosalpingography, but this is not recommended, as laparoscopy is uncomfortable to the woman and not without hazard. If hysterosalpingography shows normal tubes and no other cause for the infertility is found, and if pregnancy has not occurred in a period of 9 to 12 months following hysterosalpingography, a laparoscopic inspection of the pelvis may be made and tubal function determined.

If the oviducts are occluded, a decision has to be made whether or not surgery will be beneficial.

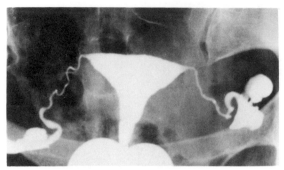

Fig. 10/2 (A) Hysterosalpingogram showing a normal uterus and tubes

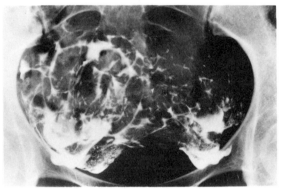

Fig. 10/2 (B) A film taken some hours later confirmed that oil was present in the peritoneal cavity and the tubes were patent

Occlusion at the fimbrial end, with or without hydrosalpinx may be found, or the block may be in the isthmus or in the interstitial position of the oviduct.

Micro-surgery to restore tubal patency is a possibility, but it must be remembered that occluded oviducts are usually caused by previous infection damage to the delicate endosalpinx, so that the pathology remains.

If tubal micro-surgery is suggested, the couple must be told of the chances of pregnancy, and more important, of their chance of having a viable child following the procedure. This is because both ectopic gestation and abortion are more frequent in women who have had tubal patency restored, than in normal woman. The mean pregnancy rate varies from about 40 per cent, if only fine adhesions have occluded the fimbrial end of the oviduct, to less than 25 per cent when interstitial or isthmal 'block' is present, to less than 10 per cent when there is a hydrosalpinx. In each case the chance of delivering a live viable baby is only 60 per cent of the pregnancy rate.

Various therapies have been suggested to complement the surgery. Hydrotubation of the Fallopian tubes using Ringer's solution or Ringer's solution with cortisone has been used widely for 15 years. In 1985, the first randomized prospective multi-centre clinical trial of the procedure showed that hydrotubation was not associated with an increased pregnancy rate.

IN VITRO FERTILIZATION AND EMBRYO REPLACEMENT

This technique is now an established method of treating tubal damage which has failed to be cured by surgery or when surgery is not possible. It is also being used, on an experimental basis, to treat immunological infertility and unexplained infertility.

The woman receives ovulatory drugs (clomiphene ± human menopausal gonadotrophin) and the development of the follicles is monitored by the measurement of oestradiol and ultrasound. When one or more follicles measures >18mm, an injection of human chorionic gonadotrophin is given to induce ovulation and, about 36 hours later, several ova are retrieved by laparoscopy. The ova are examined, treated and transferred into a culture medium for incubation. Meanwhile the male has produced a semen specimen which is treated and placed in a culture medium. About 50 000 sperms are added to each culture tube containing an ovum. About 40 hours later, the specimens are examined to see if fertilization and embryonic development has occurred. When the embryos are at the 4- or 8-cell stage, two or more are replaced (transferred) in the mother's uterus via the cervix.

The success rate, in terms of a viable pregnancy, (>20 weeks) is about 14 per cent in IVF programmes.

Endometriosis as a factor

The observation that about 40 per cent of patients with endometriosis are involuntarily infertile, and that endometriosis is the only lesion found in some 10 per cent of barren women, has led some gynaecologists to emphasize the importance of endometriosis as a factor in infertility. Whether it is a factor is unclear and recent research suggests that endometriosis may be the result rather than the cause of infertility, or the two conditions may have a common aetiology. Obviously if endometrial lesions distort or obstruct the Fallopian tubes or ovaries,

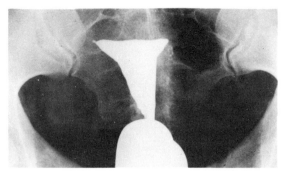

Fig. 10/3 (A) Hysterogram showing bilateral cornual block

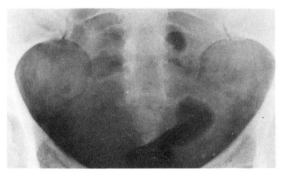

Fig. 10/3 (B) A film taken some hours later confirmed that no oil had reached the peritoneal cavity

endometriosis may be involved and should be treated. However there is much less evidence that minimal or mild endometriosis has any effect on a woman's fertility. Recent studies have shown that the same pregnancy rate is obtained whether the endometriosis is treated or not.

In such cases small areas of endometriosis are often found on the ovaries or peritoneum, and in some distortion of the oviducts may also be present. It is claimed that if these endometriotic nodules are cauterized, or less commonly excised, or, if danazol is prescribed, the pregnancy rate is increased. Two carefully designed studies of mild endometriosis (see p. 202) treated with danazol or placebo showed no increase in the pregnancy rate when the drug was used. In both cases a pregnancy rate of about 40 per cent occurred.

The reason for the relationship between endometriosis and infertility is not clear, except when distortion of the oviducts is present. Recently 'steroid profiles' taken throughout the menstrual cycles of women with known endometriosis have suggested

that the mechanisms of follicular rupture is disturbed, resulting in the failure of release of the ovum. Another theory is that endometriosis 'activates' macrophages which inhibit, in some way, egg-sperm interaction. If this work is confirmed the reason for the association between endometriosis and infertility will become more clear.

The ovarian factor

The 'ovarian factor' includes (1) defective ovarian function, (2) anovulation with regular menstruation, and (3) anovulation associated with amenorrhoea, which is discussed in Chapter 5.

In a woman who menstruates cyclically, and who is aged between 20 and 38, anovulation is rather uncommon, although it may occur from time to time. At each end of reproductive life, anovulation increases in frequency.

The absolute proof of ovulation is pregnancy. Ovulation can be inferred by observing a positive response to certain tests and procedures. These tests include (1) measurement of plasma progesterone, (2) cervical mucus quality, and (3) endometrial biopsy.

Tests for ovulation

Ovulation may be anticipated as likely to occur about 32 hours (range 24 to 56 hours) after the LH peak; about 48 hours after the oestradiol peak; and when the largest follicle, as judged by serial ultrasound, has reached 20mm in diameter.

Ovulation may be judged to have occurred in a particular menstrual cycle in several ways.

Endocrine assay for serum progesterone: The development of highly specific assays for progesterone using a competitive protein-binding technique means that the level of progesterone found in plasma may replace earlier methods of detecting ovulation. A level of plasma progesterone, late in the menstrual cycle, in excess of 30nmol/l indicates that ovulation has occurred, a level of plasma progesterone below this suggests anovulation.

Cervical mucus alteration: Ferning, or arborization, of cervical mucus is a special form of crystallization of sodium chloride due to the unopposed action of oestrogen. If a specimen of cervical mucus taken just before ovulation (between days 11 and 14) is smeared onto a glass slide (previously washed with distilled water and dried), the fern pattern appears as the mucus dries (Fig. **10/4**). Progesterone inhibits this pattern. The finding of a fern pattern in cervical mucus in the second half of the cycle is suggestive of anovulation.

Endometrial biopsy. If a biopsy shows that the luteal changes (p. 49) have failed to occur, anovulation may be suspected. However, although secretory changes usually indicate that ovulation has occurred, they may be seen in cases where the ovum was not released from the mature follicle. Diagnostic curettage (and endometrial biopsy) probably should be avoided as it may be followed by low grade pelvic infection, and has been shown to reduce the chance of conception.

Defective ovarian endocrine function

Some infertile women appear to ovulate, but the maturation of the follicle and its conversion into a functioning corpus luteum is defective. In a few instances, this defect is due to hyperprolactinaemia.

Defective ovarian endocrine function usually presents as *defective luteal function*, because this is the most significant finding. Clinically, there may be no evidence of the condition, although a few women have premenstrual 'spotting'.

Defective luteal function is diagnosed (1) by observing abnormalities in the basal body temperature chart, (2) by taking an endometrial biopsy on about day 25 of the cycle, or by measuring plasma progesterone on 2 or 3 days around day 22 of the menstrual cycle. Histological examination of the endometrium enables a histopathologist to 'date' it, in relation to the post-ovulatory day of the menstrual cycle, by evaluating the development of the glands and the appearance of the stroma. If the endometrium lags by 2 or 3 days from its expected appearance, on three or more occasions, defective luteal function may be diagnosed. The condition can be confirmed if the plasma progesterone levels are low, taken at about the same time as the endometrial biopsy. In addition, if pre-ovulation plasma oestradiol levels are low, on day 12 or 13, defective follicular maturation can be inferred.

When defective luteal function is diagnosed, serum prolactin levels should be measured two or three times during the luteal phase of the cycle, to determine if hyperprolactinaemia is present.

Treatment is not entirely satisfactory. Hyperprolactinaemia is treated with bromocriptine. If

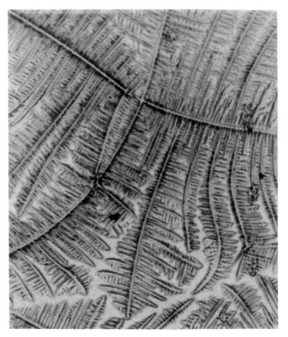

Fig. 10/4 Cervical mucus, day 19 of the cycle. Note that 'ferning' is present. Anovulation was confirmed by endometrial biopsy

the prolactin levels are within the normal range, several therapies have been suggested. These are (1) to give clomiphene 50mg, from day 5 to 10 to 'regulate' gonadotrophin release; (2) to give human menopausal gonadotrophin on days 6, 8 and 10, followed by human chorionic gonadotrophin on days 14 and 16; (3) if the plasma progesterone levels are low to give progesterone 25mg twice daily as a rectal or a vaginal suppository, or (4) to give a synthetic progestogen, such as medroxyprogesterone acetate 2.5mg daily from day 15 of the menstrual cycle.

The multiplicity of treatments, and the relatively poor pregnancy rates following any treatment, suggests that our knowledge about defective ovarian function is equally defective.

A further finding which questions whether a defective luteal phase is a cause of infertility is that the condition is found with equal frequency in fertile and infertile women.

Persistent anovulation with regular menstruation

If persistent anovulatory cycles are inferred after examination of one or more of the tests for ovulation, plasma prolactin levels should be estimated. Only raised levels indicate the use of bromocriptine. If the plasma prolactin levels are within the normal range, treatment is initiated with clomiphene 50mg daily from day 5 to 10 of the cycle. Small sub-ovulatory doses of oestrogen (ethinyl oestradiol 0.01mg) are also given from day 5 to 15 of the cycle. The oestrogen is given for two reasons: firstly this dosage stimulates LH release, and secondly it theoretically counteracts the anti-oestrogenic effect of clomiphene upon the cervical mucus.

If ovulation fails to occur on this regimen then the regimen used for the treatment of amenorrhoea is adopted.

Anovulation associated with amenorrhoea

This is considered in detail in Chapter 8. It should be stressed that provided pathological causes of amenorrhoea have been eliminated, treatment should not be given unless the woman wants to become pregnant and no other factor preventing this is present (such as oligo- or azoospermia in the man, or 'blocked' oviducts in the woman).

Unexplained infertility

Following the investigations outlined in this chapter, the cause of the infertility in 10 to 20 per cent of couples remains unexplained. The incidence of unexplained infertility depends on whether the gynaecologist includes minimal endometriosis and 'mild' pelvic infection as real causes of infertility or incidental findings during investigation. Both of these conditions are associated with the same pregnancy rate whether treated or left alone. Over a period of 3 years over half the women who have unexplained infertility will become pregnant whether 'treatment' is given or withheld. Some gynaecologists claim that, as psychological factors may be important in cases of unexplained infertility, investigation is treatment; and careful sympathetic explanation of the problem with appropriate counselling may be followed by pregnancy. The evidence is anecdotal.

As couples with unexplained infertility often seek any measure which may help the woman become pregnant, a 'last resort' is to offer gamete intra-fallopian transfer (GIFT), or *in vitro* fertilization and embryo transfer (IVF). Of the two procedures GIFT may be preferred as it is associated with a slightly higher 'take home' baby rate, it is simpler to perform, and is cheaper. After one attempt, 10 per cent of the women achieve a viable pregnancy, and this increases to 20 per cent after 3 attempts. This 'success rate' should be related to the spontaneous pregnancy rate of 50 per cent mentioned earlier.

Gamete Intrafallopian Transfer

This procedure may be used provided at least one Fallopian tube is patent and healthy. GIFT has been used to treat (1) unexplained infertility, (2) endometriosis, (3) oligospermia (with poor success) and (4) failed artificial insemination with donor sperm (AID).

The technique to obtain several ova is that used in IVF. About two hours before the ova pick-up, the man produces a semen specimen which is prepared by a 'wash and swim' technique. About 50 000 motile sperms are loaded into a special catheter, followed by two ova and a further 50 000 sperms. The whole is then injected into the fimbrial end of a Fallopian tube under laparoscopic vision.

TREATMENT

The series of investigations performed will determine if an absolute bar to conception exists, as for example azoospermia, or if no definite cause for the infertility is present. The investigations are not only diagnostic, but have some therapeutic value. This can be deduced from the fact that between 15 and 20 per cent of couples become pregnant during the course of the infertility studies. In addition to correction of defects found, advice given regarding coital technique is often helpful. Many couples are ignorant that the fertile period is around ovulation time, and that coitus at this time is more likely to result in pregnancy than concentration on the perimenstrual period.

The importance of psychosomatic factors can be deduced by the success of some gynaecologists in the treatment of infertility, which on analysis must be attributed to their psychological rapport with the patient rather than to their surgical dexterity. Drugs are of little value, but sympathy, consideration and interest can be most effective. The physician needs to be more than a medical technician, he requires to be a 'guide, philosopher and friend' to the couple – a true doctor in fact.

PROGNOSIS

Following investigations between 30 and 40 per cent

of infertile couples will achieve a pregnancy, usually within 2 years after the start of the investigative programme. This rate is increased to 55 per cent if cases where AID is used are included. However, compared with fertile couples, the couples have twice the abortion rate (300 per 1000 compared with 150 per 1000 conceptions); five times the ectopic gestation rate (25 per 1000 conceptions compared with 5 per 1000); and twice the perinatal mortality rate.

Chapter 11

Conception Control

In the past 40 years, the virtual elimination of malaria and the reduction of infectious disease, together with an increasingly powerful array of potent drugs, has enabled man for the first time to exert a significant control over death. But death control has not been matched by birth control, and the number of people born is increasing at a faster rate than ever before in the history of the world. In 1850 the world's population was estimated to be 1000 million. In the 75 years between 1850 and 1925 it doubled to 2000 million. In the 50 years between 1925 and 1975 it doubled again to 4000 million, and in the 35 years from 1975 it is likely to double again to 8000 million.

Even more important is the fact that the high birth rates are to be found exclusively in the developing countries, where the majority of the world's population is increasingly concentrated. These countries are having increasing difficulty in maintaining the per capita food supply, providing jobs for the increasing number of young people, and obtaining economic growth. The Malthusian correctives of famine, pestilence and war threaten them constantly.

In the affluent nations of the world, the problems of population increase are not national but personal, and family limitation is sought for social reasons; because an additional child would diminish materially the education of the others; because accommodation difficulties make an addition to the family undesirable; because the additional income produced by a 'working wife' improves the conditions of the existing members of the family unit. There is nothing objectionable in any of these reasons, for the determination of the size of their family is a personal, intimate decision between husband and wife, and family limitation has been practised by one method or another by families since man developed a social conscience. But neither in the developing, nor in the developed countries must a couple be *forced* to adopt

contraception, nor should they be *prevented* from adopting such measures. It is a matter for the individual conscience to decide; but equally it is a matter for Governments to supply information so that men and women can decide, and indeed if it is considered in the best interests of the community as a whole, to use propaganda to persuade them to decide to limit the size of the family. The change today is that there are methods of conception control which makes the fulfilment of the decision easy. The relative ease of modern methods of contraception has introduced the fear that fornication will be encouraged, particularly amongst unmarried teenagers. It cannot be denied that in many countries a more permissive attitude to fornication has arisen in recent years, but there is no evidence that this is due to the more ready availability of contraceptives. Whilst it is true that in the past, fear of pregnancy, fear of venereal disease and fear of social disgrace were believed to keep a girl a virgin, the young man was not expected to remain chaste, and a girl foolish enough to believe the young man was considered fair game. But to rely upon fear to maintain chastity in an age of affluence and permissiveness, is no longer a practical proposition, and a change in cultural attitudes to one in which the exploitation of another human is deplored, and socially rejected, can only come through education. The influence of freely available contraceptives in encouraging sexual permissiveness, is, at the most, peripheral and of slight importance.

There is another face to the coin. Many individual women require to prevent a further pregnancy because of temporary ill health, because of systemic disease or because of a recurrent obstetrical complication. Such individuals may seek a permanent method of birth control, such as tubal ligation; or temporary measures provided by the periodic abstinence, the vaginal diaphragm, the oral contraceptive or the intra-uterine contraceptive device.

		Rates
Group A	*Most effective*	
	Tubal ligation/vasectomy	0.005–0.04
	Combined orals	0.005–0.30
	Sequential orals	0.20–0.56
Group B	*Highly effective*	
	IUD	0.5–3.5
	Continuous progestogen	1.5–2.3
	Diaphragm or condom + cream	
	All users	4.0–7.0
	Highly motivated	1.5–3.0
	Periodic abstinence	
	All users	10.0–30.0
	Highly motivated	2.5–5.0
Group C	*Less effective*	
	Coitus interruptus	30.0–40.0
	Vaginal foam or cream	30.0–40.0
Group D	*Least effective*	
	Post-coital douche	45.0
	Prolonged breast feeding	45.0

Table 11/1 Ranking of contraceptive methods by rate of effectiveness (as calculated from unexpected pregnancies per 100 woman-years)

It has been increasingly clear that men and women, married and unmarried, who are sexually active should have the knowledge of various methods of contraception so that the person can make a reasoned choice, and be able to choose the method most suitable for the individual's particular needs. This implies that doctors should not only be informed about contraception, but able to communicate with people. Doctors must also have the knowledge to compare the reliability of various methods of contraception in preventing pregnancy. The most suitable calculation is to use cumulative pregnancy rates but most workers use the simpler, if less accurate, Pearl Index.

The index calculates the unintended pregnancy rate from the formula:

$$\frac{\text{The number of unintended pregnancies}}{\text{Total months of exposure to pregnancy}} \times 1200$$

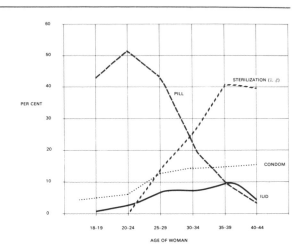

Fig. 11/1 Birth control methods, United Kingdom, 1983, by age of the woman

The result is expressed as the *failure rate per 100 woman-years*. The number of pregnancies in the numerator must include all known pregnancies, whatever the outcome.

Using the Pearl Index, the reliability of various forms of contraception can be determined (Table **11/1**). It should be noted that in certain circumstances it may be preferable to recommend a less reliable method, which is readily available and easy to use, to a more efficient but more complex method. The increasing number of nations which permit legal abortion makes this a practical proposition, as induced abortion may be used as a 'backstop' to failure of contraception. Figure **11/1** demonstrates the influence of a woman's age on her choice of contraceptive.

METHODS OF CONTRACEPTION

Coitus interruptus

Apart from abortion and infanticide, coitus interruptus (or 'withdrawal') is probably the oldest method of birth control. With the introduction of mechanical barriers and, later, of hormonal contraceptives and the intra-uterine device (IUD), its popularity has diminished, but the method is still used by men, particularly of the lower socio-economic groups and in the developing nations. The reliability of coitus interruptus, as a method of birth control, depends on the ability of the man to recognize the pre-ejaculatory phase, and his agility in withdrawing his penis from the vagina before ejaculation. Provided he has these attributes, coitus interruptus is relatively efficient. There is no evidence that it is physically or psychologically injurious.

Unfortunately the pregnancy rate is high – about 25 per 100 woman-years.

Periodic abstinence ('the safe period')

The knowledge that ovulation usually occurs 14 days prior to menstruation, that the ovum survives for 2 days unless it is fertilized and that spermatozoa survive and are able to fertilize for 4 days at the most, has been used in contraceptive methodology. If coitus is avoided from 4 days before ovulation to 6 days after ovulation, pregnancy should not occur.

Coitus at times outside this time segment can take place without too much risk of pregnancy occurring – in other words such times constitute a 'safe period'.

There are several methods of determining the duration of the safe period. The first is to record the menstrual cycle over a period of 6 months and then calculate the safe period from these data. This is the calendar method. Compliance with this method is poor and it has been largely superseded by the 'temperature' method and the 'mucus' method. In the temperature method the woman takes her basal body temperature each day. The first four days after menstruation are considered safe, but the next few periovular days are 'unsafe' and coitus should be avoided until the biphasic temperature rise has occurred (Fig. **11/2**).

In the mucus method the woman notes or feels the vulva each morning (before any sexual arousal) to detect the presence of mucus. Three types of mucus may be detected (Fig. **11/3**) and the days on which intercourse can take place safely can be determined.

In published studies, the mucus method is associated with a pregnancy rate of 20 to 30 per cent and the calendar method with one of 15 to 25 per cent. Of course, the rate is determined by the frequency of coitus, and couples who use either method but only have coitus infrequently will have lower rates.

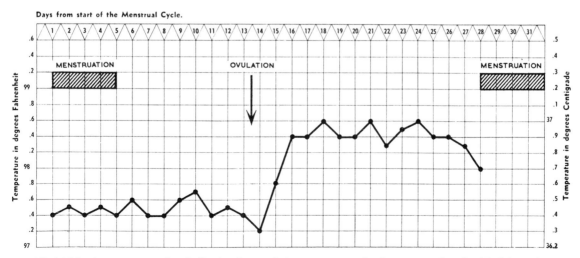

Fig. 11/2 A biphasic temperature chart indicating that ovulation was presumed to have occurred on day 14 of the cycle

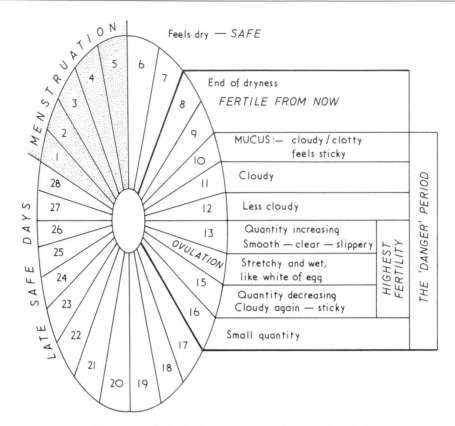

Fig. 11/3 Periodic abstinence: the mucus (ovulation) method

Mechanical barriers

These are the condom (French letter), the vaginal diaphragm (or Dutch Cap) and the sponge.

THE CONDOM

Modern condoms are made of fine latex or plastic, prelubricated by adding silicone and are individually packaged in hermetically sealed aluminium sachets. They are cheap, efficient and hardly noticeable to either sexual partner. Because they have no side-effects and a long store life, condoms are available through a variety of outlets, and for the casual copulator are an efficient method. The condom has an additional benefit. If it is used throughout each act of sexual intercourse it will diminish considerably the spread of the human papillomavirus, *Chlamydia* and the human immunodeficiency virus. The protective value of the condom in preventing the spread of sexually-transmissible diseases has led to a resurgence in its use. It is unfortunate that many sexually active young men will not use it. In principle, a condom should be worn if either partner is uncertain about the sexual behaviour of the other.

The pregnancy rate using condoms is not easy to calculate accurately, as to some extent the technique of putting a condom on the erect penis is important. The rolled condom is unrolled on to the penis, care being taken to remove air from the closed end, which may be plain or teat-ended. If air is left in, its pressure, together with that of the ejaculated semen, may be sufficient to burst the condom during active coitus. Used by motivated couples the pregnancy rate is less than 3 per 100 woman-years, but among all couples it is 4 to 6 times higher.

THE VAGINAL DIAPHRAGM, CERVICAL CAP

As its name implies, the vaginal diaphragm consists of a thin latex (or plastic) dome attached to a circular flat or coiled wire spring. The diaphragm fits across the upper vagina, precluding ejaculated spermatozoa from reaching the cervix, and is made in various sizes because of the varying capacity of different vaginas (Fig. **11/4**). The appropriate size is found by estimating the vaginal capacity during a vaginal examination and then by inserting trial diaphragms from a fitting set until the correct size is found. An arcing spring diaphragm is to be preferred as it is more likely to be inserted properly. It is also to be preferred if the woman has a retroverted uterus or a uterovaginal prolapse. The one chosen should fit snugly, the upper rim lying in the posterior vaginal fornix, the lower about 1cm above the external urethral meatus (Fig. **11/4**). The diaphragm is inserted by the patient preferably routinely each day, and removed for cleaning the next day, or at least six hours after coitus has taken place. It is usual to smear a spermicidal cream around the rim and to place a small amount on the upper surface to cover the external cervical os.

The technique a woman uses to insert and to remove her diaphragm is shown in Fig. **11/4**. Used properly the pregnancy rate should not exceed 3 per 100 woman-years.

Cervical caps are also available in some countries. These require careful insertion as the cap has to fit snugly over the cervix, consequently the pregnancy rate is higher (average 10 to 15 per 100 woman-years.).

VAGINAL CONTRACEPTIVE SPONGE

This is a polyurethane sponge, 5.5cm in diameter and 2.5cm thick, 1g of nonoxynol-9 (a spermicide) is incorporated in it during manufacture. Before insertion the sponge is moistened in water to activate the spermicide. Following ejaculation by the male, it should be left in the vagina for at least 6 hours, then removed and discarded. The pregnancy rate is between 7 and 12 per 100 woman-years.

It appears to act as much by releasing the spermicide in the vagina, as by acting as a barrier.

HORMONAL CONTRACEPTIVE STEROIDS

It has been known for over 40 years that ovulation can be suppressed if oestrogen, above a critical dose, is given to a woman over a critical period in the first half of her menstrual cycle. Unfortunately, the administration of oestrogen in this way is usually followed by episodes of irregular, unpredictable vaginal bleeding which are unacceptable to most women.

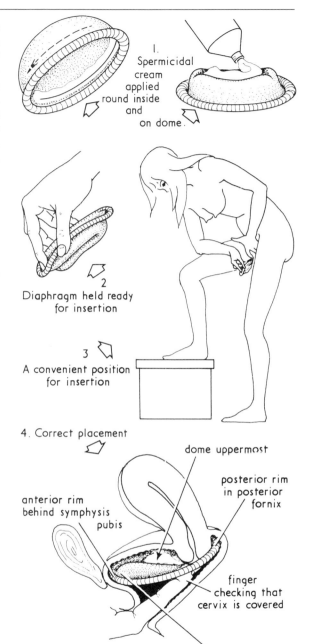

1. Spermicidal cream applied round inside and on dome.

2 Diaphragm held ready for insertion

3 A convenient position for insertion

4. Correct placement

dome uppermost

anterior rim behind symphysis pubis

posterior rim in posterior fornix

finger checking that cervix is covered

5. Removal is by hooking it out from here with a finger.

Fig. 11/4 The use of the vaginal diaphragm

However, if a progestogen – a synthetic substance which has biological effects resembling progesterone – is also given, a smaller dose of oestrogen is required to suppress ovulation and in addition predictable 'menstruation' occurs.

For centuries women have sought to escape from

the bondage of perpetual childbearing. The oral hormonal contraceptive – the Pill – was the first really effective method available to women, and has played a significant role in the current 'liberation' of women.

The steroids in oral contraceptives

OESTROGEN

The oral contraceptives available today contain either ethinyl oestradiol or its 3-methyl ether, mestranol. Mestranol is pharmacologically, and biologically, a weaker oestrogen, at least so far as suppression of ovulation is concerned. In the body it is converted into ethinyl oestradiol before acting. The best estimate is that $80\mu g$ of mestranol is equivalent to $50\mu g$ of ethinyl oestradiol, and at these doses ovulation is suppressed. However, the ability of the liver to demethylate mestranol into ethinyl oestradiol is altered when the substance is used in conjunction with a progestogen. Of the progestogens, ethynodiol diacetate inhibits the conversion by 50 per cent, lynestrenol by 30 per cent, norethisterone minimally and levonorgestrel not at all.

PROGESTOGENS

Three forms of progestogen are available: (1) those derived from testosterone by replacing the methyl group (CH_3) of the carbon 19 atom with a hydrogen atom (19-nortestosterone), (2) those derived from 17-acetoxyprogesterone and (3) the new generation progestogens, desogestrel, gestodene and norgestimate.

1. *19-nortestosterone.* These compounds act mainly as progestogens, but have a weak 'androgenic' activity, thus stimulating weight gain and reducing menstrual flow. A minute amount of the compound metabolizes in the body to oestrogen. The amount varies depending on the progestogen, ethynodiol diacetate appears to have the most oestrogenic conversion; no more than 0.02 per cent of norethisterone is converted and probably no oestrogen conversion occurs if levonorgestrel is used. If anything, norgestrel has an anti-oestrogenic effect. The 19-nortestosterones in use today are norethisterone, lynestrenol, ethynodiol diacetate and levonorgestrel.

2. *17-acetoxyprogesterone.* These compounds are pure progestogens, which have no 'androgenic' activity and do not metabolize to oestrogen. Only one, 17-acetoxyprogesterone is currently available for contraception. This is medroxy-progesterone acetate.

3. *The new generation progestogens* resemble natural progesterone in their receptor-binding properties. They have a minimal effect on lipid metabolism and do not have androgenic effects.

Formulations

ORAL HORMONAL CONTRACEPTIVES

At present several formulations of oral contraceptive pills are available.

The combined pill (monophasic)

An oestrogen and a progestogen are taken from day 5 to day 25 of the menstrual cycle. At present between 20 and 35 different competing combinations of various doses of oestrogen and various doses of different progestogens are available. This is confusing to the doctor.

Sequential pills (biphasic)

The term is a misnomer as both oestrogen and progestogen are given for 20 to 22 days. In the first 11 days oestrogen is given with a small dose of progestogen whilst in the last 10 days the dose of oestrogen and progestogen is that used in combined pills. The effectiveness of the sequential pill in preventing pregnancy is slightly lower than that of the combined pill, but the formulation is especially useful for women who have acne or scanty menstruation.

The sequential pills may be replaced by one of the combined or triphasic pills which contains one of the new generation progestogens.

Triphasic pill

In this formulation, three changes in the amount of oestrogen and progestogen are made. For the first 6 days, ethinyl oestradiol $30\mu g$ and levonorgestrel $50\mu g$ is taken. For the next 5 days, the dose of ethinyl oestradiol is $40\mu g$ and that of levonorgestrel $75\mu g$. For the last 10 days of each cycle ethinyl oestradiol $30\mu g$ and levonorgestrel $125\mu g$ is prescribed. The total dose of progestogen taken in any cycle is reduced, compared with the other two types of formulation. This is thought to be of value in reducing the lipid metabolic changes. A triphasic preparation, using norgestimate is now available.

The progestogen pill

In this formulation a low dose of progestogen is taken daily without interruption. Two types of formulation are available. In one, norethisterone is used, in the other levonorgestrel is used.

ONCE-A-MONTH PREPARATIONS

The need to take an oral contraceptive pill daily means that women have to make daily decisions to take the pill. In order to reduce the chance of omitting the pill, a study is being carried out using a single tablet of quinestrol 3mg taken on day 1 of the cycle. Quinestrol is a long-acting oestrogen which is stored in body fat and slowly released. It is used in combination with a single tablet of a short-acting progestogen which is given on the 22nd day of the cycle. Little statistical information about the value of this preparation has been published, and only one reliable report is available.

LONG-ACTING INJECTABLE PROGESTOGENS

A further development is an injectable progestogen (in most studies medroxy-progesterone acetate) which is given at 3-month intervals.

A comparison of the various formulations is made later in this chapter.

PROGESTOGEN-RELEASING VAGINAL RING

This is currently under study. The ring is made of silicone rubber containing 5mg levonorgestrel which is released at a rate of $20\mu g$ a day. The ring is inserted high into the vagina and is normally left in the vagina during menstruation. It is changed every 3 months. The absorbed progestogen alters cervical mucus and endometrial histology so that it is 'out-of-phase'. Side effects are bleeding or spotting. The pregnancy rate is about 3 per 100 woman-years.

SUBDERMAL IMPLANTS

The use of subdermal implants of a progestogen has been developed. Six silastic capsules, measuring 30mm by 2.5mm and containing 36mg of levonorgestrel each, are introduced subdermally into the anterior aspect of the forearm through a trocar. They will provide effective contraception for 3 to 4 years. Side-effects include irregular episodes of bleeding and occasional episodes of prolonged bleeding. These are experienced by about 20 per cent of women during the first year and may limit the acceptibility of the method.

Mode of action of hormonal contraceptives

The mode of action of the oral contraceptive pill depends upon the actual component steroids and the ratio between them. In all formulations the oestrogen suppresses FSH secretion and reduces the release of LH, either directly in the pituitary or, more probably, by suppressing hypothalamic FSH and LH-releasing hormones. In this way, ovulation is usually prevented, and ovarian steroid synthesis is reduced.

The progestogen (1) further suppresses LH release and prevents the 'peak' of LH which precedes, and appears essential to, ovulation, probably by blocking the positive oestrogen feedback, (2) alters the quality of the cervical mucus rendering it less penetrable to spermatozoa, (3) permits a progestogen 'withdrawal' bleed which is regular in onset, short in duration and light in quantity of blood lost, and (4) produces endometrial changes culminating in glandular exhaustion with a pseudo-decidual stromal reaction. The degree with which these changes occur depends on the type of progestogen, the ratio of oestrogen to progestogen and on the duration of unopposed oestrogen action before the progestogen is given. For example, if oestrogen is given alone for more than 10 days, and the progestogen then added, the endometrium will show a secretory pattern, but if a 19-nortestosterone progestogen is added less than 5 days after oestrogen is started the 'glandular exhaustion' pattern occurs. If the progestogen is given alone (as in the mini-pill) the effect is mainly on the endometrium.

The biochemical and physiological alterations due to hormonal contraceptives

No drug has received as much investigation as the synthetic steroids which, usually in combination, make up oral or injectable hormonal contraceptives. Of the two steroids, oestrogen seems to cause more alterations to the body's economy than the progestogens.

HYPOTHALAMIC-PITUITARY-GENITAL AXIS

As mentioned, the principal effect of hormonal contraceptives is to suppress the release of FSH and LH from the pituitary. The endometrium is also affected, probably directly by the steroids, and endometrial hypoplasia is usual. In formulations which are strongly oestrogenic (such as sequential regimens) cervical eversions may become more obvious.

BREASTS

The hormones increase the size of the breasts in some women, and have a beneficial effect on benign mammary dysplasia. There is no evidence that the use of steroid contraceptives leads to the development of mammary malignancy.

ADRENAL AND THYROID GLANDS

Serum corticosteroid binding protein and T_4 levels are raised, but there is no evidence of any disturbance to adrenal or thyroid function. The raised levels are thought to be due to an increase in serum-binding proteins.

LIVER

Oestrogen (and progestogen, to a lesser extent) stimulates liver cells to synthesize and to release into the circulation a variety of serum-binding carrier proteins so that the levels of various substances are raised, compared with those found in women who do not use hormonal contraceptives. Oestrogen also induces liver cells to secrete increased quantities of blood clotting factors II, VII, IX and X, but simultaneously increases the fibrinolytic potential of the blood.

OTHER METABOLIC CHANGES

Oestrogen (and progestogen to a lesser extent) reduces glucose tolerance, although the degree of impairment is related to the dose of oestrogen and the age and weight of the woman. About 30 to 60 per cent of women on oral contraceptives have a reduced ability to dispose of a glucose load. The impairment seems to be due to increased glucocorticoid activity induced by oestrogen.

Clinical side-effects

The reason for using hormonal contraceptives is to prevent pregnancy. The use of a birth control measure occasions feelings of relief, or guilt, depending on the cultural background of the woman. If the latter, she believes she is doing 'wrong' in hindering

a 'natural' body function; if the former, she is delighted to be spared the risk of an unwanted pregnancy. These psychological alterations make the clinical side-effects due to hormonal contraceptives difficult to assess. As Goldzieher says, 'The burden of proof must now rest on those who claim that a given symptom is attributable to the contraceptive agent rather than to coincidence or psychic induction.'

Since oestrogen is implicated in more of the biochemical changes, it is also considered to be the cause of more of the side-effects (Table **11/2**). Most of them are maximal in the first few menstrual cycles, and cease as the body adjusts to the new hormonal milieu, but a few may persist. The side-effects may be beneficial or annoying. They are discussed in alphabetical order.

ACNE

Acne is an inflammation of the sebaceous glands, associated with increased secretion of sebum. This secretion is controlled by androgens, and opposed by oestrogens. The oestrogen component of the oral contraceptive tends to improve acne; whilst 19-nortestosterone has the opposite effect because of its weak 'androgenic' component. The effect, however, depends on a variety of pre-existing factors. If a patient has severe acne, it is wise to use a sequential formulation, or a combined formulation in which the progestogen is a 17-acetoxyprogesterone.

CANCER

In primate and human studies there is no evidence that the hormonal contraceptives are implicated in the aetiology of genital or breast cancer. No increase in these malignancies has been found in women who have used hormonal contraceptives for less than 5 years, but a slight increase in incidence may occur if hormonal contraceptives are used for a longer period. The increase is very small, but it is recommended that women using hormonal contraceptives should have cervical smears taken every 2 to 3 years, and their breasts examined at the same time.

Ovarian and endometrial cancers have a lower incidence.

CARDIOVASCULAR DISEASE

Levels of HDL-cholesterol and LDL-cholesterol are

Oestrogen effects	Progestogen effects	Combined effects
Nausea and vomiting	Premenstrual depression	Tiredness
Fluid retention (i.e. transient weight gain)	Appetite increase	Irritability
	Weight gain	Breast fullness
Premenstrual tension	? Leg cramps	? Decreased libido
Headache	Reduction in menstrual flow	Rise in blood pressure
Cervical 'eversion'	Disturbance in menstrual cycle	Cardiovascular disease (dose-dependent increase)
Vaginal discharge	Acne	
Increase in menstrual flow	Greasy hair	
Venous thrombosis		

Table 11/2 The side-effects of oral contraceptives

The degree to which the side-effects are apparent depends on the oestrogen/progestogen ratio of the compound and the effect of this is on the woman's endogenous sex hormone production.

related to the increased incidence of cardiovascular disease. Higher levels of LDL-cholesterol are considered a risk factor whilst high levels of HDL-cholesterol seem protective. Oestrogen raises HDL, whilst the progestogens reduce HDL and increase LDL to a varying degree. The new generation progestogens do not alter lipid metabolism and are to be preferred where oral contraceptives containing them are available. Of the first generation progestogens, norgestrel in a dose not exceeding 150μg combined with ethinyl oestradiol 30μg alters the lipids least. Although studies in the mid-1970s (when the pill formulations contained larger daily doses of both sex hormones) indicated that oral contraceptives imposed an increased risk that the woman would develop ischaemic heart disease, subarachnoid haemorrhage or stroke, more recent studies suggest that the increased risk, which only just reaches significance, is due to cigarette smoking rather than oral contraceptives.

The annual risk of death from myocardial infarction is low amongst these women, being 8 per 100 000 annually, but higher than the 1 per 100 000 annual incidence amongst non-oral contraceptive users of the same age range.

CHLOASMA

Hyperpigmentation of the skin of the face may occur in susceptible women who have been taking a pill containing 17-acetoxyprogesterone for more than two years, and is related to exposure to the sun. Treatment is to avoid direct sunlight, to change the oral contraceptive, and in certain cases to apply 2 per cent hydroquinone ointment. Despite these measures, the pigmentation often takes up to nine months to fade.

DEPRESSION, MOOD CHANGES, REDUCED LIBIDO

It is almost impossible to make objective observations on the frequency with which depression and reduced libido are associated with the ingestion of hormonal contraceptives, as mood changes depend on a variety of external and internal stimuli, amongst which endocrine alterations may be of significance. In a study in Britain, it was found that women who had premenstrual mood changes, and had a low sexual drive before starting oral contraceptives, were more likely to develop mood changes when using the drugs. In a large series reported from California, no increase in depression or mood changes was found amongst nearly 2000 pill users when compared with 1700 controls. In a further study of 500 women, no evidence of impairment of sexuality was found. The overall findings are that it is unlikely that hormonal oral contraceptives increase depression, cause mood changes or decrease libido.

DYSMENORRHOEA

Since dysmenorrhoea is unusual in anovulatory cycles, unless menstruation is heavy and clots are expelled from the uterus, hormonal contraceptives which suppress ovulation should relieve the condition. About 65 per cent of young women have dysmenorrhoea, and in 15 per cent it is severe. Combined oral contraceptives relieve dysmenorrhoea in over 80 per cent of cases.

GALL BLADDER AND LIVER DISEASE

The incidence of gall bladder disease is reduced if women remain slim, avoid sugar, increase their intake of dietary fibre and, if they wish, drink a little alcohol. Contraceptive use may accelerate the development of gall bladder disease in susceptible women but does not increase the long-term incidence. The frequency of symptomatic gall bladder disease during contraceptive use varies directly with the dose of oestrogen in the pill, and is probably due to the effect of oestrogen on LDL-cholesterol.

A rare association between oral contraceptive usage and benign hepatocellular adenomas has been noted.

HEADACHES AND MIGRAINE

Headaches often occur amongst women who have mood changes, and tend to be worse premenstrually, perhaps because of aldosterone-induced fluid retention but there is no evidence of an increased incidence amongst women using hormonal contraceptives. Migraine may also be aggravated at this time. If a generalized migraine becomes focal, it is suggestive of vertebro-basilar occlusion and hormonal contraceptives should be abandoned.

HYPERTENSION

Hormonal contraceptives lead to a small increase in the systolic blood pressure, which is reversible. Hypertension of a greater magnitude occurs in a few women, particularly those who have a familial history, are overweight and aged 35 or more. In addition, some hypertensive women taking oral contraceptives develop an increase in the level of the diastolic blood pressure. The effect is due to oestrogen and perhaps progestogen. There is a direct relationship between the dose of oestrogen and the frequency of hypertension. The aetiology is obscure, but may be due to an alteration in the renin-angiotensin system, as both plasma renin and angiotensin II levels rise. This may cause an increase in aldosterone secretion, and vasospasm.

Amongst normotensive women, particularly those under the age of 35, the incidence is low, and the diastolic blood pressure is affected least.

Women with known hypertension, or who were hypertensive in pregnancy, are more likely to be affected and require to have their blood pressures monitored more carefully, or to use other methods of birth control, particularly if they are aged 40 years or more, as such women have an increased risk of myocardial infarction and stroke.

MENSTRUATION

Most women are culturally conditioned to believe that in the absence of pregnancy or lactation, menstruation is essential to maintain normal genital tract well-being. Menstruation informs a woman that she is not pregnant, and reassures her that she can become pregnant. In fact, menstruation is unnecessary, and in areas where protein and iron intake is low it is a cause of anaemia. Given cyclically, oral contraceptives mimic a woman's normal menstrual cycle and permit menstruation whilst suppressing ovulation. Most women appear to prefer this.

Low-dose combined oral contraceptives, using a 19-nortestosterone derivative as the progestogen, tend to produce a reduction in the quantity and duration of blood loss in over 50 per cent of women. In many the colour of the blood changes from bright red to dirty brown. Because of accumulated myths about the need for a good menstrual flow, women should be reassured that the colour of the blood loss is without danger. So-called sequential formulations are less likely to reduce blood loss, and are particularly useful for women who have very scanty periods and wish to use oral contraceptives.

For the majority of women, oral contraceptives ensure that menstruation occurs predictably on a known date. A few women, particularly in early cycles, or who are under emotional stress, develop blood spotting, or break-through bleeding, on an unpredictable day whilst still taking oral contraceptives. Spotting may be ignored unless it increases. Break-through bleeding may only occur in one cycle, but if it persists is due to insufficient progestogen. It can be controlled by increasing the quantity of progestogen in the oral contraceptive, by choosing a pill which contains a higher potency progestogen, or by giving a larger dose (i.e. two pills daily). Break-through bleeding occurs in less than 1 per cent of cycles.

A patient who has menorrhagia before choosing oral contraceptives usually has a reduced menstrual loss because of the effects of the progestogen, but may require to use an oral contraceptive with a larger than usual dose of progestogen.

About 1 per cent of women become amenorrhoeic when taking oral contraceptives. Since menstruation is of no importance, these women should be reassured that pregnancy will be prevented provided that they have not omitted to take the pill each day (one missed day is probably safe, three missed days between days 5 and 12 is hazardous), and they should recommence the next course after an interval of 7 days, if the ordinary pack is used.

On ceasing to take oral contraceptives, two things occur. The majority of women experience a delay in ovulation of up to 20 days. If the woman is attempting to become pregnant this must be taken into account; whilst if pregnancy occurs, the estimated date of delivery calculated from the last bleeding episode may be at least 2 weeks understated. Unless the patient is questioned about her use of oral contraceptives, fetal growth retardation may be erroneously diagnosed. A few women fail to menstruate on ceasing to take oral contraceptives, due to continued inhibition of the release of hypothalamic gonadotrophin releasing hormones, and, possibly, reduced ovarian responsiveness. In the majority, menstruation restarts within 3 months; but in a few cases (about 0.7 per cent) amenorrhoea persists for 12 months. If this happens, investigations should be made to find the cause of the amenorrhoea, and if pregnancy is desired, ovulation should be stimulated using clomiphene citrate.

NAUSEA AND VOMITING

Until the body adjusts to the ingestion of synthetic oestrogen, nausea, and occasionally vomiting, may occur. About 20 per cent of women experience nausea and 2 per cent vomit in the first cycle during which the pill is taken. Tolerance develops rapidly and by the third cycle fewer than 2 per cent of women have any complaint.

THROMBO-EMBOLIC PHENOMENA

Investigations in Britain and the USA have established a relationship between the use of oral contraceptives and the development of thrombo-embolism, although it appears that the relationship is influenced by the age of the woman, her weight and her consumption of tobacco. The evidence suggests that women taking oral contraceptives have 2 to 4 times the chance of developing deep venous thrombosis or thrombo-embolism compared with a woman who uses another method of contraception.

The incidence of thrombo-embolic phenomena amongst pill users is small (0.5 per 1000 users per year) and appears to be related to the dose of oestrogen in oral contraceptives. Oral contraceptives containing 30μg are associated with a reduced chance of stroke. A recent study has implicated progestogen which, if true, suggests that pills containing low doses of progestogen are to be preferred.

Even if a woman develops a thrombo-embolism, her chance of dying from the condition is low, and is less than the risk associated with pregnancy (Table 11/3).

	Age of women	
	15–34	35–49
Oral contraceptives non-users	0.2	0.5
Oral contraceptives users	1.5	3.9
Pregnancy*	9.0	26.1

*Maternal deaths 1964–66 (Rep. *Public Health and Medical Subjects* 119, HMSO, London, 1969)

Source: Vessey, M. P. and Doll, R. *Brit. Med. J.*, **2**, 651, 1969.

	Age of women			
	30–39		40–44	
	Users	Non-users	Users	Non-users
Smokers	1.6	0.2	4.1	0.6
Non-smokers	1.4	0.2	3.6	0.4

Table 11/3 Mortality per 100 000 from thrombo-embolism, in women using or not using contraceptives, who are smokers or non-smokers.

VAGINAL DISCHARGE AND VAGINITIS

An increased vaginal discharge is usual, and is due to oestrogenic stimulation of the cervical mucus-secreting cells. The symptom is more marked in women taking sequential pills, as the anti-oestrogenic effect of the progestogen is less in the first 10 days. Leucorrhoea is of little clinical importance, provided that vaginitis has been excluded. Once this has been done, the patient can be told that the leucorrhoea is a normal event and signifies nothing sinister.

Vaginal candidiasis appears to occur more frequently in women taking oral contraceptives, and a smear should be taken for culture, to exclude the presence of this condition in all women who complain of an irritant vaginal discharge.

WEIGHT GAIN

Transient weight gain is usual in the premenstrual days and is due to fluid retention; it tends to revert when menstruation starts. The degree of transient weight gain tends to be increased amongst women taking oral contraceptives. In addition, progestogens have an anabolic effect, which only becomes apparent after a few months. Weight gain may be directly due to the hormone, or to increased appetite which occurs as a consequence of relief from the fear of pregnancy. Treatment is to explain the reason for the weight gain, and to prescribe a diet high in protein, and low in fats and calories.

Benefits of oral contraceptives

1. Women using contraceptives have a greatly reduced incidence of dysmenorrhoea.

2. There is no evidence that the long-term use of the oral contraceptives reduces fertility or causes chromosomal changes in the germ cells, and indeed fertility may be temporarily enhanced for a few months after ceasing to use the drugs as coitus occurs more frequently in couples who have used oral contraceptives.

3. Benign breast disease (benign mammary dysplasia and fibroadenoma) is reduced amongst women who use hormonal contraceptives and breast carcinoma is not increased.

4. Women who use oral contraceptives have fewer benign breast tumours than those using other, or no contraceptive method.

5. In women who have several partners, oral contraceptives protect against the risk of developing pelvic inflammatory disease.

6. There is no evidence that the incidence of diabetes or of liver damage is increased.

7. The incidence of rheumatoid arthritis in the perimenopausal years is reduced in women who have taken the pill for at least five years.

8. There is a reduction in the chance of developing uterine myomata.

Fertility after discontinuation of oral contraceptives

In the first one or two cycles after discontinuing oral contraceptives, ovulation may not occur or may be delayed, but in over 95 per cent of women ovulation will recur regularly within 3 months. A few women (0.5 per cent) have post-pill amenorrhoea of at least 6-months duration. The amenorrhoea may be due to the effects of the pill, but may be due to low bodyweight, dieting or disordered eating behaviours.

Prescribing hormonal contraceptives

The majority of women prefer to use one of the modern low-dose oral contraceptives. A few women prefer to receive 3-monthly injections of the injectable progestogens, whilst women who are breast-feeding should be given the progestogen pill.

Certain women should not be given hormonal contraceptives containing oestrogen. These include women who (1) have previously developed thromboembolism or cerebrovascular insufficiency, (2) have liver disease, (3) have blood dyscrasias, (4) have severe migraine, (5) have marked hypertension, or (6) during treatment develop transient cerebral, retinal, or focal migraine attacks. These women may use progestogen-only contraceptives, either in the form of 'injectables' or of daily progestogens; or may prefer some other form of contraception.

This information should make it clear that no woman should be prescribed an oestrogen-containing hormonal contraceptive until it has been established that she has not had a deep venous thrombosis, has no blood dyscrasia, and that she does not have severe migraine. Women over the age of 25 should have their blood pressure taken before prescribing, and, a vaginal examination should be made (to exclude pelvic tumours and so that a cervical smear for exfoliative cytology may be taken).

The five-fold increase in incidence of cardiovascular disease amongst women over the age of 35, who are overweight and smoke cigarettes has led to a warning that oral contraceptives should be used with caution by such women. The correlation was obtained at a time when most oral contraceptives contained $50\mu g$ or more of oestrogen: it has not been established if such a correlation exists when oral contraceptives containing $30\mu g$ are used.

Women who are on long-term therapy with anticonvulsants or rifampicin, should use a combined pill or pills containing a total of at least $80\mu g$ of ethinyl oestradiol or use another contraceptive method because of increased hepatic enzyme activity metabolizes the contraceptive steroids more readily.

ORAL HORMONAL CONTRACEPTIVES

There are at least 25 formulations currently available. Following the reports of an association between the amount of oestrogen in the pill and thromboembolism, most formulations contain no more than $50\mu g$ of ethinyl oestradiol or mestranol, although increasingly, 30 or 35µg ethinyl oestradiol is being used. The dose of progestogen varies, but as noted earlier, the biological effects of different progestogens is so great that formulation differences are more apparent than real. Currently, the combination of ethinyl oestradiol 30µg with desogestrel 150µg causes the least biochemical and clinical alterations and is an effective protection against unwanted pregnancy. It is the most suitable oral contraceptive to use initially. Most women find the formulation satisfactory, but should break-through bleeding become a problem, a higher dose oral contraceptive can replace it.

In general it is best to become really familiar with a few formulations and to prescribe these. There appears little advantage in constantly switching the patient from one oral contraceptive to another in the hope of reducing the side-effects. Initially the patient should be prescribed the most appropriate formulation for her needs, and precautions must be instituted. For example, a few hypertensive patients develop a marked increase in the level of blood pressure when taking oral contraceptives. If they are prescribed, regular estimations of the blood pressure should be made and therapy suspended if hypertension results.

Another problem of the low-dose oral contraceptive (containing 30µg of ethinyl oestradiol) is that the dose of the progestogen (if new generation progestogens are not used) may be a factor in raising the blood level of triglyceride and reducing that of high density lipid-cholesterol. These changes may increase the risk of thrombo-embolic disease. The triphasic formulation obviates these effects. At the same time it reduces break-through bleeding and provides the same degree of contraceptive efficiency as the low-dose formulations.

When a woman starts to use contraceptives or changes to a new formulation, the British Family Planning Association recommends that she begins taking the tablets on the first day of menstruation. In subsequent cycles the pill is taken in the usual way. The advantage of this is that the couple need take no other contraceptive precautions in the first cycle; although spotting and break-through bleeding is more likely to occur.

The 'missed pill'. As the new oral contraceptives have low doses of the sex hormones, effective suppression of ovulation requires that they be taken at the same time each day. If a pill is missed for more than 12 hours the patient should take the missed pill immediately and the next pill at the usual time. If she misses two pills, these two should be taken as soon as she remembers and the next pill at the usual time. However, for safety the couple should use a barrier method for the next seven days.

The pregnancy (failure) rate amongst women using low-dose formulations is less than 0.4 per 100 women-years, but the woman must remember to take the pill at about the same time each day.

SEQUENTIAL FORMULATIONS

As the 'failure' rate is rather higher than when combined oral hormonal contraceptives are used, sequential formulations should be reserved for women who have acne and women who have scanty menstruation.

CONTINUOUS DAILY ORAL PROGESTOGENS

Small doses of progestogen (the 'mini-pill') taken daily may be prescribed to women who should avoid oestrogen-containing contraceptives, or who are breast-feeding, as oral contraceptives containing oestrogen reduce the milk supply of a few lactating women. The use of progestogen-only oral contraceptives avoids oestrogenic 'side-effects' but are associated with some degree of diminished libido. However, the main disadvantages of this type of oral contraceptive are a rather high incidence of break-through bleeding and of unpredictable menstruation, which affect over 25 per cent of women using the method, and a pregnancy rate of about 2 per 100 woman-years.

LONG-ACTING INJECTABLE PROGESTOGENS

Some women may prefer to have a single intramuscular injection at about 3-month intervals rather than have to take an oral pill each day. Most experience with injectable progestogens relates to the use of depot medroxy-progesterone acetate (DMPA) given in a dose of 150mg every 3 months. The pregnancy rate is about 1.5 per 100 woman-years, which is very acceptable, but in about 50 per cent of women menstruation is markedly disorganized. In the first 6 months of the method unpredictable uterine bleeding, or spotting, is common and although the amount lost is usually small, it may disturb the women aesthetically. This pattern affects about 50 per cent of women, whilst 30 per cent develop amenorrhoea. With continued injections, at 3-month intervals, the menstrual irregularity decreases but amenorrhoea becomes more common, so that after 12 months use about 40 per cent of women will have amenorrhoea, 40 per cent will have infrequent scanty episodes of bleeding, and 20 per cent will experience frequent or prolonged episodes of scanty bleeding. This last group is important as no effective treatment is available (although oestrogens are often prescribed). On ceasing medication, normal menstruation resumes, usually after a 3 to 9 months' delay.

A new method using a long-acting progestogen, levonorgestrel in small silastic capsules is now available as mentioned on p. 113.

POSTCOITAL CONTRACEPTION (THE 'MORNING-AFTER' PILL)

Women who have coitus infrequently, perhaps less than once a week, may prefer not to take contraceptive hormonal preparations each day. Other women who have had coitus at ovulation time without contraceptive protection may fear pregnancy.

Postcoital contraception, using hormones, may be chosen by the first group of women; and may be preferred by women in the second group rather than waiting to see if pregnancy has occurred and then requesting an abortion.

Both oestrogens and progestogens have been used. The most recent recommendation is to prescribe ethinyl oestradiol 50μg + levonorgestrel 0.50mg (Eugynon-50, Ovran). Two tablets are taken and repeated 12 hours later. Forty per cent of patients become nauseated and 15 per cent vomit so that an anti-emetic should be given at the same time as the tablets. The morning-after pill appears to lead to luteal phase dysfunction and an out-of-phase development of the endometrium, which prevents nidation. The apparent pregnancy rate following this regimen is 1.5 per cent.

Progestogens have been used to give postcoital protection in women having infrequent intercourse. Levonorgestrel in a dose of 0.8 to 1mg *taken within 3 hours of each episode of sexual intercourse* reduces the pregnancy rate to about 3 per 100 woman-years in the reported investigations.

There has been some concern that hormones used in this way may cause fetal abnormalities (or vaginal adenosis in the offspring in adolescence) should the drugs fail to prevent pregnancy. Expert opinion believes this unlikely, but abortion can be offered to women in whom the morning-after pill fails to produce menstruation.

GnRH-AGONIST ANALOGUE (LHRH-AGONIST ANALOGUE)

A GnRH super-agonist analogue has been developed which 'down-regulates' gonadotrophin receptors in the pituitary gland, so that the gonadotrophs fail to secrete gonadotrophins. This, in turn, inhibits ovulation. GnRH agonist given as a nasal spray each day has been shown (in small series) to act as an effective contraceptive. However about 20 per cent of women develop hot flushes and in 80 per cent the plasma level of oestradiol is low (< 150 pmol/litre). This level if maintained may predispose the woman to osteoporosis. The method may be of value for women unable or unwilling to use other methods of contraception.

The efficiency and reliability of hormonal contraceptives

Hormonal contraceptives are the most efficient and reliable method of temporary contraception. The combined oral contraceptive has a pregnancy rate of less than 0.5 per 100 woman-years; the sequential oral contraceptive, the progestogen pill and the injectable progestogen have a pregnancy rate of about 1.25 per 100 woman-years.

No other temporary contraceptive achieves this degree of efficiency; the closest being the IUD.

THE INTRA-UTERINE CONTRACEPTIVE DEVICE

Intra-uterine contraceptive devices, or IUDs, were introduced into clinical medicine at the end of the 19th century and again in the 1920s. Because of concern about pelvic infection and a rather high pregnancy rate, the method was largely abandoned.

In 1959 interest was revived, particularly now that the IUD could be made of polyethylene, which had a 'memory' for its shape, so that it could be straightened to introduce it into the uterus in the knowledge that it would regain its previous shape once inside the uterine cavity.

A satisfactory IUD should be easy to introduce, easy to remove, have few side-effects and should prevent pregnancy with a high degree of efficiency. These criteria have led to the development of a variety of shapes and sizes of IUD. At present only two or three are in general use and, today, devices

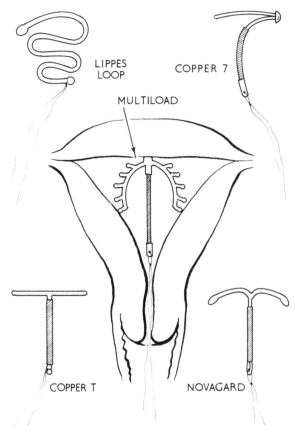

LIPPES LOOP

COPPER 7

MULTILOAD

COPPER T

NOVAGARD

Fig. 11/5 Currently used IUDs

to which copper or zinc has been added are in vogue. The addition of the metal permits a smaller device to be used which is as efficient as a large device in preventing pregnancy but has fewer side-effects (Fig. **11/5**). A disadvantage of the IUDs with added copper is that they need to be replaced after 3 to 5 years as the copper ionizes slowly.

A new IUD, shaped like a T, which contains a slowly released form of progesterone (the Prog-estasert) is now available. The IUD releases 65μg of progesterone a day which enhances the effect of the inert plastic. The device is effective for 1 year when it must be replaced. Its benefits over the IUDs with copper added have not been evaluated.

Mode of action

It is not clear just how the IUD prevents pregnancy. The current belief is that the device causes a marked allergic reaction in the endometrium, which results

in a heavy infiltration by immunocytes and macro-phages. The immunocytes infiltrate possible nidation sites, the macrophages perhaps phagocytose the impl-anting egg. Acting together they render the en-dometrium hostile, and either impede fertilization or interrupt early implanation. Copper, ionized slowly, enhances the effect, whilst the IUDs containing prog-esterone also affect the cervical mucus rendering it 'hostile' to spermatozoal penetration.

Technique of insertion

Modern IUDs, being made of polyethylene, either are dispatched in pre-sterilized packages or require to be stored in a benzylkonium (1 : 750) solution.

When a woman chooses an IUD the insertion should be preceded by counselling and discussion so that the advantages and disadvantages of the method are clearly understood (see Table **11/4**). The woman should be questioned about previous pelvic infection, as this and current menorrhagia are relative con-traindications. A pelvic examination is made to ex-clude uterine abnormalities and, when appropriate, a cervical smear is made for exfoliative cytology. The smaller IUDs (such as the Copper-7, the Copper-T and Progestasert) can be used by nullipar-ous women, and can generally be introduced without any anaesthesia.

Evaluate
* Multiparity
* Menorrhagia
* Anaemia
* Allergy to copper
* Diabetes (because of high pregnancy rate due to erosion of the device)

Table 11/4 Investigations before advising an IUD

In general IUDs should not be used by women who have not borne children. Women who have or have had several partners, or whose partner has or has had several partners should be checked for chlamydial infection before an IUD is chosen be-cause of the increased risk of developing pelvic infec-tion. If the couple has a mutually monogamous rela-tionship, an IUD is a safe choice of contraception.

The technique is relatively simple. (1) A pelvic examination establishes the position and size of the uterus, (2) a bivalve vaginal speculum is introduced, the cervix is exposed and cleaned with antiseptic, (3) the anterior lip of the cervix is grasped with a light tenaculum, and a uterine sound is introduced to

	First year	Third year
Pregnancies	2.8	5.3
Expulsions—first	10.4	12.7
—later	3.1	4.6
Removals		
Bleeding and/or pain	10.6	18.8
Other medical causes	3.4	6.6
Planned pregnancies	0.9	4.4
Other personal reasons	2.2	4.6
Percentage of patients no longer using the device	21.7	40.7

Table 11/5 Intra-uterine contraceptive device: Loop D. Cumulative results, end of first year and third year per 100 first insertions

determine the length of the uterine cavity, (4) the pre-sterilized IUD is removed from the package and loaded into the introducer, (5) the loaded introducer is inserted into the uterus to reach the fundus, (6) by manipulating the introducer and the plunger the IUD is left in the uterus, the introducer being withdrawn, (7) the thread attached to the IUD, which projects from the cervix, is cut about 3 cm from the cervix. The purpose of the thread is to enable the woman to be sure that the IUD is still in her uterus, especially after a menstrual period; it also aids its removal.

Perforation of the uterus occurs in about 1 in 1000 insertions. Most perforations are asymptomatic, and are discovered at routine examination, or abortion. If a copper device has perforated the uterus, it should be removed as it may cause an omental mass.

IUD contra-indications

* Current or previous pelvic inflammatory disease
* Known or suspected pregnancy
* History of ectopic gestation or suspected malignancy
* Gynaecological bleeding disorder before a diagnosis made
* Congenital uterine abnormalities

Side-effects

A few women complain of intermittent bleeding or of cramp-like pains in the first week after an IUD is inserted and women having an IUD for the first time should be told of the possibility. The uterine cramps usually cease within a few weeks and are not as common as abnormal bleeding. Intermenstrual bleeding, either spotting or a bloody discharge may occur for a few weeks after insertion of the IUD. The bleeding usually ceases within 2 months, but if it persists may necessitate removal of the IUD. About 5 per cent of users require to have the IUD removed on account of bleeding or pain. Most women experience a slight increase in menstrual blood loss, and menstruation tends to last longer. It is scanty at first and then becomes heavier. If menstrual bleeding increases after prolonged use of an IUD, the device should be removed, although it can be replaced with a new IUD if the woman wishes to continue with this form of contraceptive.

Pelvic infection is the most serious side-effect, fortunately it occurs infrequently in the absence of pre-existing pelvic infection. Copper-containing IUDs seem less likely to be associated with pelvic infection than other IUDs. The infection rate with non-copper IUDs is less than 2 per 1000 insertions, but is twice that of women who use other kinds of contraception, or no contraception. Women who have had several sexual partners or whose sexual partner has had several sexual partners have an increased risk (>4 per 1000 insertions). For these women the IUD is not a first choice of contraception. This also applies to women who are under the age of 25 and who are nulliparous.

In most women tubovarian infection is preceded by a prodromal period of 2 to 5 weeks during which time the woman complains of vague lower abdominal pains, dyspareunia and pelvic tenderness. Should this symptom complex occur the IUD should be removed, as it must be should overt pelvic infection occur.

About 5 per cent of women expel the IUD, usually during one of the first three menstrual periods after insertion (Table 11/5). If this occurs a larger device should be inserted.

Ectopic gestation is also twice as likely to occur amongst women who have an IUD, compared with women who use no contraceptives, the rate rising from 1 in 200 conceptions to 1 in 100 conceptions.

Efficiency

The pregnancy rate using an IUD is about 2 per 100 woman-years. If a woman becomes pregnant with an IUD in the uterus, it should be removed if this can be done easily. If it cannot be removed easily the obstetrician should not continue pulling the thread. He should inform the woman that she can have an

Method of contraception	Age Group in years			
	15–29	30–34	35–39	40+
None (i.e. pregnancy related deaths)	6.4	13.9	20.8	22.6
Legal abortion < 12 weeks	1.5	1.7	1.9	1.2
Oral contraceptives				
Non-smokers	1.4	2.2	4.5	7.1
Smokers	1.6	10.8	13.4	58.9
IUD	1.0	1.4	2.0	1.9
Barrier methods	1.5	3.6	5.0	4.2
Barrier methods plus abortion if failure	0.2	0.3	0.3	0.2

Table 11/6 Estimated annual deaths associated with fertility control per 100 000 fertile women. This includes pregnancy related deaths if no contraceptive method is used or if the method fails to prevent pregnancy (Data from Tietze C., *Fam. Plan Perspect.* **9**, *74.1977*)

abortion induced, or can elect to continue with the pregnancy. If she chooses this course, it is proper to tell her that she has a 30 to 50 per cent chance of aborting spontaneously and that there is an increased risk of the abortion being a septic one, compared with spontaneous abortions in other pregnant women. The ectopic pregnancy rate is also raised, from 1:200 to 1:100 gestations. Because of this a pregnancy occurring to a woman using an IUD must be carefully checked (using ultrasound, when available) to detect if the pregnancy is intra-uterine or ectopic.

Some doctors use an IUD as a method of post-coital contraception. The pregnancy rate is less than 1 per cent if the IUD is inserted within 5 days of periovulatory intercourse.

Over 80 per cent of women choosing an IUD still have it in utero after 12 months, and 70 per cent continue to use the method for 24 and 36 months.

THE BENEFIT : RISK ASSOCIATION OF CONTRACEPTIVES

All contraceptives carry some risk, and so does pregnancy, although in this case the risk varies depending on the nutrition of the mother, the availability of obstetric care and her motivation to use the services provided.

An analysis made in the USA, where the maternal

mortality is low, is shown in Table **11/6**. Where no contraceptive is used, the death rate is that associated with pregnancy and childbirth. Traditional methods include coitus interruptus, the 'safe period' and the use of a diaphragm and condoms. The mortality associated with traditional methods together with that of legal abortion when pregnancy occurs, is shown in the last line of Table **11/6**.

An analysis, made in Britain, also computed the benefits and risks of various forms of contraceptives and is shown in Table **11/7**.

PERMANENT METHODS OF BIRTH CONTROL

In recent years increasing numbers of men and women having achieved their desired number of children, choose to have a permanent method of birth control. For men vasectomy is available; for women tubal ligation or hysterectomy are choices.

Vasectomy

Vasectomy is now accepted as a highly effective, easily performed, permanent method of conception control. The operation is easy to perform but does require considerable motivation to induce men to accept it. This motivation must be linked with information, so that the many verbalized and non-verbalized questions asked by prospective clients are answered. Health workers must avoid the trap of assuming that the intelligent are necessarily more accurately informed about their reproductive system. Even amongst intelligent people, vasectomy is confused with castration, and a hidden fear is that a man's sexual powers will be reduced postoperatively. He needs reassurance that the operation will in no way affect his sexual desires or his sexual performance. Concern may also be expressed about the dangerous accumulation of spermatozoa distal to the cut vas deferens. The physician must explain that the accumulation of spermatozoa is minimal, and that most of the quantity of the ejaculate derives from secretions of the accessory glands. He may also explain that as spermatozoa accumulate in the testicles, spermatogenesis almost ceases, and macrophages eliminate sperm in the epididymis and tubules but the synthesis of androgens continues. The most successful method of convincing a prospective client is for him to meet a man who has had a vasectomy performed, and who is satisfied with the result.

Condition	Oral contraceptives	Diaphragm and IUD
All 'strokes'	45	9
All thrombo-embolisms	91	20
Idiopathic deep thrombosis or pulmonary embolism	45	5
Acute myocardial infarction:		
Patients aged 30–34	6	2
Patients aged 40–44	57	10
Gall bladder disease	183	118
Cervical 'eversion'	539	249
Benign breast disease	119	277
Benign ovarian disease	138	201

Table 11/7 Non-obstetric morbidity and contraceptives (Hospital admissions per 100 000 women aged 15–45 per year) (Data from Vessey M. and Doll R.)

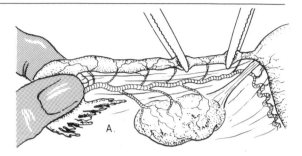

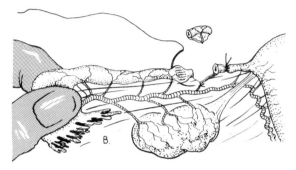

Vasectomy does not increase the risk of developing cardiovascular disease, cancer, prostatic disease, erectile failure or autoimmune disease. Psychological effects are unusual if the man has been prepared for the procedure and is anxious for the operation.

Following vasectomy a man is not immediately sterile, as spermatozoa in the epididymis proximal to its division are still potent. Until the spermatozoa have been ejaculated, pregnancy may occur, so that other methods of contraception must be continued until only non-motile spermatozoa or azoospermia are found in a seminal analysis. This takes, on average, about 12 ejaculations.

As mentioned, vasectomy should be considered a permanent method of contraception. Reversal using microsurgery is possible but difficult and the pregnancy rate following reversal is less than 50 per cent.

Tubal ligation

The name tubal ligation is a misnomer, as most surgeons remove a segment of the tube, ligating each cut end or use a metal clip to occlude the oviduct.

Laparoscopic tubal 'ligation' has largely replaced laparotomy. Under laparoscopic observation a metal clip or a 'ring' is applied to the isthmus of each oviduct. These methods have replaced diathermy to the oviducts. In other cases a portion of the oviduct is excised through a small suprapubic incision (a mini-laparotomy) or through a normal suprapubic incision if preferred (Fig. **11/6**).

The failure rate is between 2 and 4 per 1000

Fig. 11/6 Method of tubal excision and ligation. (A) The oviduct is drawn taut and an area is isolated by two clamps. (B) A wedge has been removed from the tube. The uterine side of the tube has been clamped and tied using an unabsorbable suture. The lateral side has been clamped but not yet tied

operations, and depends, to some extent on the experience of the surgeon. Women choosing tubal 'ligation' should be aware of the failure rate before the operation. The mortality rate is less than 6 per 100 000 operations.

As the operation should be considered to produce permanent sterility it should only be performed after full discussion with the woman, and preferably with her husband as well. At present there is some confusion in law whether a woman may have a tubal ligation (or a man a vasectomy) without the consent of the other marital partner. Until this is resolved written consent of both partners (assuming the woman is currently married) should be obtained.

Provided the woman understands the permanent nature of the operation, and has made her own choice to have it, adverse reactions are unusual, over 99 per cent of women expressing themselves as satisfied that they chose to have the operation.

It is important for the doctor to find out, as best he can, that the woman has made an informed decision. It is preferable, if there is any doubt, to avoid performing tubal ligation immediately after childbirth, as about 5 per cent of women regret their decision, and seek re-anastomosis of the oviduct, compared with less than 1 per cent when tubal ligation is done at other times.

Recent developments in microsurgery have made it possible to re-anastomose tubes ligated or clipped in the isthmial area, with some success; about 60 per cent of women treated in this way later conceive and deliver a live baby provided the re-anastomosis is performed by an experienced surgeon in a centre which does the operation frequently. The results of re-anastomosis performed by less experienced surgeons are much less satisfactory. Fallopian tubes occluded by laparoscopic electrocautery are irreversibly damaged.

Because of the increasing costs of being in hospital, a trend has occurred to perform laparoscopic sterilization on patients who are 'day cases'. These patients should be told that severe postoperative pain is usual for up to 6 hours. Most patients complain of continuing abdominal pain or discomfort and shoulder-tip pain. These symptoms usually cease in 24 hours but may persist for up to 7 days, as may abdominal discomfort, bloating and tiredness.

Chapter 12

Abortion

Abortion means the expulsion of a fetus before it reaches viability. The World Health Organization has recommended that a fetus shall be considered viable when the gestation period is more than 22 completed weeks, or the fetus weighs 500g or more. Australia and several states of the USA have adopted this criterion, but Britain and most other nations continue to contend that viability occurs at the 28th week of pregnancy or if the fetus weighs 1000g or more. In Australia, it is held that if the expelled fetus weighs less than 400g it is an abortus; if between 400 and 999g it is an 'immature infant'. Occasionally the euphemism 'miscarriage' is used, particularly by non-medical people, as synonymous with abortion, the latter term implying a 'criminal' abortion.

FREQUENCY

Most textbooks claim that between 10 and 15 per cent of clinically diagnosed pregnancies end as an abortion. Recent investigations in which pregnancy was diagnosed within 21 days of conception by measuring beta HCG and an ultrasound examination was made at 8 weeks' gestation, indicate that the abortion rate is higher, probably over 33 per cent, but 22 per cent occur before the pregnancy can be diagnosed clinically, so that the clinical abortion rate is about 11 per cent.

Abortions occur more frequently as the woman grows older. Among women aged > 30 years about 3 per cent abort; the rate doubles if the woman is aged 30 to 34 and trebles if she is 35 or older. Abortion also increases with increasing gravidity. About 6 per cent of first or second pregnancies terminate as an abortion; with third and subsequent pregnancies the abortion rate increases to 16 per cent.

Sixty-five per cent of abortions of clinically diagnosed pregnancies occur between the 6th and 10th week of pregnancy.

Abortion is not the only cause of bleeding in early pregnancy, although it accounts for 95 per cent of cases. Rarer causes are ectopic gestation (1 per cent), cervical eversion (1 per cent), endocervical polyp (1 per cent), hydatidiform mole (0.1 per cent), and cervical carcinoma (0.05 per cent).

AETIOLOGY OF SPONTANEOUS ABORTION

The causes of abortion can conveniently be divided into three groups – ovofetal, maternal and paternal (Table **12/1**). In the early weeks (0 to 10) of pregnancy, when most abortions occur, ovofetal factors predominate, but in the later weeks (11 to 19) maternal factors become more common and the fetus is often born apparently normal, although too immature to survive.

Ovofetal causes

Careful studies of abortuses show that in about 60 per cent of cases the ovum is defective and has failed to develop, or the fetus is malformed (Fig. **12/1**). In

Fetal or ovular	*Percentage*
Defective ovofetus	60
Defective implantation or activity of trophoblast	15
Maternal	
General disease	2
Uterine abnormalities	8
Psychosomatic	?15

Table 12/1 Aetiological factors in 5000 abortions

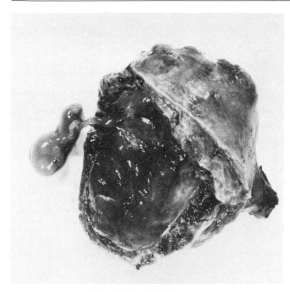

Fig. 12/1 Blighted ovum

many cases the defect occurs before or at the time of conception, and chromosome studies of first trimester abortions show that between 20 and 40 per cent have chromosomal abnormalities. As the defect affects all parts of the ovum, the trophoblast does not implant adequately, and is unable to synthesize progesterone in adequate amounts.

Maternal causes

General maternal disease, especially acute fevers, favour abortion by the transplacental passage of viruses or bacteria, or by the general metabolic effects of pyrexia and diminished oxygen release through the placenta.

Local disorders of the genital tract, such as retroversion, myomata and developmental defects were, at one time, considered to be important causes of abortion. It is now known that only when the retroverted uterus is fixed in the pelvis, or when the myomata distort the uterine cavity, do these conditions increase the risk. Developmental defects are relatively uncommon, and of them a bicornute uterus may cause abortion, especially after the 12th week of pregnancy. Another cause of late abortion is cervical incompetence which may be due to a congenital weakness, but is usually due to previous rough dilatation of the cervix. Cervical incompetence accounts for no more than 1 per cent of all abortions, and is considered further on page 135.

Psychosomatic causes

It is known that environmental stress operating through the cerebrum affects the secretion of substances by the medial eminence of the hypothalamus. This area is richly supplied with nerves which are in intimate contact with the pituitary portal vessels. The hypothalamus secretes several pituitary hormone-releasing factors, which are carried by the portal vessels to the pituitary where they regulate the release of the various pituitary hormones. These in turn may affect uterine function. Stress may affect uterine activity, and may lead to abortion. This is most clearly seen in some patients who habitually abort, and the only common factor in the success of the many treatments offered is the interest shown in the patient by the physician.

Paternal causes

Since the paternal spermatozoon gives to the ovum half of its chromosomes, defects may result in abortions, particularly if both partners share many common HLA antigen sites.

MECHANISM OF ABORTION

The immediate cause of the abortion is the separation of the ovum by minute haemorrhages in the decidua. The altered uterine environment stimulates the onset of uterine contractions, and the process of abortion begins.

Before the 8th week the ovum, covered with villi and some attached decidua, tends to be expelled en masse. If the internal os dilates but the external os of the cervix fails to dilate, the sac may be retained in the cervix (cervical abortion).

Between the 8th and the 14th week, the mechanism may be as described, or, more commonly, the membranes rupture expelling the defective fetus, but the placenta is only partially separated and protrudes through the cervical os into the vagina, or remains attached to the uterine wall (incomplete abortion). This type of abortion is attended by considerable haemorrhage.

After the 14th week, the fetus is usually expelled, followed by the placenta after an interval. Less commonly, the placenta is retained. Bleeding is not marked and the process of abortion resembles a 'miniature labour'.

VARIETIES OF ABORTION

For descriptive purposes the abortion is classified according to the findings when the patient is first seen, but obviously one kind may change into the next with the passage of time. The following clinical types are recognized (Fig. **12/2**):

Threatened abortion, inevitable abortion, incomplete abortion, complete abortion, missed abortion.

Any of the above types, but usually the inevitable or incomplete types, may be complicated by infection, when the term *septic abortion* is used.

Recurrent abortion (or habitual abortion) indicates that the woman has had three or more known successive abortions, and *therapeutic abortion* indicates that the pregnancy was terminated legally for a specific medical indication. *Induced* or *criminal abortion* indicates that the abortion was induced illegally for social reasons.

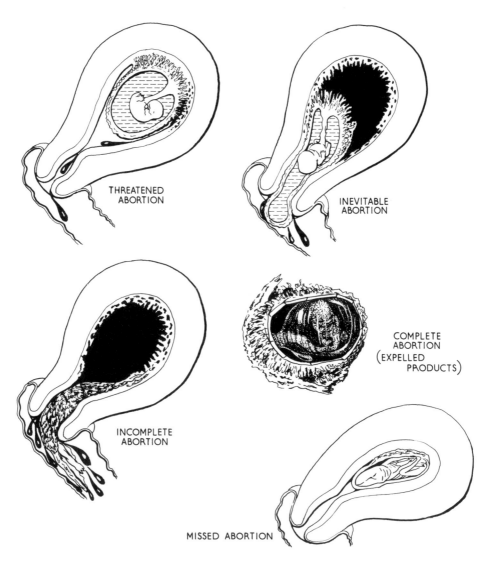

Fig. 12/2 The types of abortion which may be seen

THREATENED ABORTION

An abortion is presumed to threaten when a woman who is known to be pregnant develops vaginal bleeding during the first 28 weeks of pregnancy, whether this bleeding is associated with uterine contractions or not. Threatened abortion affects about 10 per cent of all pregnancies. A few patients bleed slightly at the time of the first missed period when the trophoblast is implanting deeply, and this is called implantation haemorrhage. It may be difficult to distinguish this type of bleeding from threatened abortion, but in the former the amount is slight, the colour bright red, and the bleeding settles quickly.

Threatened abortion is diagnosed by (1) determining that the patient is pregnant, (2) determining that the bleeding is coming from inside the cervix, (3) deciding that the uterine contractions, if present, are only slight and that the cervix is not dilated. It is sometimes advised that a speculum or bimanual examination should not be carried out on a patient threatening to abort, as this may precipitate the abortion or introduce infection. This is bad advice, and provided the examination is done gently, no harm will result, and an occasional mistake in diagnosis will be avoided. To avoid infection, the speculum should be passed and the bimanual examination performed with attention to aseptic technique.

If possible an ultrasound examination (using a modern sector or curvilinear transducer) should be made, particularly if the pregnancy has reached the 7th gestational week. The echogram may show (1) a normal sized sac and a fetus whose heart is pulsating, (2) an empty sac, (3) a missed or an incomplete abortion. Examination of the adnexae may show a mass indicative of a tubal (ectopic) pregnancy, particularly if a transvaginal probe is used.

Treatment

Traditionally a woman who is threatening to abort and whose fetus is alive is put to bed, although there is no objective evidence that bed rest has any value. Nor are drugs, hormones or sedatives of any value except as a placebo. If the echogram shows a normal-sized sac (for gestational date) and a live fetus the pregnancy will continue in 97 per cent of cases, and the woman can be reassured. However, about 5 per cent of the pregnancies will be curtailed and a preterm baby will be delivered. If the echogram shows an incomplete or a missed abortion, curettage should be performed.

INEVITABLE ABORTION

The abortion becomes inevitable if, in addition to the signs described in threatening abortion, the uterine contractions become increasingly painful and strong, and lead to dilatation of the cervix. The patient complains of severe colicky uterine pain, and vaginal examination shows a dilated os with some part of the conception sac bulging through. This sequence may follow signs of threatened abortion, or, more commonly, may occur without warning, the whole process being speeded up. Quite soon after the onset of the symptoms, the abortion occurs, either completely, when all the products of conception are expelled, or incompletely when either the pregnancy sac, or placental tissue, remains in the uterine cavity, or distends the cervical canal. This last can produce considerable shock, even in the absence of marked haemorrhage.

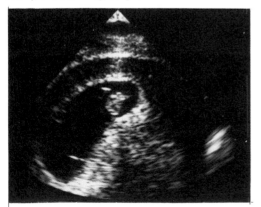
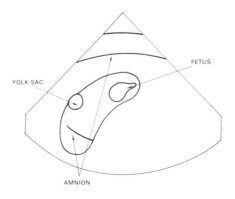

Fig. 12/3 Ultrasound scan showing yolk sac and amnion

INCOMPLETE ABORTION AND COMPLETE ABORTION

The majority of patients present with an incomplete abortion. The amount of bleeding may have been considerable, associated with cramp-like uterine contractions and the patient claims that she has passed 'something'. This may mean that all the products of conception have been passed and the uterus is empty (complete abortion) or it may mean that only part has been passed (incomplete abortion). If the obstetrician has not had the opportunity to examine the expelled tissues he should consider the abortion to be incomplete and curette the uterus. However, an empty uterus, as shown by ultrasound, obviates the need for this invasive procedure.

Treatment

Unless the patient has aborted completely when seen, or the abortion is imminent, she should be transferred to hospital. Whilst waiting for the arrival of the ambulance, morphine 15mg or pethidine 100mg should be given if the patient is in pain. A sterile vaginal examination must be made, as placental tissue distending the cervix can cause considerable shock. Any tissue in the cervix should be removed with the finger or a sponge forceps, and if the patient is bleeding heavily, ergometrine 0.5mg should be given intramuscularly. Once this has been done, her condition usually improves and evacuation of the uterus can be completed by curettage in a calm and deliberate way when convenient.

In hospital, treatment is conservative only if the abortion is proceeding quickly and with minimal blood loss. On admission, the general condition of the patient is assessed and compatible blood obtained. A vaginal examination is carried out and if products of conception are distending the cervix, these are removed with a sponge forceps or the finger. Pethidine 100mg or morphine 15mg is given intramuscularly to relieve the pain, and ergometrine 0.25mg intravenously to control the bleeding.

If the entire products of conception are not rapidly expelled, active intervention is required and the sooner the uterus is emptied, the better. Evacuation of the pregnant uterus should be done with care, as in unskilled hands damage can easily occur. Under general anaesthesia the patient is examined, and if the cervix is sufficiently dilated to admit a finger, this is used to detach any remnants of placental tissue. It is by far the safest instrument! In cases in which the cervix is insufficiently dilated to admit a finger, the suction curette or a sponge forceps and sharp curette may be used. If the sponge forceps is chosen it is introduced until the tip reaches the endometrium at the fundus, and then the two jaws are opened and closed again whilst rotating the forceps (Fig. 12/4). In this way products of conception are grasped without danger to the myometrium. Finally the uterine cavity is curetted. A large sharp curette, used gently, is safer than a blunt curette used roughly. Towards the end of the operation ergometrine 0.25mg is given intravenously and intramuscularly.

After a complete abortion (or one which has been completed by curettage) the bloody discharge diminishes and ceases in about 10 days. When placental remnants have been left in the uterus, bleeding continues beyond this time, varies in severity from day to day, and may be accompanied by periodic uterine cramps. Examination shows a bulky uterus, with a patulous os. Careful curettage should be performed in these cases, and all tissue examined histologically in case the rare choriocarcinoma is present.

Following an incomplete or a complete abortion a woman who is Rhesus negative should be given an injection of anti-D immunoglobulin, and a Kleihauer test should be performed to determine the amount of fetal blood in her circulation.

SEPTIC ABORTION

Infection of the uterus may occur with any abortion, but is usually found in association with incomplete abortion and most frequently after an induced abortion, particularly if this was done in an inappropriate place by a relatively unskilled person. As countries alter their laws to permit legal abortion, the number of illegally induced abortions are reduced, and septic abortion becomes less common. For these reasons the incidence of septic abortion varies considerably, depending on the kind of patient treated, and figures varying from 3 to 30 per cent of all abortions have been reported, the mean being 9 per cent.

In countries which have 'liberalized' their laws on abortion, the number of septic abortions has fallen considerably suggesting that most of those reported in the past occurred following induced abortion inexpertly performed with poor control of infection.

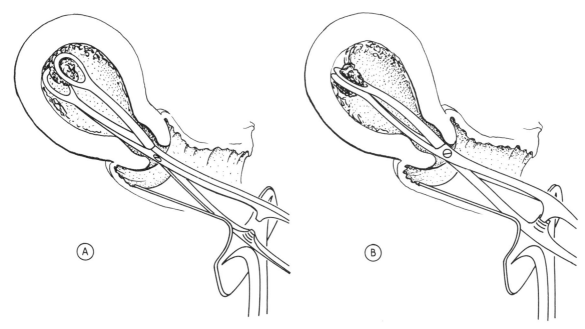

Fig. 12/4 The use of sponge forceps for clearing placental tissue from the uterus

Pathology

In 80 per cent of cases the infection is mild and is localized to the decidua. The organisms involved are usually endogenous, and are most commonly anaerobic streptococci, staphylococci or *E. coli*. Their virulence is low. In 15 per cent of cases the infection involves the myometrium with spread to the tubes and pelvic cellular tissues or pelvic peritoneum. In 5 per cent of cases there is generalized peritonitis or vascular collapse. The last is most often due to the release of endotoxins by *E. coli* or to the growth of *Cl. welchii*.

Clinical features

The first sign is pyrexia, the degree of which may not be related to the severity of the infection. Associated with this is a tachycardia. If the pulse rate is faster than 120 per minute, spread beyond the uterus has usually occurred. In infections localized to the endometrium, an offensive vaginal discharge is common, but this is less marked in spreading infections. Examination shows a boggy, tender uterus and evidence of extra-uterine spread may be apparent. Diagnosis is by finding in a case of abortion, whether threatened, incomplete or complete, two of the following: a temperature in excess of 37.8°C (100°F), a foul smelling pink discharge, a leucocytosis in excess of 15 000 or extra-uterine spread of infection.

Investigations

A high vaginal, or cervical, smear is taken and if the temperature exceeds 38.4°C (101°F) a blood culture is also made. In severe infections, urinalysis, serum electrolyte and fibrinogen studies are also undertaken.

Treatment

Antibiotics are given to combat the infection. The precise antibiotic chosen will depend on knowledge of the prevalence of bacterial resistance in the area and on the result of the bacteriological examination of the smears. As about 60 to 70 per cent of pathogens are Gram-negative, amoxycillin 500mg three times a day and metronidazole 1g 12-hourly (for 2 doses) should be given. An alternative is to give cefoxitin 2g 6-hourly.

If infection with *Cl. welchii* is suspected anti-gas gangrene serum is given.

Twelve hours after starting antibiotics, or sooner if haemorrhage persists or increases, the uterine contents are evacuated. If the gestation is less than 12 weeks this is done by curettage; after 12 weeks' gestation an oxytocin infusion is set up unless the cervix is sufficiently dilated to permit curettage. Early emptying of the uterus reduces the risk of haemorrhage and removes necrotic tissue which acts as a culture medium.

In a few cases of septic abortion, where for some reason curettage is contra-indicated, hysterectomy can be life-saving. Clinical deterioration, if associated with a large tender uterus, is the main indication, but individualization is essential.

In about 3 to 5 per cent of all cases of septic abortion, endotoxin shock occurs. It is a consequence of septicaemia caused by Gram-negative organisms, and has a mortality of between 30 and 80 per cent.

ENDOTOXIN SHOCK

Excluding haemorrhagic shock, endotoxin shock is the most common type of shock found following abortion, and has a mortality of from 30 to 80 per cent. In most cases the shock is associated with septicaemia due to Gram-negative organisms, especially *E. coli*, but it may be due to *Cl. welchii*. These bacteria release an endotoxin which is carried in the lipopolysaccharide fraction of the blood. In the initial stages, the endotoxin is neutralized by the phagocytes, but eventually the protection fails and shock develops. The pathology of the shock is not clear, but there is intense vasoconstriction of the post-capillary vessels, so that blood flows into the capillary bed and does not return to the heart. In addition there may be occlusion of central veins in the liver (and possibly pulmonary capillaries) by small thrombi. The effect of these changes is that there is pooling of blood in the venous system, a reduction of the return of venous blood to the heart, a reduced cardiac output, an increase in peripheral vascular resistance and poor effective tissue perfusion. In addition, the Gram-negative endotoxins may act directly on the blood vessels and the heart, and release substances (e.g. serotonin, histamine and catecholamines) which profoundly affect the cardiovascular system. These effects are magnified if the woman has hypovolaemia. If the infection is due to *Cl. welchii* haemolysis may occur and anuria may result from the deposition of blood pigment which blocks the renal tubules.

Diagnosis and investigation

The onset of endotoxin shock is usually sudden with pyrexia ($38.4°C$ or more), rigors, nausea and occa-

sionally diarrhoea. The systolic blood pressure falls to below 80mmHg and remains low despite adequate transfusion. Tachycardia and hypoventilation occur. The patient's skin becomes cold and clammy, with mottled patches of cyanosis. She may be mentally alert initially but becomes confused and lethargic if treatment is not instituted. Normally there is a leucocytosis but leucopenia may result. It is a grave prognostic sign, as is the development of a subnormal temperature.

The investigations listed under septic abortion must be made, and a pelvic x-ray taken to exclude a foreign body.

Management

General

The patient is best treated in a special unit where haemodynamic studies, serum electrolytes and blood gas estimations can be made. Since there is a failure of venous return in endotoxin shock, the most reliable estimate of cardiac competence relative to the circulation is to measure the central venous pressure by inserting a polythene catheter into the superior vena cava, via the antecubital or external jugular vein. Blood pressure estimations alone are unreliable guides.

Specific

Because the principal physiopathological disorder is an intense vasospasm in the capillary bed with markedly deficient tissue perfusion, treatment is urgent. Assessment of progress cannot be made with accuracy by measuring the pulse rate or blood pressure, so that monitoring by determining the central venous pressure and the urinary output are mandatory. With these indices constantly under observation, specific measures to treat endotoxin shock are initiated.

1. If clinical observation or a diminished pulse pressure together with a central venous pressure deficit indicates a deficient circulating blood volume, the hypovolaemia is corrected by blood transfusion. The observed blood lost is replaced and an additional 1000ml is given, followed by low molecular weight dextran or Hartmann's solution (Ringerlactate) until the central venous pressure is maintained at between 10 and 15cm H_2O. Low molecular weight dextran has the theoretical advantage that it reduces aggregation of erythrocytes (sludging) in the capillaries and improves tissue perfusion, particularly

of the kidneys, while Hartmann's solution is identical electrolytically with extracellular tissue fluid.

2. Antibiotics are administered in large doses. Most cases of septicaemic shock are due to *E. coli* or Gram-negative anaerobes. For this reason current opinion recommends the use of gentamicin (3 to 5 mg/kg body-weight/day divided into 3 doses) and clindamycin (20mg/kg body-weight/day) orally. If Gram-negative anaerobic septicaemia is suspected or proved, metronidazole or tinidazole 2g should be given in a single dose. If *Cl. welchii* infection is suspected, gas gangrene antiserum is given.

3. Since the main problem is an intense vasospasm, additional measures are initiated to reduce the effect of the vasospasm and to improve myocardial contractility.

  a. Chlorpromazine 50mg intramuscularly is given every 6 hours. The drug reduces shock, prevents shivering and may cause some degree of vasodilatation by its alpha-adrenergic receptor blocking effect.

  b. Dexamethasone 20 to 50mg intravenously is given 4- to 6-hourly for 24 hours. The drug, in pharmacological doses, is thought to enhance cellular vitality, to improve venous tone and to increase cardiac output.

4. If the above measures fail to relieve the hypotension and peripheral failure in 4 to 8 hours, despite a normal central venous pressure, isoproterenol 4mg per kg body-weight is infused intravenously, at a rate of 0.1 to 0.2mg per hour. The drug is a beta-adrenergic receptor stimulator which increases myocardial contractility, and improves tissue perfusion by causing vasodilatation in the capillary bed. An alternative treatment which is under investigation is to give an infusion of naloxona (30 μg/kg/hr) for 8 to 16 hours.

Additional measures

Urinary output

If the urinary output falls below 20ml per hour despite correction of the hypovolaemia, 100ml of 20 per cent mannitol may be given intravenously. This may be repeated after 2 hours if the urinary output remains less than 50ml per hour, but if the second infusion is not effective, there is no point in persisting with this line of therapy, and renal dialysis may be required.

Digitalis

Because digitalis improves myocardial function, some authorities recommend that 0.25mg is given intravenously, followed by 0.25mg intramuscularly until digitalization is effected. There is some dispute of the value of the drug in a relatively young woman who develops endotoxin shock in obstetrics, and digitalis should not be given if hyperkalaemia is present.

Acidosis

Provided that the serum potassium levels can be maintained, increasing acidosis measured by blood gas estimations should be corrected by the use of sodium bicarbonate. The quantity required is calculated from the formula: weight in kg × base deficit in mEq/litre × 0.2. Usually between 100 and 200mEq of bicarbonate is required and should be given rapidly over a 15-minute period.

MISSED ABORTION

In a few cases, the dead embryo and placenta are not expelled spontaneously, and a condition of missed abortion occurs. If the embryo dies in the early weeks, it is likely to be blighted and multiple haemorrhages occur in the choriodecidual space. These bulge in mounds into the empty amniotic cavity, whilst on the maternal side layers of blood clots are deposited. This condition is known as a *carneous mole* (Fig. **12/5**). When the fetus dies at a later period of pregnancy, and is not expelled, it is either absorbed or becomes mummified and thin, the liquor amnii is largely absorbed and the placenta becomes thin and adherent.

Clinical aspects

The patient usually has a history of a threatened abortion which settles down, but the symptoms of pregnancy disappear and the uterus fails to enlarge or may become smaller (Fig. **12/6**). Sooner or later an intermittent brown discharge recurs. The immunological test for pregnancy will remain positive so long as placental tissue survives, but eventually all the trophoblast dies and the test becomes negative. The diagnosis is not usually confirmed for 21 days or so, by which time most cases will have terminated by a spontaneous abortion. The diagnosis can be established earlier if ultrasound is available, as a distinct pattern appears in cases of missed abortion.

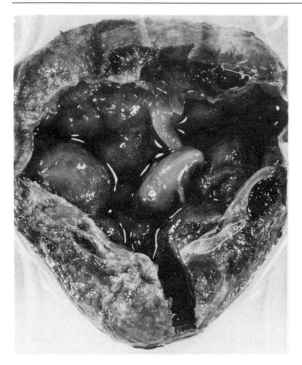

Fig. 12/5 Carneous mole – a small fetus can also be seen in the centre

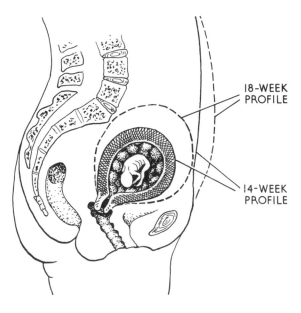

Fig. 12/6 Missed abortion. The duration of the pregnancy is 18 weeks but the uterus has failed to enlarge beyond the size of a 14-week gestation. Note that the abdomen is flat

18-WEEK PROFILE

14-WEEK PROFILE

Treatment

There is no urgency in treating missed abortion, but if after a reasonable time spontaneous abortion of the products of conception has not occurred, treatment may be instituted. If the size of the uterus is less than 12 weeks, evacuation is made per vaginam with an aspiration curette or with a sponge forceps and curette after cervical dilatation. The operation is messy and laborious, and should continue until the uterus is empty. Blood loss can be reduced by setting up an oxytocin infusion before starting the dilatation of the cervix. If the uterus is larger than 12 weeks in size it should be stimulated to expel the fetus by giving the patient an intravenous infusion of prostaglandin $F_{2\alpha}$ or E_2 or by using pharmacological doses of oxytocin infused intravenously.

An alternative is to insert vaginal pessaries of prostaglandin E_2 (20mg) high up the vagina each 3 to 6 hours, depending on the strength of the uterine contractions.

The side-effects of prostaglandin are nausea and vomiting in 80 per cent of women and diarrhoea in 70 per cent.

RECURRENT (HABITUAL) ABORTION

Only a few women have the misfortune to abort successively. It has been calculated that after one abortion the risk of another abortion is 20 per cent, after two abortions 25 per cent and after three abortions about 30 per cent. A woman who has three or more successive abortions is referred to as a 'recurrent aborter.' She has a 30 per cent chance of aborting the next pregnancy. Recurrent aborters are also said to be at greater risk of delivering a preterm baby (before the 37th week) if they escape aborting once again. If the abortions occurred in the first quarter of pregnancy, there is no increased risk of delivering a preterm baby. Women who have recurrent second quarter abortions, and those whose next pregnancy reaches 20 weeks, have a 70 per cent chance of delivering a term baby.

The aetiological factors in recurrent abortion vary with the population surveyed and to some extent with medical fashion. Two series of over 100 recurrent aborters reported from the USA and Norway offer some idea of the aetiology (Table **12/2**), and indicate possible approaches to investigation and treatment.

RECURRENT ABORTERS

Possible aetiology	% of abortions occurring	
	≤ 12 week	> 12 week
Unknown	55	35
Uterine malformations or abnormality	10	10
Cervical incompetence	3	30
Chromosome abnormality	< 5	< 4
? Endometrial infection	15	15
Endocrine dysfunction	3	3
Systemic disease	1	1
? Sperm factors	3	1
? Immune factors	?	1

Table 12/2 The aetiology of recurrent abortion

Investigation of recurrent abortion

A full medical and obstetrical history may disclose systemic disease or suggest cervical incompetence. A vaginal examination may show uterine myomata, or evidence of cervical incompetence. A hysterogram should be performed to exclude uterine malformations (bicornute uterus, a subseptate uterus or submucosal myomata). If endometrial infection is considered to be a factor, endometrial tissue cultures should be set up for the isolation of urealyticum and *T. gondii*. Not all workers believe that endometrial infection is a cause of recurrent abortion. Endocrine dysfunction, for example hypothyroidism should be excluded, and in certain cases chromosomal studies made on both parents, although the value of this has not been established. If the two parents share several HLA sites, the fetus might provide an insufficient stimulus for the mother to produce blocking IgG. This antibody is thought to be a major factor in preventing the fetus from being rejected. Some women who have recurrent abortions lack circulating blocking IgG antibodies, as measured by a mixed lymphocyte reaction test. If these women are injected with allogenic (paternal) leucocytes or compatible leucocyte rich erythrocyte transfusions (obtained from a donor or the husband) prior to the woman's becoming pregnant, abortion may not occur and a viable infant may be born.

Conversely, a strong blocking antibody response may be found in women who have an autoimmune disease, especially systemic lupus erythematosis (SLE). SLE must be excluded before donor leucocytes are injected or transfused, as the autoimmune disease may be aggravated. If SLE is identified, small doses of aspirin (75mg a day) or corticosteroids

may permit the pregnancy to continue to fetal viability. In these women, pregnancy complications, especially pregnancy-induced hypertension, are more likely than in other pregnant women. Immunotherapy must still be considered experimental until long-term follow up of mothers and their babies has been undertaken.

Cervical incompetence

About 20 per cent of habitual aborters will be found to have cervical incompetence. This is diagnosed by evaluation of the following criteria, (1) a history of two or more abortions, occurring after the 14th week of pregnancy, and usually starting with painless leaking of liquor amnii, (2) the easy passage through the cervix of a Hegar sound, size 9, when the patient is non-pregnant, and the absence of internal os 'snap' on its withdrawal, (3) the finding in pregnancy of a gradual and painless dilatation of the internal os until it is more than 3cm dilated. Recently, ultrasound has been shown to enable the obstetrician to make the diagnosis at an earlier stage than the clinical finding described in (3), and should be used increasingly in these cases.

When cervical incompetence is thought to be the cause of the habitual abortion, a soft unabsorbable suture, such as Mersilk 4, is placed around the cervicovaginal mucosa, or submucosally, at the level of the internal os and this is tied (Fig. **12/7**). The patient remains in bed for 3 to 5 days and then can go home, but should rest adequately through the remainder of the pregnancy. The use of progesterone during and after the operation has no valid basis. The operation should not be done if there is infection or if the membranes have ruptured. Should abortion become inevitable despite the suture, it must be cut; otherwise it is left until about 7 days before term, when it is divided and the patient permitted to deliver vaginally.

The treatment of recurrent abortion

If a specific cause for recurrent abortion is found treatment can be given. Uterine myomata may be extirpated by myomectomy; cervical incompetence treated as described; endometrial infection treated with doxycycline or trimethoprim-sulphamethoxazole; and endocrine dysfunction with appropriate substitution. Chromosomal abnormalities are untreatable but over half of the patients will subsequently deliver a live child. Women with diagnosed

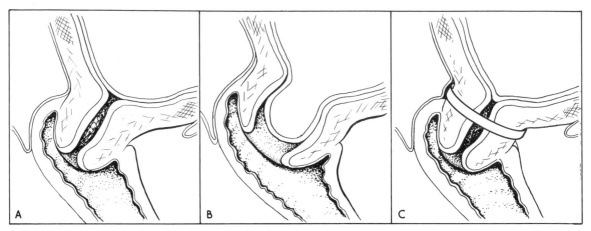

Fig. 12/7 Cervical incompetence. (A) Normal cervix at 16 weeks; (B) Incompetent cervix at 16 weeks; (C) 'Cerclage' with an unabsorbable suture

SLE may produce a viable infant if treated during pregnancy with corticosteroids or aspirin, although the results are unimpressive. If the woman is found to have an apparent immunological cause for recurrent abortion, prepregnancy treatment with paternal or donor leucocytes may be effective, but this approach is still experimental. In over 50 per cent of patients, no aetiological cause is found. For these patients 'tender loving care' and supportive psychotherapy is associated with the birth of a live baby in over 80 per cent of cases.

In all cases the patient should be given an adequate diet, stop smoking and once she becomes pregnant should avoid all travel, discontinue coitus and should go to bed for 2 hours each afternoon. The results from this regimen are as good as those following the use of hormones, vitamins, metallic chemicals, thyroid extract or acupuncture, and are far less expensive and time-consuming.

THERAPEUTIC ABORTION

In the past 20 years, legally induced abortion has become possible in many countries, although the regulations permitting legal abortion vary considerably. In some countries abortion may be performed legally in the first 28 weeks of pregnancy; in others the operation may only be performed in the first 20 or 24 weeks. In addition, in countries where abortion is illegal, large numbers of women obtain an 'illegal' abortion. The purpose of legalizing abortion was to enable all women, irrespective of social or economic status, to obtain an abortion performed by a trained health professional in hygienic surroundings; and to obtain counselling before and after the operation. To a large extent these objectives have been met.

The indications for therapeutic abortion are listed in Table **12/3**. Over 95 per cent of abortions are performed for social or psychiatric reasons. Most of these could have been avoided if one or other of the couple had used a reliable (or any) contraceptive.

The future

Experience in Britain suggests that after a few years of liberal abortion laws, the number of abortions starts to decline, as more women use contraceptives. Nonetheless, in all nations, induced abortion con-

* *Social*

* *Psychiatric:* severe neuroses, psychoses

* *Medical*
    Severe cardiac disease, heart failure
    Severe chronic renal disease, renal failure
    Malignant disease, especially breast or uterine cervix

* *Fetal*
    Viral infections
    Haemolytic disease
    Genetic defects
    Congenital defects incompatible with normal life (e.g. anencephaly, spina bifida)

Table 12/3 Indications for therapeutic abortion

tinues, and will continue to be one of the most usual methods of birth control. In time, with better sex education and a wider availability of contraceptives, the prevalence of induced abortion will drop. Until this happens, medical attendants must seek to deal with the problem in an unemotional way. Women rarely seek abortion without considerable thought and are, in general, receptive to counselling during this period. It is the duty of the doctor to give information and advice about contraception, so that recurrent therapeutic abortions are avoided.

Technique

Abortion is safest if performed between the 6th and 10th week of pregnancy. Before the 6th week the embryo is so small it may be missed during suction curettage; after the end of the 10th week it is larger and more cervical dilation is required, so that complications may occur.

A plasma radio-receptor assay of HCG, or the measurement of the β-subunit of HCG, enables the physician to diagnose pregnancy from the time of the first missed period, whilst the usual immuno-assays are not positive until about 14 days later.

If either assay is positive, the uterus can be emptied at 6 to 7 weeks gestation using a narrow plastic 'curette', attached to a 50ml syringe. Alternatively the woman can place 15 methyl $F_{2\alpha}$ (or E_2) prostaglandin tablets high in her vagina at short intervals.

If the assays are not available, and the woman believes she is pregnant, suction-curettage can be used – the method of so-called 'menstrual regulation'.

The technique is safe. When 'menstrual regulation' is used only one woman in every 250 000 treated dies – and this rate is 3 times lower than that following an injection of penicillin.

Pregnancy can be diagnosed 42 days after the menstrual period by immunological tests for urinary HCG (and within 10 days of conception using a radioimmunoassay for the β-subunit of HCG). Between diagnosis and the end of the 10th (or perhaps 12th) gestational week, the uterus can be evacuated easily and safely by the vaginal route. The use of a hollow flexible plastic, glass or metal curette attached to a suction apparatus is associated with the lowest mortality (less than 1:100 000 abortions) and morbidity (2 to 3 per 1000 abortions). The procedure is called suction (or aspiration) curette.

Abortion after the 12th week of pregnancy is more safely effected by the use of prostaglandins than by the other methods of intra-amniotic or extra-ovular 20 per cent NaCl, or dilatation and curettage.

Experience using prostaglandins indicates that the extra-ovular use of PGF_2 produces fewer side-effects (nausea, vomiting, gastro-intestinal upsets and fever) than intra-amniotic injection. Other studies have shown that prostaglandin in the form of PGE_2 is effective in inducing second quarter abortions given in the form of vaginal pessaries placed in the posterior vaginal fornix. The dose of PGE_2 is initially 10mg, repeated after one hour and, following this, 20mg is given every 2 hours until the woman aborts. Unfortunately about half of the women are nauseated or vomit. These side-effects can be reduced by giving anti-emetics. More recently, a new method, which is as effective in inducing abortion but has fewer side-effects has been developed. This is a silastic device impregnated with 11mg of 15 methyl PGF_2 methyl ether. The device is introduced high into the vagina and ensures a steady release of prostaglandin. Abortion occurs in over 90 per cent of cases in a mean time of 15 hours.

Progesterone antagonists

These drugs, notably mefepristone, occupy progesterone binding sites in the endometrium, which prevents the early pregnancy being maintained. Mefepristone (400 to 800mg daily for 4 days) given in the first 10 days after the expected menstrual period has failed to begin will provoke uterine bleeding in all pregnant women, and abortion in about 85 per cent. In one-fifth of women the bleeding is heavy for 2 to 6 days, and in a quarter painful uterine contractions occur. If mefepristone fails to induce an abortion, the uterus should be evacuated using a suction curette. The drug can also be used in combination with a prostaglandin analogue, when the abortion rate increases to 95 per cent. The incidence of diarrhoea, vomiting and abdominal pain is less than if only a prostaglandin is used.

A few skilled experienced gynaecologists claim that vaginal evacuation (at least between weeks 13 and 16) is as safe as the use of prostaglandins, and that the procedure is less psychologically disturbing to the woman. The cervix is dilated and the fetus removed by crushing and tearing using an ovum forceps and a large curette.

Whatever method is used to evacuate the uterus it is important to remember that ovulation is likely to recur as early as 21 days after the abortion in over 70 per cent of women. In view of this, contraception should be instituted within the first two weeks after pregnancy termination.

The sequelae of induced abortion

If the abortion is performed in a well-equipped clinic or hospital by a trained surgeon, complications are few. Less than 1 per cent of women develop infection or post-abortal haemorrhage requiring a curettage. The mortality from induced abortion is less than 1 per 100 000 (when abortion is performed before week 13) and rises to 12 per 100 000 (when the abortion is performed after the 13th, gestational week).

The effect of abortion on future fertility and obstetric success

Provided the abortion is performed in an appropriate place by a skilled gynaecologist and, preferably, before the 12th week of pregnancy, it is not associated with any reduction in fertility or any increase in spontaneous abortion, preterm birth or fetal loss in a subsequent pregnancy. However, recurrent induced abortions may increase the risk of fetal loss in a subsequent pregnancy.

Chapter 13

Infections of the Genital Tract

The fact that the genital tract, apart from the lowest third of the vagina and the vulva, derives from the Mullerian duct and has anastomosing systems of arteries, veins and lymphatics, means that infections of individual organs, although they occur, are less frequent than a generalized infection of the genital tract. One example of infection of a single organ is the inflammatory enlargement of the ovary (acute oophoritis), which uncommonly is a sequel to mumps contracted in the reproductive years.

In most cases infection starts in the uterus, or the cervix, and spreads upwards to involve the oviducts (salpingitis), the ovaries and the pelvic peritoneum. The precise diagnosis may be difficult, and the conditions are usually diagnosed, less precisely, as acute pelvic inflammatory disease (PID).

As there is a direct connection between the exterior and the peritoneal cavity, pelvic infections would be more serious and more frequent were it not that (1) the vulval cleft is normally closed and the vaginal walls are in apposition, (2) the vaginal acidity is a bar to bacterial growth, and (3) the endometrium is shed each month during menstruation. For these reasons pelvic inflammatory disease is rare in a virgin (the exceptions being pneumococcal peritonitis in children, and pelvic tuberculosis in adolescents), and most infections are introduced as a result of coitus, illegally induced abortion, or childbirth.

Infection following coitus is usually due to gonococci or to *Chlamydia*, whilst that following abortion is usually due to streptococci, staphylococci or to anaerobes. In many cases the infection is polymicrobial.

It is easier to understand pelvic inflammatory disease if its development following (1) gonorrhoea, (2) non-gonococcal genital infection (usually *Chlamydia*), (3) septic abortion and (4) pelvic tuberculosis are considered separately. The symptoms associated with each type of infection are similar in many cases, but vary considerably in severity. For a diagnosis of acute PID to be made clinically, the patient must have lower abdominal pain and tenderness, pelvic tenderness, usually a profuse vaginal discharge and pyrexia. Even using these criteria, PID is overdiagnosed and laparoscopy may be required to establish a diagnosis.

If laparoscopy is used routinely to confirm a clinical diagnosis of PID, no evidence of pelvic infection is found in 35 per cent of patients.

With these reservations, PID annually affects about 1 per cent of women aged 15 to 34, peaking at 2 per cent in women aged 17 to 24. The widespread use of antibiotics has reduced the number of cases of severe pelvic infection and particularly severe, chronic genital infections, but low-grade or asymptomatic infections seem to be occurring more frequently.

GONORRHOEA

The incidence of gonorrhoea appears to be rising, particularly amongst urbanized female adolescents, and this is related in turn to the greater permissiveness of sexual behaviour in recent years. Gonorrhoea is an acutely infectious disease, caused by an intracellular diplococcus, *N. gonorrhoeae*. The bacterium is very susceptible to its environment and is killed by drying, seldom surviving outside the body, in natural conditions, for more than a few hours. Copulation with an infected partner is the most usual and important mode of transmission of the disease, although the conjunctival sacs of newborn infants whose mothers have untreated gonorrhoea may be infected during childbirth.

Symptoms first appear in the female after an incubation period of 3 to 7 days, during which time the bacteria multiply in the urethral glands, Bartholin's glands and the crypts of the endocervix. The vagina is not invaded, as the gonococcus does not appear able to penetrate stratified squamous epithelium, and its metabolism is disturbed by the vaginal acidity. The initial symptoms are dysuria, frequency, and a purulent discharge per vaginam. If the discharge is present in considerable amount, it is suggestive that a co-existing trichomoniasis is present. The severity of these early symptoms varies, and in 50 to 80 per cent of infected women they may be so mild as to be ignored. Whatever the mode of onset, the symptoms subside fairly rapidly; but in an untreated patient viable bacteria persist in the endocervix, Bartholin's glands and the paraurethral glands. These micro-organisms are capable of infecting a new sexual partner, or of spreading from the primary sites to involve the oviducts.

The diagnosis is made in the acute case by studying the symptom complex and by examining stained smears of the urethral and cervical discharge, when the typical intracellular diplococci will be seen. At the same time a culture should be set up by inoculating the exudate on to Thayer–Martin medium. If the exudate has to be sent to a distant laboratory it should be inoculated on to a transport medium, called Transgrow. This medium maintains the viability of the organism for 48 hours. In the subacute and chronic cases, the diagnosis is much more difficult.

Treatment

The treatment of gonorrhoea is under constant review. A problem is that concurrent chlamydial infection occurs in 25 to 50 per cent of women. If the two infections are not treated simultaneously pelvic inflammatory disease is likely to occur later due to *Chlamydia*.

Because of the frequent association of gonorrhoea and *Chlamydia*, the Centre for Disease Control in the USA recommended in 1987 that all cases of gonorrhoea receive amoxycillin 3g with probenecid 1g followed by a 7-day course of tetracycline 500mg orally 4 times a day or doxycycline 100mg orally twice a day for 7 days. Other recommended treatments are (1) clavulanate-potentiated amoxycillin 1 tablet 3 times a day for 7 days; (2) co-trimoxazole 9 tablets in one dose daily for 3 days. This dose of co-trimoxazole is accompanied by minor neurological side-effects which may reduce compliance.

When the above regimens fail to eliminate gonor-

rhoea, as judged by smears taken from the urethra, the cervix and the anus 7 days after completing treatment, ceftriaxone 250mg or spectinomycin 2 to 4g by deep intramuscular injection should be chosen. It must also be remembered that the patient may have contracted syphilis at the same time, and investigations to determine this point must be made; however, serological flocculation tests for syphilitic infection do not become positive for 6 to 8 weeks after infection.

Spread

Acute gonorrhoea, although inconvenient, is of little clinical importance, and is fortunately confined to the primary infected sites in most cases. But if the disease spreads beyond these sites serious consequences may result, particularly the development of salpingitis and, later, sterility. The spread may be downwards from the duct of Bartholin's gland to involve the gland itself causing an acute Bartholinitis, but more frequently is upwards from the infected endocervical crypts. The gonococci pass up through the cervix and the uterine cavity, and lodge in the mucosal crypts of the oviduct, where, finding a suitable environment, they multiply (Fig. **13/1**). This spread usually occurs postmenstrually when the alkaline blood permits growth and migration of the bacteria more readily. The spread may occur in the month after an untreated infection, or may be delayed for several months.

Acute salpingitis

The rapid growth of the organisms within the cells of the mucosa of both oviducts reproduces the acute stage of the primary infection. A large amount of infected mucus is secreted, together with a fibrinous exudate which produces agglutination of the mucosal folds of the endosalpinx, and of the oviduct itself, at one or more locations. In some cases the infected exudate spills into the peritoneal cavity, causing a pelvic peritonitis. The normal response to infection occurs, and lymphocytes are mobilized and attack the invading gonococci. The oviducts become enlarged, oedematous and inflamed, and the typical symptoms of acute salpingitis result. These are (1) severe bilateral, lower abdominal pain and tenderness, (2) spasm of the abdominal muscles, (3) fever (usually more than 38.0°C), often with rigors, (4) leucocytosis (usually exceeding 20 000 per ml). On examination the lower abdomen is acutely tender

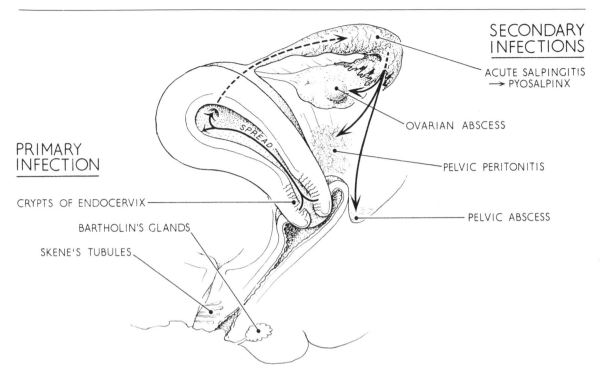

Fig. 13/1 Diagram of route of spread of gonococcal infection

on either side; on pelvic examination movement of the cervix to both sides produces pain; and bi-manual palpation, through the fornices, is excruciatingly painful. In particularly virulent infections, abscess formation may occur, pus collecting in the tube to form an acute pyosalpinx, or in the utero-rectal pouch to form a pelvic abscess. In many cases the diagnosis may be difficult. To avoid unnecessary anxiety, and possible improper treatment, the use of the laparoscope to visualize the genital organs and confirm, or exclude, acute salpingitis is justified.

Treatment of acute salpingitis requires admission to hospital for bed rest until the temperature settles and the pain disappears. Pelvic infection due to gonorrhoea requires large doses of an appropriate antibiotic. If penicillin is chosen, aqueous procaine penicillin G 4.8 million units intramuscularly or amoxycillin 3g or ampicillin 3.5g is given, and with each, probenecid 1g is also given. Either regimen is followed by amoxycillin 0.5g orally 3 times a day for 10 days. Other antibiotics chosen are tetracycline 250mg intravenously 4 times a day until improvement occurs followed by ampicillin 0.5g orally 3 times a day to complete 10 days therapy. If no

improvement occurs, a careful clinical reassessment must be made, and if it is thought that the infection is due to penicillinase-producing *N. gonorrhoeae*, spectinomycin 2g intramuscularly twice a day is given for 3 days, or cefoxitin 2g as a single intramuscular injection with probenecid 1g by mouth is chosen. In the first days only fluids are given, and the physician remains constantly alert for evidence of bowel obstruction. Surgery is rarely necessary, and may be hazardous, the indications being (1) no response to adequate antibiotic therapy, (2) rupture or probable rupture of a pyosalpinx, (3) intestinal obstruction, (4) pelvic abscess formation, and (5) doubt about the diagnosis, particularly confusion with acute appendicitis. If a laparotomy is performed and acute salpingitis found, the abdomen should be shut and surgical extirpation of the tubes avoided. The symptoms usually disappear rapidly in uncomplicated cases treated adequately, but in many instances the infection of the tubal mucosa has so disturbed the function of the tubes that fertility is markedly reduced.

The patient must be kept in hospital during the 'subacute stage' and examined vaginally at 5-day intervals to determine if pus has collected in the uterorectal pouch. Should a pelvic abscess develop, an incision is made through the posterior vaginal fornix and a drain inserted. This is termed a posterior colpotomy. If treatment is inadequate or is not given chronic salpingitis results. This is considered later in the chapter.

NON-GONOCOCCAL GENITAL INFECTION (NGGI)

Non-gonococcal pelvic infection, usually due either to *Chlamydia trachomatis*, *Mycoplasma hominis* or to mixed aerobic and anaerobic organisms accounts for at least half the cases of acute salpingitis.

Between 5 and 10 per cent of healthy women will be found to have chlamydial infection of the endocervical cells, and between 30 and 50 per cent will have circulating antichlamydial antibodies, indicating previous subclinical infection. It is clear that NGGI has replaced gonorrhoea as the most common cause of pelvic infection in many countries. In about 20 per cent of women who have cervical infection caused by *Chlamydia*, spread occurs and endometritis or salpingitis develops. This may be symptomless or symptomatic. Symptomatic chlamydial pelvic infection affects about 2 per cent of women each year, the peak incidence being to women under the age of 25. Because of the possible serious consequences to women, including sterility, caused by NGGI, it is important to educate the public that the disease will only be contained if men and women who have several sexual partners resort to 'safe sex'. Safe sex implies limiting the number of sexual partners and using condoms if either partner is uncertain whether the other has chlamydial infection.

The initial infection is sexually acquired and involves the endocervix or the urethra. It is usually symptomless. Occasionally dysuria occurs, or a yellowish, mucopurulent cervical discharge is detected. If a swab is taken, the cotton wool bud is stained yellow.

If spread occurs the route followed is similar to that following gonococcal infection. The presence of *Chlamydia* may be confirmed by tissue culture of endocervical cells or by a monoclonal antibody test on material obtained from the cervical canal. This test may be used to screen women and men who are at higher risk of NGGI.

Chlamydial pelvic infection, unless treated, causes damage to the Fallopian tubes in 10 per cent of cases. If a second infection occurs, the proportion who develop tubal damage increases to 25 per cent; and after a third infection to over 50 per cent. This indicates that chlamydial pelvic infection is a significant cause of infertility and of ectopic gestation. For this reason, if chlamydial infection is suspected, or if a woman's sexual partner has NGGI, the woman should also be treated, even if swabs from the endocervix fail to show *Chlamydia*. Treatment is to take doxycycline 100mg twice a day for 7 to 10 days.

A major problem in non-gonococcal salpingitis is the difficulty in determining the infective organism, and often several organisms (including anaerobes) are involved. Laparoscopy during an acute attack, with culture of the peritoneal exudate, may help to identify the infective organisms, but this is often impracticable and a treatment regimen active against a broad range of micro-organisms is chosen. In severe cases the patient requires admission to hospital and one of the following drug regimens is prescribed: (1) doxycycline 100mg intravenously twice a day *plus* metronidazole 1g orally, rectally or intravenously for at least 4 days and then both drugs orally for 6 more days; (2) cefoxitin 2g intravenously every 12 hours for 4 days. Doxycycline is then given orally in a dose of 100mg twice daily for 6 days; (3) clindamycin 600mg intravenously twice a day *plus* gentamicin 1.5mg/kg intravenously three times a day for at least 4 days, then clindamycin 450mg by mouth for 6 days; (4) clavulanate-augmented amoxycillin tablets, 1 tablet three times a day for 7 days; (5) trimethoprim-sulphamethoxazole 9 tablets daily for 3 days.

In less severe cases the patient may be ambulant and doxycycline and metronidazole may be given orally in the dose previously recommended; or the treatment recommended for gonococcal infection (p. 141) may be prescribed.

POST-ABORTAL PELVIC INFECTIONS

Bacteria introduced during the performance of an illegally induced abortion (or uncommonly during a spontaneous abortion) or at childbirth, can readily cause infection of the reproductive tract. The bacteria are usually staphylococci, streptococci, *E. coli* or anaerobes. The micro-organisms enter the tissues through lacerations in the cervix, or more frequently through the disturbed placental bed. The infection may be confined to the cervix (acute cervicitis) or the endometrium (acute endometritis). In these cases

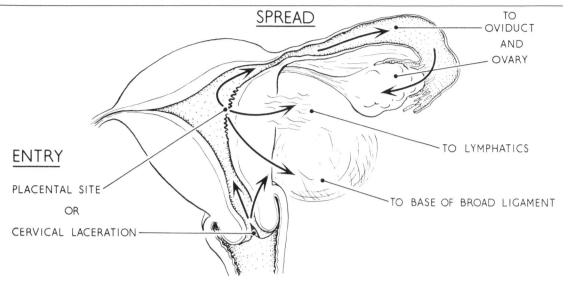

SPREAD

TO OVIDUCT AND OVARY

TO LYMPHATICS

TO BASE OF BROAD LIGAMENT

ENTRY

PLACENTAL SITE

OR

CERVICAL LACERATION

Fig. 13/2 Diagram of route of spread of pyogenic infection

the patient will feel unwell and an offensive sero-sanguinous discharge per vaginam will be noted. Examination may or may not show a tender uterus, and if it does, it is suggestive that the organisms have spread to involve the myometrium, causing a myometritis.

In a more virulent infection, the organisms may spread through the myometrium and invade the uterine lymphatics. They are carried to the tubes and ovaries, causing an acute salpingitis, identical with that due to gonorrhoea; or to the extraperitoneal tissues in the bases of the broad ligaments, causing a pelvic cellulitis, or parametritis (Fig. 13/2).

Acute pelvic cellulitis may also follow if infective organisms reach the parametrium through cervical lacerations, produced by damage in attempting to induce an abortion or at childbirth. The bacteria multiply in the cellular tissues of the parametrium, and a marked inflammatory reaction occurs. Depending upon the degree of virulence and resistance, the infection either resolves, healing without trace, or with residual fibrosis and scarring; or abscesses form. The symptoms and signs rarely appear until 7 to 10 days after the initial infection, and consist of fever, tachycardia, malaise and a dull aching pain deep in the pelvis. If an abscess forms, rigors occur. A vaginal examination shows that the uterus is involved in a firm, indurated tender mass, which extends to the pelvic wall and pushes the uterus to the contralateral side.

Infection may be due to streptococci, to staphylo-cocci or, increasingly frequently, to anaerobes. Because of this, a high vaginal (or a cervical) swab should be taken for bacteriological investigation.

Treatment is to give large doses of antibiotics, and ampicillin or amoxycillin remain the most useful. Once an 'antibiotic cover' has been made, in cases of incomplete abortion, the remaining products of conception should be evacuated from the uterus (Chapter 12).

If the infection is thought, or proved, to be due to anaerobes, metronidazole 2g orally (or parenterally) is the treatment of choice; (some authorities give clindamycin as well).

In all cases of acute pelvic infection, if the patient's temperature does not begin to fall within 48 hours, the antibiotic should be changed. If the symptoms increase in severity despite this, and the patient becomes increasingly toxic and the pelvic masses larger, the development of an acute tubo-ovarian abscess must be suspected. This is a serious complication and two approaches are suggested. The first is to perform a posterior colpotomy and insert a drain. The second, which is recommended by some authorities, is to perform a total hysterectomy and bilateral salpingo-oophorectomy. The protagonists of this approach point out that the pelvic organs are invariably functionally damaged by the infection, and the patient treated conservatively has a long period of ill health, eventually requiring surgery in most cases. The antagonists point out that the operation is associated with a higher mortality, even if the morbidity is lower. The matter has not yet been settled, but only involves a very small percentage of patients who develop acute pelvic infection. If the woman has an intra-uterine device in her uterus, this should be removed.

OTHER CAUSES OF PELVIC INFECTION

Pelvic infection may follow gynaecological operations and occur in association with cases of cervical cancer. The infection usually presents as a pelvic cellulitis, although abscess formation may occur. Treatment is that described already.

DIFFERENTIAL DIAGNOSIS IN ACUTE PELVIC INFECTIONS

Four conditions require to be considered, (1) tubal pregnancy, (2) acute appendicitis, (3) acute pyelonephritis, and (4) an infected ovarian cyst.

Tubal pregnancy

A period of amenorrhoea is usual, vaginal bleeding common and on examination a unilateral adnexal mass is palpable, the cervix being tender when moved to one side only. The fever, if present, is less than 38°C (100.4°F), and the leucocytosis is less than 20 000 per ml. If any doubt exists, laparoscopy should be made.

Acute appendicitis

The pain starts as a general abdominal pain, and settles in the right iliac fossa, which is the area of greatest tenderness. Usually no history of pregnancy, abortion or gonococcal infection is obtained.

Acute pyelonephritis

The symptoms of frequency and dysuria, and the presence of tenderness in the loins, suggest pyelonephritis, which may be confirmed by an examination of the urine.

Infected ovarian cyst

Although rarely encountered, an infected ovarian cyst gives rise to a tumour in the same region of the abdomen as acute salpingitis, the symptoms are identical and the differentiation may be difficult. If the patient has never been pregnant, has no signs of abortion, denies gonococcal infection, and has no evidence of vaginal discharge, the diagnosis of an infected ovarian cyst is more likely.

It should be added that acute pelvic infection is overdiagnosed when only the clinical findings are evaluated. To avoid this, many gynaecologists now routinely examine the pelvis of a suspected case of acute salpingitis (or more widespread pelvic infection) using a laparoscope, before reaching a diagnosis and prescribing treatment.

CHRONIC PELVIC INFECTION (PELVIC INFLAMMATORY DISEASE)

Chronic pelvic inflammatory disease (PID) or chronic pelvic infection seems to be occurring with greater frequency. The condition may be so mild as to be symptomless. In these cases laparoscopy (often made during infertility investigations) may show some pelvic adhesions which distort the oviducts. In other mild cases the endosalpinx is damaged, the oviductal endothelial folds being agglutinated and functionally inadequate, or the oviducts are blocked by adhesions. Adhesions may involve the ovary and the fimbria of the oviducts. However, not all cases of diagnosed PID cause tubal damage or block. After one attack of PID about 12 per cent of women will be made infertile; after 2 attacks, 24 per cent and after 3 attacks 54 per cent will be infertile. In more severe infections, there is more obvious pathology and the condition is often symptomatic. The infective agent or agents may cause the development of a 'pus tube' (pyosalpinx) or a hydrosalpinx which may develop either initially or following a pyosalpinx. In other

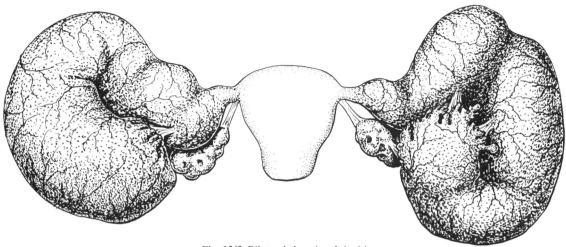

Fig. 13/3 Bilateral chronic salpingitis

cases the infection involves the pelvic connective tissue causing chronic pelvic cellulitis.

The symptoms vary in severity and include chronic, vague pelvic pain which is intermittent or constant. It is often worse perimenstrually. A second common complaint is deep dyspareunia. The symptoms are not specific for chronic pelvic infection, and may be due to psychosomatic conditions (see p. 62). However, the latter should never be diagnosed until the organic causes have been excluded.

PYOSALPINX

Pyosalpinx, or chronic 'pus tube', forms as a result of blockage of the lumen of the oviduct at the fimbrinated end and at one or more points along the tube. This occurs in the acute phase and the exudate accumulates, distending the tube to a greater or lesser degree (Fig. 13/3). Since the inflammatory process extends through the wall of the oviduct, adhesions to surrounding structures are usual and

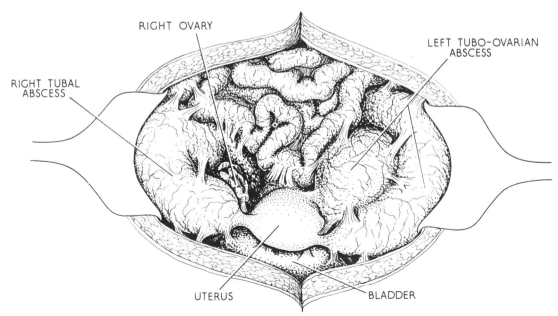

Fig. 13/4 Bilateral pyosalpingitis – the appearance at operation

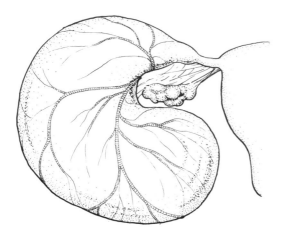

Fig. 13/5 Hydrosalpinx. Note the 'retort'-shaped distension of the oviduct

may be considerable (Fig. **13/4**). The distension flattens the normal complex folds of the tubal mucosa, and the inflammatory process thickens the wall of the tube; the stroma and muscle layer being infiltrated with lymphocytes and plasma cells. In many instances the ovary is involved to form a chronic tubo-ovarian abscess. The condition usually remains quiescent, although not symptomless, but acute exacerbations may occur. These may be due to reinfections, or to an increase in the virulence of residual bacteria lying in the wall of the pus tube. The exacerbation may occur months, or years, after the initial infection, when all the symptoms and signs of acute pelvic infection are superimposed upon the underlying mild symptoms, the patient becoming seriously ill.

HYDROSALPINX

Hydrosalpinx is the end-result of a 'burnt out' pyogenic salpingitis, which was of low virulence but high irritation, and produced large quantities of clear exudate within the closed portion of the tube (Fig. **13/5**). The enlargement of the tube may be marked, and it is typically retort-shaped. Adhesions may or may not be present. The walls of the tube are thin and translucent, and the contents a clear watery sterile fluid.

The symptoms of chronic salpingitis are varied, and most patients complain of a chronic aching in the lower abdomen, which is worse pre-menstrually and

after exertion; but a variety of complaints, varying from general ill health, lassitude and irritability to menstrual disturbances (usually polymenorrhoea) and dyspareunia may be encountered.

Abdominal examination usually discloses no abnormality, but vaginal examination may show a generalized tenderness or a smooth cystic enlargement of the adnexae. Laparoscopy may be required to make a diagnosis.

TREATMENT OF PID

The treatment depends on the severity of the symptoms and on the clinical findings. If the tubal enlargement is minimal, and the patient anxious to have further children, plastic surgical operations to restore tubal patency are sometimes advocated, although the results are poor. If the symptoms persist and the masses are large, surgery is required. Unfortunately, the operation in general requires to be radical, although it is usually possible to conserve at least part of one ovary. As the original infection involves both tubes, a bilateral salpingectomy and total hysterectomy should be performed. In general, surgery should not be undertaken until the temperature has been normal for 3 weeks, there is no leucocytosis, and antibiotics have been given pre-operatively.

CHRONIC PELVIC CELLULITIS

This condition may be a sequel of acute pelvic cellulitis (acute parametritis), and results in thickening and fibrosis of the parametrium so that the uterus is more or less fixed. Occasionally the inflammatory process involves the uterosacral ligaments, or extends forwards into the connective tissue beside the bladder (Fig. **13/6**). Chronic pelvic cellulitis may accompany chronic salpingitis, in which case the symptoms and signs are overshadowed by those of the latter condition; or it may occur in the absence of salpingitis. In this event the infecting organisms are usually pyogenic bacteria, and small abscesses are likely to be found in the fibrosed connective tissue.

Symptoms

The symptoms of chronic pelvic cellulitis are therefore variable. The most common complaint is a

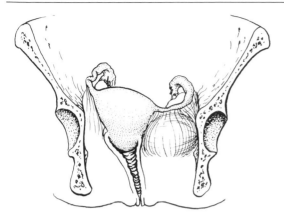

Fig. 13/6 Diagram of chronic pelvic cellulitis

chronic deep pelvic ache, often localized to one side, and accompanied by sacral backache. Dyspareunia on deep penetration of the penis is frequent, and may be so severe as to prevent coitus. Pelvic examination shows that the uterus is drawn to one side, tender and relatively fixed in position.

Treatment

Treatment is difficult, but some patients respond to deep pelvic short wave diathermy, and if this fails hysterectomy often results in cure. Unfortunately despite physiotherapy and surgery, many women continue to have chronic pelvic pain.

TUBERCULOUS INFECTION OF THE GENITAL TRACT

The incidence of tuberculosis of the genital tract varies very considerably with the social status of the patient and her environment. Where the incidence of pulmonary tuberculosis is high, and where the initial infection is acquired in adolescence, tuberculosis of the genital tract occurs in 5 to 10 per cent of patients who have the pulmonary form of the disease, and accounts for 2 to 5 per cent of all cases of pelvic infection. The value of prophylaxis can be seen from the Australian experience, where an intensive programme for the control of tuberculosis has been in operation for years. In Australia pelvic tuberculosis accounts for less than 0.2 per cent of all cases of chronic pelvic infection. Prophylactic control is not the only factor, however, as in East Asia, where prophylactic control is rudimentary but where the

initial pulmonary infection is usually acquired in childhood, the incidence of pelvic tuberculosis is low. The reason is that the tubercle bacillus spreads to the genital tract in the post-primary haematogenous phase of the disease. If this phase coincides with, or follows, the increased growth of blood vessels supplying the oviducts which occurs at puberty, bacilli are carried to these organs and multiply in their tissues. In East Asia the spread precedes this growth phase, and the pelvic organs are usually spared.

The disease may be limited to the oviducts, or bacilli may be spread to the endometrium by direct continuity via the lumen of the oviducts, or by the anastomosing lymphatics. The oviducts are always infected, and the endometrium frequently; but the cervix, vagina and vulva are only rarely involved, and then by ascending infection contracted from a male who has urogenital tuberculosis.

Pathology

The gross findings are variable, and depend upon the duration of the disease and the host's resistance to infection. The oviducts may appear normal, or red and swollen, often being kinked and irregular, although, for some reason, the fimbriated end remains patent. In advanced disease they become markedly thickened and multiple adhesions form, so that the condition is identical with chronic salpingitis. On microscopy, typical tubercles are found. The uterus is usually normal in size, and uterine tuberculosis only diagnosed by histological and bacteriological examination of curettings.

Symptoms

In many cases, there are no symptoms and the disease is discovered during the investigation of an infertility problem, as in 70 per cent of women with pelvic tuberculosis, primary infertility occurs. In more advanced disease, which is uncommon today, disturbances of menstruation occur and chronic pelvic pain is usual.

Diagnosis

In countries where epidemiological studies have shown tuberculosis to be common and where prophylactic measures are not undertaken, pelvic tuberculosis should be sought in all women presenting with primary infertility, once the male factor has been eliminated. As well as this, tuberculosis should be suspected in any virgin who has symptoms and signs of chronic pelvic infection. Diagnosis is made by examining the debris obtained from a careful curettage, both histologically after staining with Ziehl–Neelson's method, and by inoculating some of it in culture media and into a guinea pig. Some authorities recommend using progestogens in suspected cases for 3 months prior to the curettage. The drugs produce a pseudo-pregnancy which prevents the cyclic shedding of the superficial endometrial layers. This enhances the development of tubercles in the endometrium, and their more ready detection.

Treatment

The treatment of choice is medical, surgery being reserved for cases which fail to respond to medical treatment or in which there are large pelvic masses. But in no case should surgery be performed if there is active disease elsewhere in the body, or until medical treatment has been given for at least 12 weeks. Medical treatment is that of tuberculosis in other organs, combinations of streptomycin, rifampicin, isoniazid (INAH) and para-aminosalicylic acid (PAS) being given.

Chapter 14

The Vulva

The majority of patients attending a physician because of symptoms or signs relating to the vulval area, complain of an itchy vulva; only a few attend because of a lump, an ulcer or pain. The lump may be due to infection, or rarely to a benign or malignant tumour. These matters are considered in this chapter; but because of its frequency, pruritus vulvae, or the itchy vulva, is discussed first.

ANATOMICAL CONSIDERATIONS

The anatomy of the vulva has been described in Chapter 2, and only the salient points of clinical interest are repeated here. The lateral boundaries of the vulva are formed by the labia majora, which are two large skin folds containing sebaceous glands and adipose tissue, and which have hair follicles on their outer surface. In the reproductive years they hide the labia minora, which are delicate folds of skin containing some sebaceous glands but no adipose tissue. Anteriorly the labia unite to form the prepuce of the clitoris, and posteriorly to form the fourchette. The cleft between the labia minora is the vestibule, which contains the clitoris, the external urethral meatus, the vaginal introitus and the hymen (Fig. 14/1). Lateral to the hymen and deep to the entrance of the vagina are two collections of erectile tissue, the vestibular bulbs. Embedded in the posterolateral part of each bulb is Bartholin's gland, which

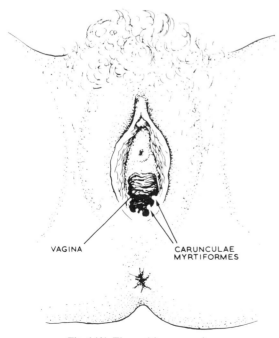

Fig. 14/1 The multiparous vulva

VAGINA

CARUNCULAE MYRTIFORMES

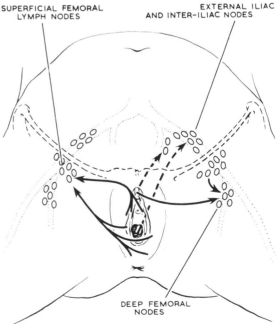

Fig. 14/2 Lymphatic drainage of the vulva

SUPERFICIAL FEMORAL LYMPH NODES

EXTERNAL ILIAC AND INTER-ILIAC NODES

DEEP FEMORAL NODES

is connected to the vestibule, between the hymen and the fourchette, by a duct. This duct may become infected, and an abscess may form in the gland.

The vulval arterial blood supply comes from the internal pudendal arteries and the external pudendal arteries; and the venous drainage is from large plexuses to veins which accompany the arteries.

The lymphatic drainage is more complex. The drainage of the anterior part of the vulva is to the superficial femoral nodes; but some of the lymphatics draining the clitoris run directly to the external iliac nodes and the interiliac nodes deep in the pelvis. The drainage of the posterior part of the vulva is to the superficial inguinal and the superficial femoral nodes. Both groups of lymph channels anastomose with those of the opposite side, and with the lymphatics of the lower third of the vagina which drain to the external iliac nodes (Fig. **14/2**).

THE ITCHY VULVA (PRURITUS VULVAE)

At least 1 woman in 10 who attends a gynaecologist complains, amongst other things, of itchiness of the vulva. The reason for this high incidence remains obscure, but there is evidence that psychosomatic factors play an even greater part here than in the aetiology of other skin disorders. That is not to say that itchiness of the vulva is caused solely by psychosomatic factors, and these should only be incriminated when organic causes have been eliminated. Itchiness of the vulva and a need to scratch, are probably due to the release into the tissues of histamine-like substances, mediated perhaps by an underlying vascular instability. It is known that the skin of the vulva, and the underlying vascular connections, are unstable and influenced greatly by the emotions. Thus sexual frustration, anxiety and marital disharmony frequently are manifested as pruritus vulvae, and the itch is worse at night when there are no distractions for the mind. Itching leads to scratching; and scratching an unstable epithelium causes a variety of histological patterns which have confused pathologist, dermatologist and gynaecologist alike, and have been invested, quite undeservedly, with sinister malignant potentialities. The effect of the female sex hormones on the vulval skin adds a further complication, particularly after the menopause, when because only minimal quantities of oestrogen are produced, the vulva tends to become atrophic, and the epidermis thin. A final complication is that the vulval skin being a part of the integument, is liable to be affected by skin diseases which are general in distribution.

With this introduction, it is possible to suggest a classification of possible causes of pruritus vulvae (Table **14/1**).

1. *General skin diseases*, such as psoriasis, leuco-
derma, lichen planus, intertrigo and scabies may cause vulval itching. Similarly, fungal skin infections, particularly tinea, may be accompanied by pruritus vulvae, although the itch is generally intercrural rather than vulval. Threadworms and whipworms cause anal itching, but occasionally they migrate on to the vulval skin and lead to vulval itching.

2. *General diseases*. The main general disorder causing pruritus is diabetes, particularly if glycosuria is present. As well as itching, the vulva becomes swollen and dark red in colour. There is some evidence, too, that pruritus vulvae may be a manifestation of deficiency diseases, particularly in old age when the stimulating effect of oestrogen on the vulval epithelium is absent.

3. *Allergic dermatitis*. Sensitivity to soaps, to chemical contraceptive creams, and to other contact allergens may cause an itchy vulva. In recent years a new allergen has appeared. Some women are allergic to

		Percentage of cases
1.	*General skin diseases* (psoriasis, leucoderma, lichen planus, intertrigo, scabies) *NB* Threadworms cause *anal* itching.	5
2.	*General diseases* (diabetes, ? deficiency diseases)	5
3.	*Allergic dermatitis*	5
4.	*Vaginal discharges* Trichomoniasis Candidiasis	50
5.	*Psychosomatic conditions*	35

Table 14/1 The itchy vulva: aetiology

certain detergents used to wash pantihose, and the garment itself, by keeping the vulval area moist, may aggravate the condition.

4. *Vaginal discharge*. About half the cases of pruritus vulvae are due to vaginal discharges containing *Trichomonas vaginalis* or *Candida albicans*. The itchy area is at the introitus as well as further out on the vulva.

5. *Psychosomatic causes*. These operate either alone, or permit the itchiness from the other causes to be brought more prominently to the cerebral cortex. Mental anxiety and sexual frustration may manifest themselves, as has been noted, by an intense vulval itchiness. This is relieved by scratching, but scratching irritates the unstable vulval epithelium and causes further itching, and a 'vicious' circle is initiated.

HISTOPATHOLOGY: CHRONIC VULVAL EPITHELIAL DYSTROPHIES

In most cases a biopsy of the vulva of a patient complaining of pruritus vulvae of less than 6 months duration will show a normal skin (Fig. **14/3**). However, if the pruritus vulvae has persisted for longer,

a variety of epithelial changes may be found. It is proposed to avoid all the terms used in the past, and to call these changes chronic vulval epithelial dystrophies, as has been suggested by Jeffcoate. Within this term various patterns of epithelial change may be found, and the patterns may interchange in the same patient at different times; or different areas of the vulva may show different patterns at the same time.

Atrophic dystrophy (lichen sclerosis)

This may be found in young women when the condition has been called lichen sclerosus et atrophicus, or in old women when it has been called senile vulvitis. Clinically the skin is pale, and a biopsy shows that the horny layer is unchanged or hyperkeratinized, but there is marked thinning of the epidermis and the disappearance of the rete pegs. The subepidermis is oedematous and some degree of hyalization occurs, whilst deep to this collections of round cells are found (Fig. **14/4**).

Hypertrophic dystrophy (squamous cell hyperplasia)

Previously this pattern was called chronic dermatitis

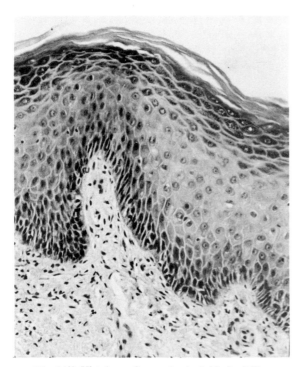

Fig. 14/3 Histology of normal vulval skin (× 160)

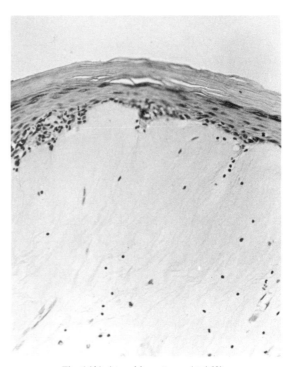

Fig. 14/4 Atrophic patterns (× 160)

or neuro-dermatitis, and the 'infection' was suggested by the presence of plasma cells in the dermis. Clinically the vulva looks red and is thickened with exaggeration of the skin folds, but in moist areas where maceration of the horny layer occurs, 'white patches' may be seen. The histological examination shows that the epidermis is thickened and the papillae elongated and oedematous, but the rete pegs retain a finger-like shape. The dermis is oedematous and contains variable numbers of plasma cells, and

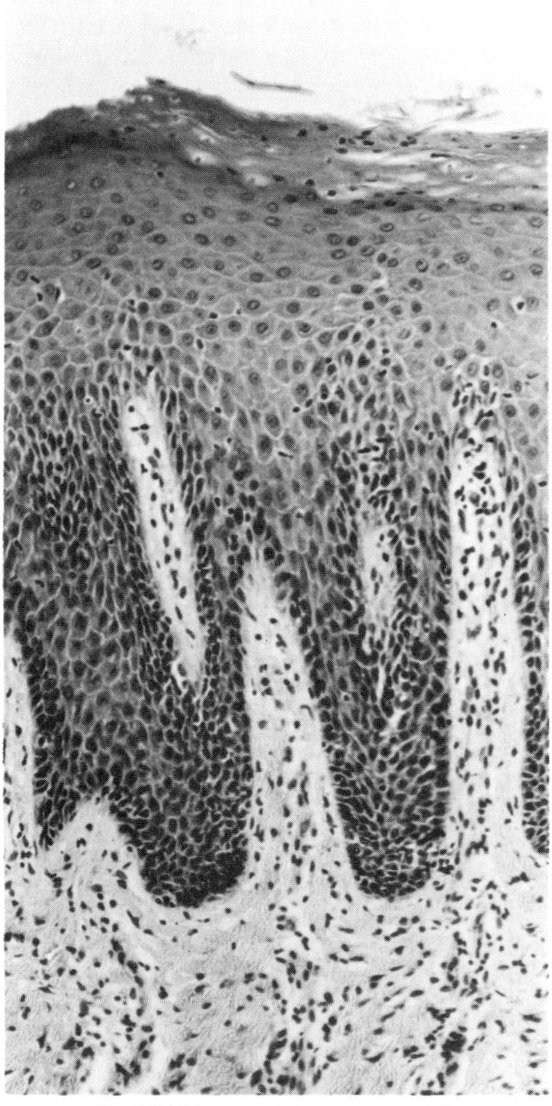

Fig. 14/5 Hypertrophic patterns (× 160)

sometimes collagen. The elastic fibres usually have disappeared (Fig. **14/5**).

Mixed dystrophy

In this pattern, atrophic and hypertrophic areas are found in the skin and both features may be found in the same lesion. All three patterns may show cellular dysplasia, to form the dysplastic pattern of vulval dystrophy.

Dysplasia (vulval intraepithelial dysplasia)

On clinical inspection the vulva may be red, white or pale, and the diagnosis is therefore a histological one. On section, there may or may not be an overgrowth of the horny layer. The Malpighian layer is thickened with lengthening of the rete pegs, which have abnormal shapes and often show denticulate processes. The basal cells of the epithelium are disorderly, showing atypical activity and pleomorphism. The subepithelial zone is usually hyalinized and elastic fibres are absent (Fig. **14/6**). Dysplasia is the only dystrophic pattern which may lead, in a few cases, to carcinoma of the vulva.

INVESTIGATION OF PRURITUS VULVAE

Firstly, general skin diseases, including leucoderma and fungal infections, must be excluded, by examining the naked patient in a good light and inspecting the interdigital folds of the hands and feet. In order to decide if the condition is pruritus vulvae, a careful determination of the extent of the itching area is necessary. If the itchy area is predominantly anal or intercrural, the cause is probably threadworms, tinea or intertrigo.

However, if the main, or only, area of itchiness is vulval, it is necessary to search diligently for an underlying cause, such as glycosuria, contact allergic 'dermatitis' and local fungal infections. (1) Repeated smears should be taken from the vulva and vagina, and cultured for the presence of trichomonads and of *Candida albicans*. (2) The urine should be examined for albumin and sugar. (3) A 2-hour postprandial, or a fasting, blood sugar should be obtained. (4) In elderly women a test for achlorhydria, should be made. About half of the patients will have achlorhydria. (Achlorhydria is generally accepted to be an auto-immune phenomenon, but its relation to vulval dystrophia is unclear.) (5) Sero-

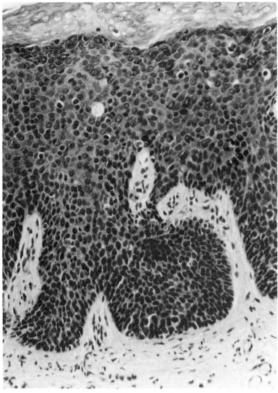

Fig. 14/6 Dysplasia (× 160)

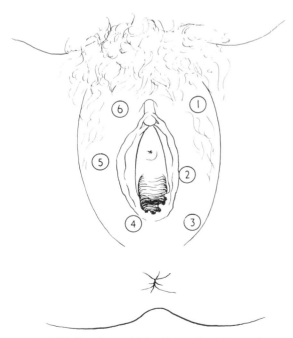

Fig. 14/7 Sites from which a biopsy should be made

logical tests for syphilis and a full blood count should be taken when required. (6) A careful history should seek evidence of drug sensitivity and contact allergies.

If the pruritus has persisted for more than one year, multiple biopsies using a dermatome (Fig. **14/7**) should be made irrespective of the probable aetiological factor, the age of the patient, or the appearance of the vulva.

TREATMENT

Four principles should be stated: (1) Treatment should be medical rather than surgical, unless biopsies show dysplasia. (2) Possible aetiological factors detected should be treated aggressively. (3) 'Instant' cure is rare, and the patient must be informed that she will require to persist with treatment for a considerable period. (4) The longer the duration of the pruritus before treatment, the longer it takes to effect a cure.

1. Treatment is primarily medical. Whilst most gynaecologists would agree that pruritus of short duration should be treated medically, some believe that a simple vulvectomy is the preferred treatment of pruritus of longer duration, and particularly when the vulval skin is altered in colour; firstly because it removes the itchy area, and secondly because it removes a 'pre-cancerous lesion'. The evidence on both points is unconvincing. It has been shown repeatedly that if a simple vulvectomy is performed, pruritus recurs in at least 50 per cent of cases, and the mutilating operation causes introital dyspareunia, or apareunia, in 30 per cent of cases. Since dysplasia is the only dystrophy liable to be followed by vulval carcinoma, surgical excision of skin showing other patterns of epithelial disorder is unnecessary, and does not cure the patient as the same, or another, dystrophic pattern recurs in the new vulval skin in about 60 per cent of cases. For these reasons vulvectomy is contra-indicated in most cases of pruritus vulvae, except when dysplasia or malignancy is found in the biopsy. If dysplasia is found, partial or simple vulvectomy is indicated, and the excised skin must be carefully examined histologically for evidence of malignancy. Another possible indication for vulvectomy is in the elderly woman who no longer practises coitus, and who is not relieved by medical treatment. However, even in this instance, recurrence of pruritus is frequent after vulvectomy.

2. Treat aetiological factors. Trichomoniasis is treated by oral metronidazole; candidiasis by intra-vaginal fungicidal pessaries, and fungicidal ointment or cream to the vulval skin; anaemia is corrected by oral iron and, if indicated, vitamin B_{12}; achlor-hydria is treated by administering dilute hydro-chloric acid three times a day with meals; fungal infections in other areas, particularly hands and feet, are treated by local applications of the appropriate fungicide. Soap should not be used when washing the vulva, and vaginal douches should be avoided.

3. Treatment required over a prolonged period. The co-operation of the patient is needed, as treatment must be continued over a long period, and during this time efforts should be made to uncover any psychological upsets which may have precipitated the itching. Because of the scratch-itch-scratch cycle, local application of an antihistamine, or a cortisone ointment is required. An alternative is to apply 2% testosterone propionate in petroleum jelly. The patient is instructed to apply a small amount of the ointment and smooth it gently into the vulval skin, rather than scratching when an episode of itching occurs. Even if no fungal infection has been found, on empirical grounds a fungicidal ointment may be applied, alternating with the other chosen ointment. As well as this, a sedative should be given, and adequate rest at night ensured.

Using these methods, complete cure, or cure with intermittent relapses, will be obtained in at least 90 per cent of cases. The risk of malignancy developing in atrophic or hypertrophic patterns of chronic vulval epithelial dystrophy is negligible, and even if dysplasia is found the risk is only in the order of 10 per cent. But this small risk means that those patients whose symptoms are not completely cured must be kept under careful observation (even if a vulvectomy has been performed) and vulval biopsies should be performed at intervals if necessary.

Vulval atrophy

Most cases of vulval atrophy occur in postmeno-pausal women and, in many instances, pruritus vul-vae is also present. Vulval atrophy may occur in younger women, and can cause marked distress, par-ticularly as coitus becomes painful or impossible. A number of the women have impaired glucose toler-ance and this should be investigated.

The treatment of vulval atrophy is to avoid wear-ing pantihose, as these garments prevent ventilation and absorb moisture. An anti-pruritus ointment may be prescribed, but the results are not good. Some success has been obtained using an ointment contain-ing 2% testosterone propionate. A small amount of the ointment is rubbed gently into the affected area three times a day.

If the woman is postmenopausal and has evidence of vulval atrophy, as well as pruritus, a mixture of dienoestrol cream and 1% hydrocortisone cream alternating with testosterone ointment may provide relief of the symptom.

CARCINOMA OF THE VULVA

This malignancy accounts for about 3 per cent of genital tract cancers, and occurs most often in post-menopausal women, although it may arise in women of all ages. The invasive lesions may be preceded by an intra-epithelial stage, but since the vulval epi-thelium in these women is particularly unstable, dysplasia, intra-epithelial carcinoma and invasive car-cinoma may be found in different areas of the same vulva. It is for this reason that multiple biopsies must be taken in all cases of pruritus vulvae of long duration. However, less than 10 per cent of cases of dysplasia dedifferentiate further to become malign-ant. It has been observed that women with a vulval carcinoma are likely (in 10 per cent of cases) to have coincidental malignant disease elsewhere: this sug-gests a genetic influence.

PATHOLOGY

Pre-invasive carcinoma. The vulval skin is usually normal, but may be red or white. On histology, the dysplasia and cell pleomorphism involves the whole thickness of the epidermis. The rete are large and elongated, and there is a complete loss of cellular polarity (Fig. **14/8**).

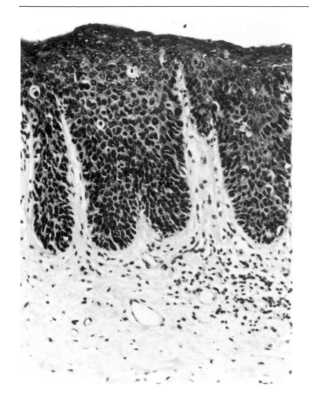

Fig 14/8 Pre-invasive carcinoma of the vulva (× 160)

Squamous cell carcinoma. (Fig **14/9A** This malignant neoplasm accounts for 95 per cent of cases. The colour of the vulva may be white, or red or pink, and the appearance of the skin is thickened, or cracked and atrophic. By the time the patient seeks help, the gross appearance is usually one of an ulcer with raised edges and a necrotic base, but occasionally it is nodular or papillomatous. The growth is usually found on the labium majus (50 per cent of cases) or the labium minus (25 per cent), in most instances in the anterior half of the vulva. In a few cases multiple growths are found. On histology the lesion is identical with skin cancer in any other location; irregular masses of pleomorphic cells invade the stroma, and there is a tendency for epithelial pearls to form (Fig. **14/9B**).

CLINICAL ASPECTS

Pre-invasive carcinoma. Occasionally the patient has no complaints, but usually she consults a physician because of an itchy vulva. The vulval skin may be normal or thickened in appearance, and pink, red, or whitish in colour. Diagnosis can only be made by multiple biopsies, and if these confirm that no areas

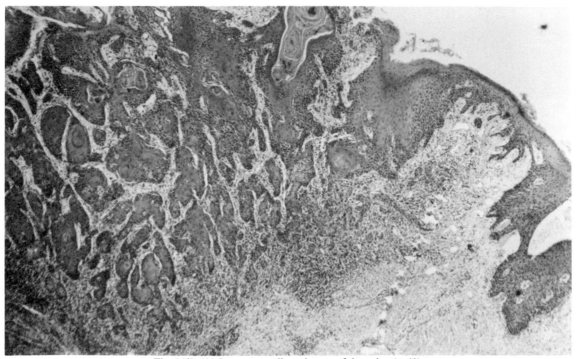

Fig. 14/9 (A) Squamous cell carcinoma of the vulva (× 40)

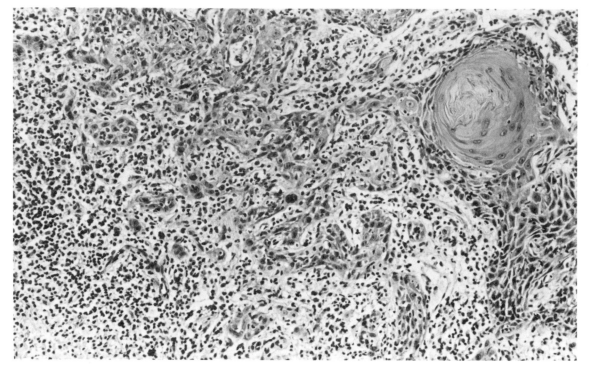

Fig. 14/9 (B) Note the epithelial pearl (× 160)

of invasive carcinoma are present, total vulvectomy without lymphadenectomy is the preferred treatment. A careful follow-up must be instituted for the rest of the patient's life, as the disease may recur in the new vulval skin.

Squamous cell carcinoma. In half the cases of vulval malignancy the patient's attention is drawn to her vulva by the presence of a lump, or a painful ulcer. Most of these women have no symptoms of vulval itching, but in a few a history of pruritus vulvae of short duration is obtained, suggesting that the symptom is caused by the carcinoma and is not its antecedent. In the other half of cases the main complaint is of pruritus vulvae, usually of more than 6 months' duration. The matter is put in better perspective if it is understood that carcinoma of the vulva will be found in fewer than 5 per cent of women who consult a physician because of pruritus vulvae of more than six month's duration.

The lesion presents as a hard nodule, or an ulcer with a sloughing base and raised edges, or as a discharging papillomatous mass, which is hard and friable and bleeds easily. Its size is variable (Fig.

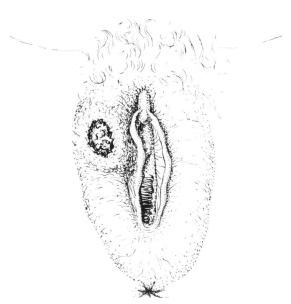

Fig. 14/10 (A) Drawing of a vulval carcinoma in the anterior part of the vulva

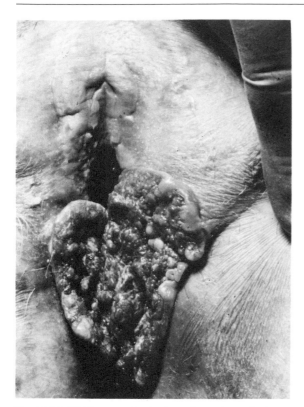

Fig. 14/10 (B) Photograph of a large fungating vulval carcinoma arising in the posterior part of the vulva. (By courtesy of Dr Malcolm Stening.)

14/10). In the early stages it is small, and the prognosis is directly related to the size of the lesion when first seen. The tumour spreads directly to the vagina, the urethra and the anus; but more sinister is lymphatic spread, which may involve nodes on the same or the opposite side, and is already present in 50 per cent of cases when first seen. If the deep nodes are involved, the prognosis is poor.

Until recently the accepted treatment was to perform a radical vulvectomy and a bilateral dissection of the inguino-femoral nodes (Fig. **14/11**). This approach is now questioned as the morbidity is high (wound necrosis, over 30 per cent; leg oedema, 20 per cent). In place, it is suggested that a more appropriate treatment is simple vulvectomy with irradiation of the inguinal nodes using modern radiotherapeutic techniques. Patients who have large palpable nodes at presentation are probably incurable, but chemotherapy followed by radiotherapy with or without surgery may help.

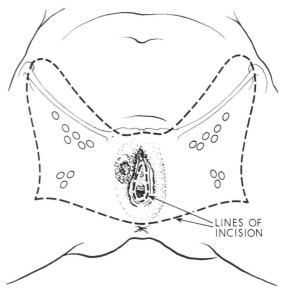

Fig. 14/11 Extent of operation of radical vulvectomy

OTHER VULVAL CONDITIONS

INFECTIONS OF THE VULVA

The skin of the vulva, being frequently subjected to chafing and friction, is liable to become infected by any of the common skin pathogens.

Infection of the hair follicles, causing boils or carbuncles, is fairly common, particularly when the standard of hygiene is low. Multiple superficial ulcers are occasionally encountered, especially in debilitated patients, and are due to staphylococcal infection. The vulva is exquisitely tender, and the ulcers are shallow and have a grey, discharging base. Treatment of acute bacterial vulvitis is to apply soaks of 1:1000 potassium permanganate solution, or preferably of 1% chlorhexidine cream if this can be done without undue discomfort. Simultaneously, sulphonamides or the appropriate antibiotic are given orally or intramuscularly.

Chancroid is due to infection with *H. ducreyi* and leads to superficial ulcers on the labia, fourchette or peri-anal areas of women, 3 to 7 days after infection. The ulcers are multiple, less than 2cm in diameter and have ragged edges. In about 50 per cent of women inguinal lymphadenitis occurs. Laboratory diagnosis is difficult. Currently the recommended treatment is to prescribe erythromycin 500mg four times a day, or co-trimoxazole 2 tablets twice daily for 10 days. Chancroid is uncommon in temperate countries but is being reported more frequently.

Fungal infections, usually due to *Candida albicans* (candidiasis) are frequent, and may occur alone or in association with diabetes, as the glycosuria encourages the fungus to grow. In diabetic vulvitis, the area is oedematous, wrinkled and dusky-red in colour. Treatment is to cleanse the vulva with water after each micturition and, after drying the area, to apply an antifungal ointment, and also to use antifungal pessaries (see p. 165). Because *Candida* grows well in hot, moist areas, a woman who develops vulval candidiasis should not wear nylon pantihose. She should wear cotton panties or no underwear at all. She should also avoid douching and the use of 'feminine vulval deodorant sprays', as these do not help the condition and may cause an allergic vulval reaction.

Genital herpes

Herpetic infection of the genital area, usually ulcers, are becoming increasingly common and afflict women more than men, because the herpes simplex virus (most frequently Type 2, but also Type 1) grows better in warm moist areas, such as the vulva and cervix. Epidemiological studies in the USA in the late 1970s showed that about 16 per cent of sexually-active females and males had antibodies to herpes simplex virus type 2 (HSV2). Of these people only a quarter had had any symptoms, but they were potentially infectious to their sexual partner.

Before the ulcers develop, the woman may feel an itching or burning sensation. Small blisters then appear which ulcerate rapidly. The ulcers are multiple, shallow and exquisitely painful. The surrounding tissues become oedematous and secondary infection may occur, aggravating the oedema and pain.

Specific treatment is unsatisfactory. Idoxuridine and photodynamic dyes are no more effective than placebo. Topical acyclovir (5% ointment applied 4-hourly) or oral acyclovir (200mg every 4 hours for 5 days) reduces the healing time, the duration of the vesicles and viral shedding of first episodes of herpes but does not seem to be as effective in preventing or treating recurrent herpes. If the woman has recurrent episodes of herpes more often than once a month, prophylactic acyclovir may be tried. But the drug is expensive and long-term use has not been evaluated.

Local relief may be obtained if the area is painted with 1% aqueous gentian violet or washed with very dilute potassium permanganate solution, until the ulcers heal in 7 to 14 days. The woman needs analgesics, and a local analgesic ointment may relieve her discomfort.

The virus also enters the myelin sheath of the sensory nerves supplying the vulva, where it lies dormant in the sacral neurones for weeks or months, when for some reason it may be reactivated, and travels back to the skin, with a recurrence of genital herpes. A single recurrence occurs in about 50 per cent of women, and between 1 and 5 per cent have frequent recurrences, often more than 6 times a year. When ulceration is present the disease is contagious, and coitus should be avoided.

BARTHOLINITIS

Infection of Bartholin's gland and duct is not uncommon, and is usually due to *E. coli* or staphylococcal infection, but may follow gonorrhoea. In the acute stage, both duct and gland are involved. If untreated, the infection may subside or an abscess may form. Occasionally a chronic enlargement of the duct follows an inflammatory conglutination of the duct epithelium. The patient complains of acute discomfort, and a reddened swelling appears beneath the posterior part of the labium majus. The surrounding skin and subcutaneous tissues become indurated and oedematous.

Treatment in acute bartholinitis is bed rest, analgesics and the administration of a broad-spectrum antibiotic. If an abscess has formed, surgery is necessary. Marsupialization of the abscess is preferable to simple incision. It is performed by excising an elliptical piece of the vagina and abscess wall just inside the hymenal ring, and suturing the vaginal and abscess walls together to maintain patency of the cavity. This then slowly heals. In other cases, the acute phase subsides without surgery, and a chronic retention cyst forms. Since this can easily become reinfected, it should be excised intact.

BENIGN TUMOURS OF THE VULVA

Since the tissues of the vulva are covered by epithelium, and contain sebaceous glands, sweat glands and hair follicles in a matrix of adipose and connective tissue, benign tumours may arise from any of these tissues. The commonest benign swellings are sebaceous cysts, lipomata and fibromata; but melanoma, haemangioma, and endometrioma and others may occur. If the tumour causes symptoms, treatment is surgical excision. A number of women develop vulval varicose veins which are most noticeable during pregnancy, but which rarely cause symptoms in the non-pregnant. Symptomatic veins are treated by the injection of sclerosing fluids.

GENITAL WARTS (CONDYLOMATA ACUMINATA)

Genital warts are caused by one or more types of the human papillomavirus (HPV). The disease is sexually transmitted and the types of HPV which are most likely to be a factor in cervical or vaginal neoplasia are 6, 16, and 18. The primary infection may occur on the vulva, the vagina or the cervix. Vulval infections may spread to the vagina and vaginal infections to the cervix. Vulval warts usually present as cauliflower growths of various sizes, but may be undetectable clinically. They may occur on any part of the vulva and involve the anal area. Usually they are multiple. Vaginal and cervical warts may be obvious on inspection, but often can only be detected using a colposcope. In Europe about 8 per cent of men aged 16 to 35 have evidence of HPV infection, based on swabs taken from the penis, and 16 per cent of women of the same age range have evidence of cervical infection. This observation is important because of the evidence that HPV is a factor in the development of cervical intraepithelial neoplasia and cervical cancer (see p. 173). For this reason a cervical smear should be taken from any woman who presents with vulval warts.

Vulval warts are treated by trimming away excess vulval hair and applying podophyllin to the wart. As podophyllin burns normal skin, the application must be made carefully. Two choices are available: (1) The doctor may apply 20 per cent podophyllin in benzoin tincture to each wart. The mixture is allowed to dry, and washed off 8 hours later by the patient. (2) The patient is given 0.5 per cent podophyllin in ethanol (or preferably the more expensive but less toxic podophyllotoxin). She applies this to each wart twice a day for three days.

If these treatments fail to cure the warts after several applications, the warts should be treated by cryosurgery or electrocautery. An alternative treatment is to vaporize each wart using a CO_2 laser. Vaginal and cervical warts have to be treated by laser, cryosurgery or electrocautery. In pregnancy podophyllin is contra-indicated as it may be absorbed and reach the fetus, which suggests that CO_2 laser may be the preferred treatment in this situation.

GRANULOMATOUS INFECTIONS OF THE VULVA

In the following discussion three diseases, usually transmitted during coitus, are described. The first, *syphilis*, has a world-wide distribution and its incidence appears to be increasing, particularly amongst urban-dwelling young females. The second, *lymphogranuloma venereum*, is fairly common amongst the indigenous population of most tropical areas, as is the third, *granuloma inguinale*, but the incidence of this disease is decreasing.

SYPHILIS

Syphilis is due to the invasion of tissues by *Treponema pallidum*, usually introduced during coitus. Following an incubation period of 10 to 90 days, but usually of 14 to 28 days, a small papule appears at each site of inoculation. In the female this is usually on the vulva, but the vagina or the cervix may be infected. The papule rapidly enlarges to an oval lesion of variable size, the centre of which becomes eroded and granulomatous. The edges of the eroded area are sharp, and beyond this a thickened and indurated zone occurs, hence the name *hard chancre*. The lesion is painless, and the symptoms so slight that often the chancre is not noticed by the patient, or if noticed is considered to be a small 'sore'. Ordinarily the primary lesion disappears in 21 days or so. The secondary and tertiary manifestations of syphilis are not confined to the genital tract, and are dealt with in textbooks of medicine, but it is to be remembered that only if the disease is treated early is cure certain. A sore on the vulva, a roseolar skin rash on the chest and back or a sore throat, persisting for more than 21 days, merits investigation to exclude syphilis before any treatment is instituted. This is particularly important in the female, as not only can she infect her male partner, but the treponema passes through the placenta, and may infect her unborn child.

Diagnosis

The diagnosis of the primary state is made by detecting the spirochaete, *T. pallidum*, in a smear obtained from the chancre and examined under dark ground illumination through a microscope. The chancre must first be cleansed with a swab and then its edge and base scarified with a scalpel so that exudate appears before the specimen is taken. The diagnosis in the later stages of the primary lesion, and in suspicious secondary lesions, is serological, and by 6 weeks after the initial infection a flocculation test which detects reagin. The VDRL or Rapid Plasma Reagin (RPR) test is positive in all infected patients. The tests are also positive in other closely related diseases, such as yaws and some chronic diseases. Following adequate treatment, the tests take from 6 to 12 months to become negative. Because of these problems, if there are no other diagnostic signs indicating syphilis, the presence of the infection must be confirmed by making a specific test to detect anti-treponemal antibodies. The most commonly used test is the Fluorescent Treponemal Antibody Test (FTA-ABS).

Treatment

Penicillin is specific in the treatment of early syphilis. The addition of other drugs adds no benefit and may increase the hazards. For primary syphilis one of the following may be chosen: (1) Procaine penicillin 1.0 mega-units daily for 10 to 14 days, (2) PAM 2.4 mega-units initially, followed by 9 weekly injections of PAM 1.2 mega-units.

If the patient is unable to tolerate penicillin, tetracycline 250mg by mouth 6-hourly for 30 days is given.

Following treatment the patient must remain under observation with clinical and serological examination every 2 months for 6 months, then every 3rd month for a further 18 months. Re-treatment is required (1) if evidence of clinical progression or relapse occurs, (2) if a previously non-reactive test becomes reactive, or (3) if a rise in titre occurs. It is probably wise to make serological tests annually for life.

LYMPHOGRANULOMA VENEREUM

Lymphogranuloma venereum is caused by a substrain of *Chlamydia trachomatis*, and is usually acquired during coitus. It begins as a small papule on the vulva after a short incubation period, and this is followed by rubbery enlargement of the inguinal lymph nodes, which may undergo necrosis and abscess formation. These finally heal leaving puckered scars. The lymphatic obstruction may produce massive vulval swelling; whilst lymphatic extension of the disease to the vulva, vagina, or rectal areas can lead to ulceration, fibrosis and strictures of the vagina or rectum. The treatment of the disease is to give tetracycline in the dosage recommended for the treatment of syphilis.

GRANULOMA INGUINALE

This disease is caused by a small bacterium, *Donovania granulomatis*, which develops within mononuclear cells. It is probably transmitted by coitus, but the disease is not very contagious. Granuloma inguinale is primarily a disease of mucous membranes, small papules coalescing and breaking down to form irregularly shaped ulcers in vulval regions. The edges of the ulcer are thick and uneven, and often surrounded by small papules which have, as yet, not broken down. The base of the ulcer is dark red granulation tissue. The ulcers are itchy and painful, but involvement of the inguinal lymph nodes is uncommon. The vulva becomes swollen, often massively. The diagnosis is made by demonstrating 'Donovan bodies' in the mononuclear cells obtained by cutting into the infected tissue. Treatment is to give 10 to 20g of tetracycline over 10 days; or 40g of streptomycin over 20 days.

Chapter 15

The Vagina

Apart from infections and prolapse, diseases of the vagina are relatively uncommon. Occasionally its walls are distended by a cyst of one of the vestigial structures, usually Wolffian duct in origin. The cysts are small, occasionally multiple, and arise in the lateral or anterolateral vaginal wall. If they cause symptoms, treatment is surgical excision, otherwise they may be left alone. Tumours may arise from each of the layers which make up the vagina, and may therefore be papillomata (which are often multiple), fibromata, angiomata or lipomata. Malignant neoplasms are very rare, primary carcinoma of the vagina forming only 1 per cent of genital malignancies. Secondary malignancies occur rather more frequently, and usually the primary lesion is a cervical carcinoma, an endometrial carcinoma or a choriocarcinoma, although in advanced disease, metastases from any organ may be found. Treatment of malignant neoplasms is unsatisfactory, whether radical surgery, irradiation or chemotherapy is used, and fewer than 30 per cent of patients survive 5 years.

VAGINAL DISCHARGES

The vagina of the adolescent and adult woman in the reproductive years is lined by a layer of stratified squamous epithelium, 10 to 30 cells thick; the thickness, activity and glycogen content being controlled principally by the variations in the level of circulating oestrogens. Oestrogen acts as an enzyme, causing an increase in the RNA content of the cell and the synthesis of protein and glycogen. The glycogen is formed only in the superficial cells. Once these cells have been exfoliated, the glycogen is converted into lactic acid by the lactobacilli of Döderlein, which are normal vaginal inhabitants. By this means, the acidity of the vagina is maintained, during the re-productive years, at a pH of between 3.5 and 4.5. In addition to the lactobacilli, the vagina harbours large numbers of bacteria, mainly staphylococci and micrococci, *Gardnerella*, bacteriodes, bacteria of faecal origin, aerobic streptococci, beta-haemolytic streptococci and vaginal yeasts. These bacteria are non-pathogenic and are normal vaginal inhabitants. Only in certain circumstances, due to a change in vaginal acidity, epithelial resistance or damage, do the vaginal flora become pathogenic. For example, before puberty and after the climacteric, when oestrogen production is low, the vaginal epithelium tends to be inactive, and only a few cell layers thick. The cells are of the intermediate or parabasal types, contain no glycogen, and Döderlein's bacilli are absent, so that the pH rises to between 6 and 7 (Fig. **15/1**). The relatively inactive epithelium of a postclimacteric woman is prone to infection, whilst the many-layered acid vagina of a young woman is resistant to many pathogens.

It appears that a considerable number of women harbour potential pathogens in their vaginas. In studies of unselected women in Britain, Sweden and the USA, 2 to 20 per cent had symptomless trichomoniasis infestation, and 5 to 30 per cent

	per cent
Lactobacilli	80–90
Staphlococci, micrococci	50–70
Ureaplasma	40–50
Anaerobes	20–50
Streptococci	20–30
Gardnerella	10–30
E. coli	5–15
Candida sp	5–15
Bacteroides	5–10
Trichomonads	3–7

Table 15/1 Normal vaginal flora

VAGINAL :—				
OESTROGEN	EPITHELIUM	GLYCOGEN	pH	FLORA

	OESTROGEN	EPITHELIUM	GLYCOGEN	pH	FLORA
NEWBORN	+	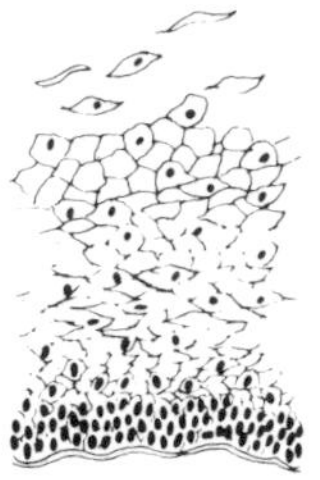	+	ACID 4—5	STERILE ↓ DÖDERLEIN'S BACILLI SECRETION ABUNDANT
MONTH-OLD CHILD	–	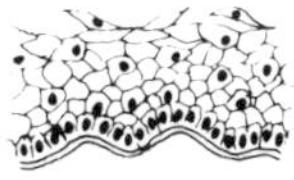	–	ALKALINE >7	SPARSE, COCCAL AND VARIED FLORA. SECRETION SCANT
PUBERTY	APPEARS	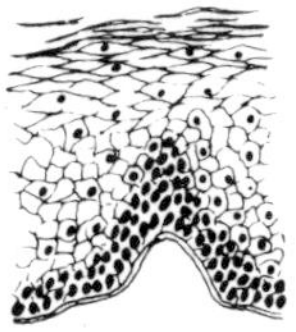	– ⟶ +	ALKALINE ↓ ACID	SPARSE, COCCAL ↓ RICH BACILLARY
MATURE	+ +	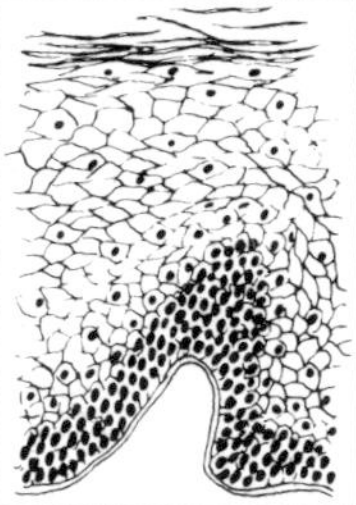	+	ACID 4—5	DODERLEIN'S BACILLI SECRETION ABUNDANT
POST MENOPAUSE	+ ⟶ –	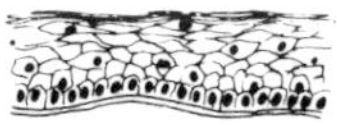	–	NEUTRAL OR ALKALINE 6 — >7	VARIED DEPENDENT ON LEVEL OF CIRCULATING OESTROGEN SECRETION SCANT

Fig. 15/1 Changes in the vaginal epithelium and acidity related to the woman's age

harboured *Candida albicans*. The prevalence of both conditions increases with age during the reproductive years. These organisms cause symptoms in only a few women.

Normally the vagina is kept moist by a transudate from capillaries in the vaginal wall together with a smaller quantity of secretions from Bartholin's glands and the endocervix. The vaginal fluid also contains vaginal exfoliated epithelial cells, aliphatic acids, carbohydrate and the micro-organisms mentioned earlier. During the menstrual cycle, the quantity of the secretions varies, and is related to the oestrogen production. The peak is reached at ovulation, when a much greater exfoliation of the vaginal epithelial cells occurs, so that some women notice a vaginal discharge only at this time. The cervical secretions and vaginal transudation are also affected markedly by emotional stress, and a physiological vaginal discharge, or leucorrhoea, is a frequent complaint in such women. Sexual stimulation, with or without coitus, is also a potent stimulant to an increased vaginal discharge.

PHYSIOLOGICAL VAGINAL DISCHARGE: LEUCORRHOEA

As mentioned, the volume of vaginal secretions varies considerably, and when increased may cause concern to the woman. In these cases, the discharge is called 'leucorrhoea', which is defined as any white non-bloody, non-infected vaginal discharge. When a patient presents with leucorrhoea, the physician must exclude the presence of pathological vaginal discharges by clinical and laboratory investigations. These are discussed later. Treatment is only required for women who become distressed by what they perceive as excessive quantity, imagined odours or itching. Reassurance that the discharge is physiological is the primary treatment; and an acid vaginal jelly (Acijel) may be prescribed if reassurance is insufficient. Antibiotics should not be prescribed, as they aggravate rather than relieve the discharge, nor should specific fungicides be prescribed.

DISCHARGE DUE TO PATHOGENS: VAGINITIS

On the other hand, an irritant discharge from the vagina often indicates a true vaginitis due to pathogens, and is a common complaint. The three principal types encountered are (1) trichomoniasis, (2) candidiasis (or monilial) vaginitis and, (3) non-specific bacterial vaginitis (amine vaginosis).

In many cases the diagnosis can be made in the

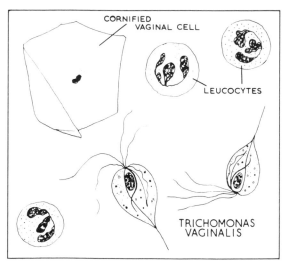

Fig. 15/2 *Trichomonas vaginalis*

doctor's surgery, office or the outpatient clinic. Fifty years ago, when women often presented after the vaginitis had been present for some weeks a clinical diagnosis was possible. Today, with earlier presentation, the clinical signs are usually non-specific. However, if the doctor has a microscope, a diagnosis can be made in about half of the cases. A vaginal swab is taken. Part is mixed on a slide with two drops of saline, and part is mixed on a second slide with two drops of 10% potassium hydroxide (KOH). The saline preparation is viewed under a microscope when the trichomonal flagellates may be seen moving, or thrashing their tails (Fig. **15/2**). The saline preparation may also reveal vaginal epithelial cells with serrated borders, suggestive of non-specific vaginitis (see Fig. **15/4**). The latter is also suggested if the vaginal discharge or the KOH preparation has a strong fishy smell. (This is called the amine test.) The KOH preparation is examined under the microscope when the hyphae of *Candida albicans* may be seen (Fig. **15/3**). Culture is needed only when microscopy fails to establish a diagnosis. In this case a further vaginal swab is sent to a laboratory in a transport and culture medium such as Transgrow.

Trichomoniasis

The *Trichomonas vaginalis* parasite is a flagellate, $20\mu m$ long and $10\mu m$ wide, with four anterior flagellae and a long tail membrane. It is a little larger than a pus cell and about half the size of an exfoliated superficial vaginal cell (Fig. **15/2**). It is the cause of vaginitis in about 50 per cent of women complaining of an irritating vaginal discharge, but is also found in the vaginal secretions of about 10 per cent of symptomless women. It seems, therefore, that it only becomes pathogenic when a change in the vaginal resistance and acidity is brought about. This may occur during and after menstruation, after sexual stimulation and after illness. At these times the vaginal secretions increase, and the pH of the vagina is raised to 5.5 to 6.5, at which level the trichomonads thrive. The flagellate is readily transferred between coital partners, but in the male is usually symptomless. It is possible that the organism is initially introduced into the vagina during coitus, although rarely the condition has been found in presumed virgins. Once introduced, the flagellate shelters at the bottom of the crypts of the velvet-like vagina, and only manifests itself when a change in vaginal acidity occurs.

Clinical features. When the environmental conditions are appropriate, a rapid multiplication of the flagellates leads to overt trichomoniasis, and the parasites may invade the urethra, Skene's tubules or even Bartolin's gland. Thus urethritis may occur as well as vaginitis.

The primary complaint of the patient is a moderate to profuse discharge, accompanied by itching and irritation inside and around the vaginal introitus. Typically the discharge is greenish in colour and frothy, but this is of little diagnostic value.

Diagnosis. The diagnosis should be confirmed in all cases by examining a drop of vaginal discharge, mixed with a drop of warmed saline, under the microscope without staining, when the motile trichomonads will be seen. However, for greater accuracy, a sample of the vaginal discharge should be added immediately to a test tube of Kupferberg's medium, which is then incubated. At the same time, a smear should be stained with Gram's stain and examined to exclude a coincident gonococcal infection.

Treatment. The development of the drug metronidazole has simplified the treatment of trichomoniasis. Metronidazole is given in a dose of 200mg three times daily for 7 days orally. An alternative is to give a single dose of tinidazole 2g. The sexual partner is also treated. These therapies cure 90 per cent of cases, but if symptoms persist and the flagellates are again found, a second course is given after an interval of 7 days. A further vaginal examination is made 2 months after treatment is concluded, and if vaginal swabs are found to be positive on culture, treatment must be repeated. Side effects are minimal, although a few patients complain of nausea. Alcohol should not be consumed during treatment.

The itching is generally relieved by metronidazole, but local antipruritic ointments may be prescribed, or natamycin ('Pimafucin', BDH) pessaries introduced into the vagina daily for 20 days. Natamycin pessaries should also be used in the first 12 weeks of pregnancy (when metronidazole is possibly contra-indicated), or if metronidazole fails to cure the patient.

Candidiasis or monilial vaginitis

This form of vaginitis is caused by a yeast-like fungus, *Candida albicans*, which infects vaginal epithelial cells, particularly in its germination stage (Fig. **15/3**). In this stage *Candida albicans* develops spores and long threads (hyphae). Inside the cell it may lie

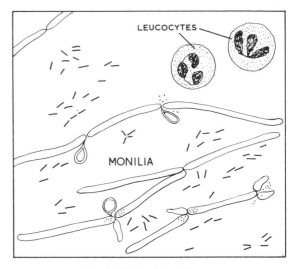

Fig. 15/3 *Candida albicans*

dormant until environmental conditions encourage germination. Its growth is normally kept under control by the vaginal flora, but if vaginal acidity rises it may produce symptoms. For these reasons, monilial vaginitis is found in diabetics, during pregnancy when glycosuria is common and there is much vaginal glycogen, and following the use of 'broad spectrum' antibiotics, or corticosteroids. *Candida albicans* is found in the mouth of 10 per cent of healthy women, in the anogenital region of 15 per cent, and in the vagina of 10 to 25 per cent. At least two-thirds of vaginal infections are symptomless. It is likely that most vaginal infections spread from the intestinal tract, but in some cases *Candida* is transmitted sexually.

Clinical findings and diagnosis. The main complaint is severe pruritus, which may affect the whole vulval area and is associated with a vaginal discharge. The male partner may complain of postcoital irritation of his penis and foreskin in some cases. In the female the discharge is typically thick and cheesy, and adheres to the vaginal wall in plaques, but frequently the characteristic findings are absent. If the diagnosis is uncertain after the KOH procedure, a vaginal swab should be sent to the laboratory. The swab should be kept moistened, and inoculated as soon as possible into a tube containing Sabouraud's medium. After 48 hours at room temperature, any yeast-like organisms present will appear as brown or brown-black colonies growing in the medium.

Treatment

Several drugs are available to treat vaginal candidiasis. No one seems superior to any other. Because of problems of patient compliance, the trend has been to reduce the duration of the course of treatment. Most of the drugs are imidazole derivatives. They include clotrimazole, econazole, isoconazole and micronazole. They are given as a vaginal pessary or a cream (using an applicator) placed high in the vagina. The duration of treatment is a single application; or a 3- or 6-day course depending on doctor and patient preferences. The imidazole derivatives have largely replaced nystatin pessaries, which needed to be used for at least 7 days, and messy gentian violet (2% in water) vaginal paintings.

Some women prefer oral treatment. For them fluconazole 150mg as a single tablet or ketoconazole 200mg twice a day for 5 days should be prescribed.

One course of any of the medications cures between 85 and 95 per cent of patients.

Relapsing or recurrent candidosis

Between 5 and 15 per cent of patients have repeated attacks of candidosis, often more than four times a year. Most are relapses of the initial infection, possibly because of a reduced local host defence against *Candida*. The attacks may cause a considerable disruption to the woman's personal and sexual life. Treatment is difficult. A recent suggestion is that prophylactic ketoconazole 100mg by mouth daily for 6 months may protect against relapses. Because ketoconazole may cause liver damage (1:15 000 in people usually aged 50 or more) some doctors recommend that the woman has liver function tests made periodically. During treatment about 10 per cent of women complain of nausea. Hygienic measures should also be adopted although their value has not been tested. Tight jeans or pantihose should be avoided as they reduce the circulation of air around the vulvo-vaginal area. As the intestinal tract may be a source of reinfection, women should pay attention to hygiene. They should wipe the area from front to back after defaecation and should avoid introducing a finger into the vagina which may be contaminated by anal touching.

Non-specific vaginitis (amine vaginosis)

Occasionally the normal bacterial inhabitants of the vagina become pathogenic and induce a low-grade non-specific vaginitis, which may be impossible to differentiate clinically from leucorrhoea. In some cases the discharge is thin, greyish in colour and has a disagreeable 'fishy' odour. The precise cause is not known, but in a large proportion of cases, the low-grade Gram-negative pathogen, *Gardnerella vaginalis* (*Haemophilus vaginalis*) may grow on culture. In other cases, Gram-negative anaerobic bacilli, staphylococci and rarely, *Mycoplasma hominis* are grown. Whether *G. vaginalis* is the cause of the vaginal discharge is uncertain, as up to 30 per cent of women harbour the organism in their vagina. It is probable that an interaction occurs in some circumstances between *G. vaginalis* and anaerobes which leads to the offensive vaginal discharge. Because of this uncertainty, the terms 'non-specific vaginitis' or amine vaginosis have been coined.

The clinical suspicion of anaerobic vaginosis may be confirmed by taking a vaginal swab and smearing half on a slide for Gram staining and the remainder on a second slide, with a drop of saline added for a wet-mount preparation. The Gram stain will show Gram-variable coccibacilli (pepper and salt) attached to vaginal epithelial cells and the wet mount may show vaginal epithelial cells with a serrated edge due to the adherence of organisms. They are called 'clue cells' (Fig. **15/4**). Metronidazole or tinidazole in the dose recommended for the treatment of trichomoniasis appears to be the most effective drug; preferably using the seven-day course which is more effective. Other less effective treatments are sulphathiazole vaginal cream (Sultrin or Triple-sulphonamide vaginal cream) inserted high in the vagina twice daily for 7 days, and an acid jelly (Acijel) used in a similar manner.

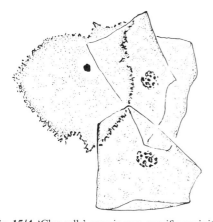

Fig. 15/4 'Clue cells', seen in non-specific vaginitis

VULVO-VAGINITIS IN ADULTS

Occasionally, a woman with trichomoniasis or candidiasis may develop a secondary vulvitis, due to staphylococcal infection, which probably occurs from scratching. The vulva is spotted with exquisitely painful superficial ulcers which stand out on the swollen labia. Treatment is to paint the vulval lesions with 1% aqueous gentian violet, to give analgesics and to diagnose and treat the vaginitis.

CHEMICAL OR ALLERGIC VAGINITIS

These conditions are less common today as more women use oral rather than vaginal contraceptives, and now that douching has been generally discarded. Treatment consists of ceasing to use the chemical or allergen, and the administration of antihistamines orally.

ATROPHIC 'VAGINITIS'

This is not really a true vaginitis, but an inflammatory reaction occurring in a vagina whose mucosa has degenerated and become ulcerated owing to inadequate oestrogenic stimulation. It is discussed in Chapter 29.

OTHER CAUSES OF VAGINAL DISCHARGE

These include a foreign body (such as a forgotten tampon), 'cervicitis' and malignant conditions of the cervix or corpus uteri.

CARCINOMA OF THE VAGINA

This is a very rare form of genital tract carcinoma. It is usually treated by radiotherapy but the results are poor. Recently a few cases of vaginal adenosis and clear cell adenocarcinoma of the vagina have been reported. Most of the patients are post-pubertal and investigation shows that their mothers were prescribed large doses of stilboestrol in the pregnancy which resulted in the birth of the patient. The girl complains of a mucoid vaginal discharge. Clear cell adenocarcinoma is treated by radiotherapy but the results are rather unsatisfactory.

Chapter 16

The Cervix

The cervix is that part of the uterus which lies below the histological internal os. In this area the proportion of muscular tissue diminishes and that of connective tissue increases rapidly. The cervix is therefore predominantly composed of connective tissue which constitutes 80 per cent of its volume, muscle fibres and blood vessels constituting 10 per cent each. It is barrel-shaped and is penetrated by the cervical canal. The lower half of the cervix projects into the vaginal vault (Fig. **16/1**). The arterial blood vessels are continuations of the uterine arteries, and the veins drain into the uterine venous plexus. The lymphatic system in the cervix is of great importance, particularly in respect of the spread of carcinoma. A fine plexus of lymphatics lying beneath the cervical epithelium combines into lymphatic channels in the stroma. These channels interconnect and are linked to the paracervical lymph nodes, and then to those of the internal iliac chain, the obturator fossa and the sacral chain.

The cervical canal is lined with columnar mucin-secreting epithelium. Its walls are convoluted into a complex of epithelial-lined crypts and tunnels which invaginate the stroma, and are separated by epithelial-covered ridges of stroma (Fig. **16/2**). In the past the crypts and tunnels have been considered to form the cervical 'glands'. The columnar epithelium extends on to the vaginal portion of the cervix to a varying degree beyond the slit-like external os, and then merges imperceptibly, or is transformed suddenly, into the stratified squamous epithelium which covers the vaginal portion of the cervix (Fig. **16/3**). The position of the squamo-columnar junction is determined by the volume of the cervical stroma, and this in turn is dependent on the influence of oestrogen and probably, synergistically, of progesterone. Oestrogen causes softening of the cervical connective tissue by altering the structure of collagen, and binds water in the ground substance

which surrounds the stromal cells. This increases the volume of the cervix, and the clefts and tunnels of the cervical canal unfold to some extent so that the squamo-columnar junction appears to move outwards on to the vaginal portion of the cervix, causing an eversion. The eversion of the columnar epithelium therefore occurs at times of maximal hormonal influence, and is particularly likely to arise in the female fetus in the last weeks of her mother's pregnancy; in the pubertal girl at the time of the first few ovulatory periods; and finally in pregnancy. During the first pregnancy, eversion is likely to be maximal, but it may also occur in subsequent pregnancies.

In the different environmental conditions of the

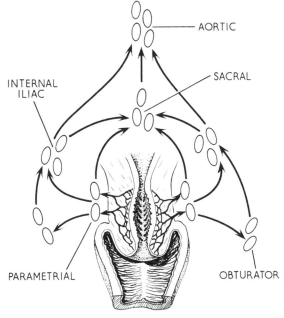

Fig. 16/1 Coronal section of the cervix and upper vagina showing diagrammatically the lymphatic drainage

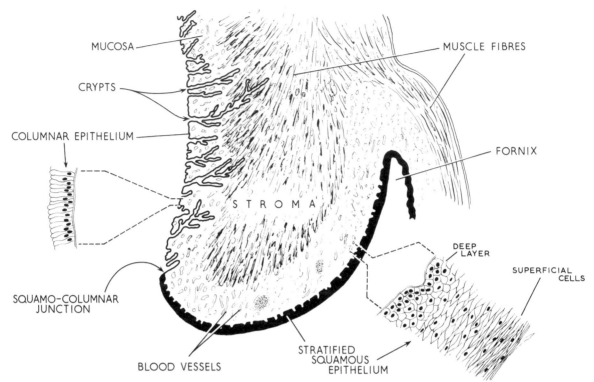

Fig. 16/2 The structure of the cervix. Note particularly the abrupt transition from columnar to squamous epithelium at the squamo-columnar junction

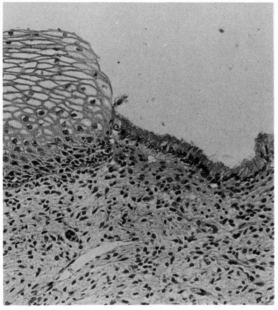

Fig. 16/3 The squamo-columnar junction. Note the abrupt transition from columnar to squamous epithelium (× 160)

vagina, squamous metaplasia of the exposed columnar epithelium occurs, starting from the outer edge and moving inwards in tongues of cells towards the cervical canal. The metaplasia is apparently permanent, and forms a 'transformation zone' of squamous epithelium which lies between the original, or native, squamous epithelium of the vaginal portion of the cervix and the columnar epithelium of the cervical canal (Fig. **16/4**). The transformation zone is the area in which cervical carcinoma usually develops. As squamous metaplasia proceeds, small collections of columnar epithelium may be buried under the surface and, continuing to secrete mucin, may form small retention cysts (Nabothian follicles) (Fig. **16/5**).

ECTROPION OR EVERSION OF COLUMNAR EPITHELIUM

The degree of eversion of the columnar epithelium, the degree of squamous metaplasia and the position of the squamo-columnar junction, depend on local

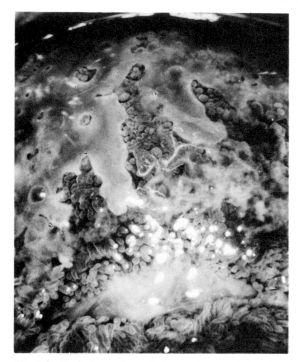

Fig. 16/4 Typical transformation zone. The cervical os is at the lower side of the illustration. Pearly tongues of new metaplastic squamous epithelium are appearing in the upper portion of the cervix below the original squamo-columnar junction. The grape-like structures are collections of columnar epithelial cells (colpophotograph)

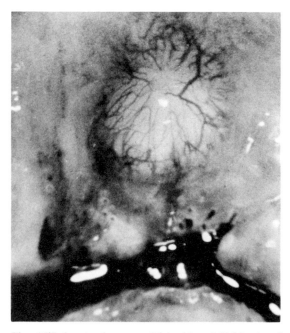

Fig. 16/5 A retention cyst (Nabothian follicle) viewed through the colposcope

tissue conditions as well as hormonal influences. Thus on vaginal examination a zone of variable size of exposed columnar epithelium is visible upon the vaginal portion of the cervix. This is called an 'ectropion' or 'eversion'. If a bivalve speculum is used to expose the cervix and opened widely, the slit-like external cervical os is stretched, and a larger amount of columnar epithelium of the cervical canal becomes visible; when opened only to expose the lips of the cervical os, less columnar epithelium is visible, which is entirely ectopic in nature, and indicates the *real* rather than the *apparent* degree of eversion of columnar epithelium (Fig. **16/6**).

In the past this physiological eversion was considered pathological and called a 'cervical erosion', which is false for there is no discontinuity of epithelium; or 'chronic cervicitis' which is equally erroneous for no infection is present. But because of these concepts, and the belief that 'chronic cervicitis' led to carcinoma, innumerable eversions have been subjected to chemical and electrical cauterization.

Anecdotal 'evidence' suggests that 'erosion' is a cause of backache, of deep dyspareunia, of cystitis and of pelvic pain. Careful investigation shows that none of these symptoms are more commonly found in women with a cervical eversion than in women with a 'normal' cervix. Cervical eversion is found more often in women taking oral hormonal contraceptives and may cause increased mucorrhoea.

In most instances the discovery of an ectropion is not an indication for treatment, although a cervical smear should be taken for exfoliative cytology, if this has not been done within the previous year. In a few cases when the mucorrhoea from the exposed cervical cells is excessive and distressing to the patient, the ectropion may be cauterized by linear strokes of a heavy-duty cautery. The strokes should encompass the width of the ectropion, but should not extend further up the cervical canal. Many gynaecologists have replaced electrocautery with cryosurgery as the latter is almost painless. A probe of appropriate size and shape is applied to the cervix, and freezing is started. Within seconds the probe adheres to the cervix. Freezing is continued until the edge of the 'ice-ball' extends about 2mm beyond the margin of the eversion. Thawing is then permitted and the probe removed. Cryosurgery is also used to treat dys-

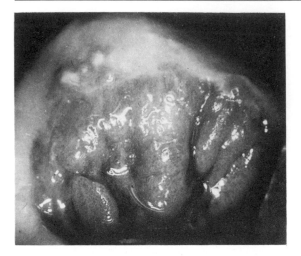

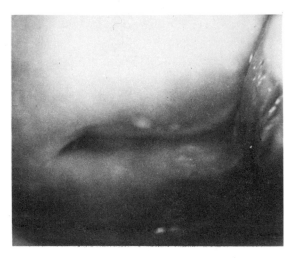

Fig. 16/6 In the top illustration the cervix has been exposed with a bivalve vaginal speculum. The bottom illustration shows the same cervix after closing the speculum. All the columnar epithelium has now disappeared inside the cervical canal, and the Nabothian follicles now lie at the external cervical os. The eversion was only apparent, not real

columnar epithelium. These methods should be reserved for selected symptomatic cases, and should replace all chemical methods, which are inefficient and of little value. Following treatment an increased amount of vaginal discharge (which is often blood-stained) persists for about 3 weeks. Vaginal antiseptics, enzymes or hormonal suppositories are of no value in speeding up the healing process, and should not be used.

CHRONIC CERVICITIS

A number of authorities consider that chronic non-specific infection of cervical crypts forms a clinical syndrome of undetermined aetiology. The main symptom is a mucopurulent vaginal discharge, but it is postulated that other, rather non-specific, symptoms may be present, such as deep pelvic pain, dyspareunia and backache. If mucopurulent cervical discharge is present endocervical cells should be obtained and tested for the presence of *Chlamydia* using a fluorescent monoclonal antibody technique. If *Chlamydia* are found doxycycline 100mg twice a day for 7 to 10 days should be prescribed. In other cases if the condition is considered to be a true entity, which causes the symptoms, treatment is indicated. This is by cauterizing the affected area of the cervix with an electric cautery or freezing the area with cryosurgery. Following either method, the dead tissue sloughs off over a period and is replaced by metaplasia of cell remnants. The postoperative symptoms of vaginal discharge is less after cryosurgery, and the cure rate higher than when diathermy is used.

OTHER BENIGN CERVICAL CONDITIONS

Acute cervicitis

The condition probably occurs more often than it is diagnosed. The usual organisms involved in the infection are sexually transmitted, gonococci and *Chlamydia* predominating. In most cases the infection is symptomless, but in some a mucopurulent discharge leads the patient to seek medical help.

Acute cervicitis may follow trauma to the cervix during childbirth, and may form a part of puerperal infection. In most cases the acute cervicitis is found incidentally.

plasia of the cervix, and some cases of carcinoma-in-situ. In these cases, freezing for 3 minutes is followed by thawing for 5 minutes and then freezing is repeated.

Another method is to use a CO_2 laser under colposcopic vision, a method which may prove better than cryosurgery or electrocautery. It is believed that the thermal destruction of tissue leads to complete squamous metaplasia within 10 days, and clinically there is a rapid disappearance of the ectopic

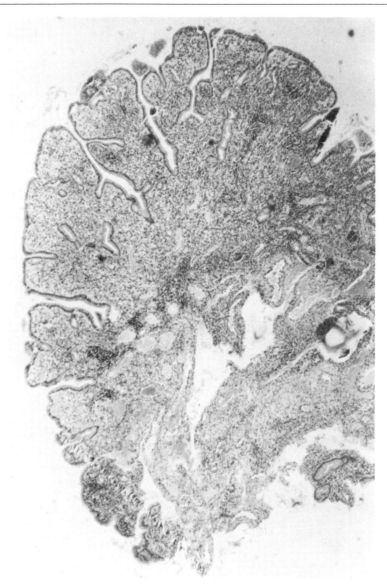

Fig. 16/7 A cervical polyp ($\times 40$)

Ulcers of the cervix

These are rare and may be malignant, tuberculous, syphilitic, traumatic (especially after 'criminal' abortion) or due to the chronic granulomata. Diagnosis is made following biopsy, and treatment is directed to the underlying cause.

Benign tumours of the cervix

The most common cervical tumour is the cervical polyp, which occurs as a result of localized hyperplasia of the stroma and epithelium covering a ridge between two clefts in the cervical canal. The polyp is covered with columnar epithelium which in some areas, particularly at the tip, may undergo squamous metaplasia, or may be rubbed off leaving an ulcerated area. The core is made up of stroma which is often congested, and infiltrated with leucocytes (Fig. **16/7**). The main symptom is intermittent vaginal bleeding, often occurring post-coitally. The diagnosis is made by inspection of the cervix, when the reddened polyp will be seen. Treatment is to avulse the polyp by twisting its long pedicle, but if the patient is over the age of 35 and has had abnormal bleeding, a diagnostic curettage and exfoliative cervical cytology should also be performed to exclude malignant disease of the uterus. The polyp should be submitted for histopathological examination to ensure that malignant change has not occurred, although this is rarely found.

Other tumours which may be encountered are papillomata, fibromata, myomata and endometriomata. Papillomata arise in the squamous epithelium of the vaginal portion of the cervix and may resemble condylomata acuminata, but the latter are associated with similar lesions in the vaginal and vulval epithelium. Papillomata are uncommon and usually appear in pregnancy, regressing after delivery, so that conservative treatment is indicated initially. As they are caused by the genital wart virus, they should be treated using cautery, cryosurgery or laser vaporization. Fibromata and myomata are also rare, and if causing symptoms should be removed surgically.

THE SQUAMOUS EPITHELIUM OF THE CERVIX

The ready accessibility of the cervix, and the comparative frequency of malignant change, has led to a considerable study of the squamous epithelium by exfoliative cytology, colposcopy, histology and tissue culture. From these studies it has become apparent that in certain women the cervical epithelium is particularly unstable. This instability appears to occur mainly (but not exclusively) in women who have had sexual intercourse with several men in adolescence and suggests that a sexually transmitted infection, such as wart virus or herpes simplex virus, type 2, may be of significance in causing the later occurrence of instability.

The normal squamous epithelium is stratified, and separated from the underlying stroma by an apparent basement membrane. Superior to the basement membrane is a layer of basal cells from which all other cells differentiate. Above the basal cell layer are five or six layers of deep prickle, or parabasal cells, and superficial to them the cells differentiate into intermediate (superficial prickle cells)

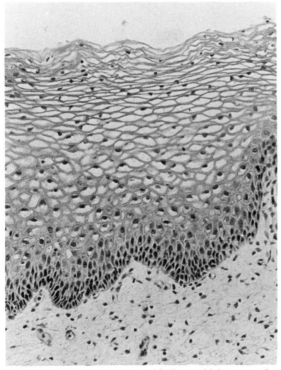

Fig. 16/8 Normal squamous epithelium which covers the vaginal portion of the cervix (× 160)

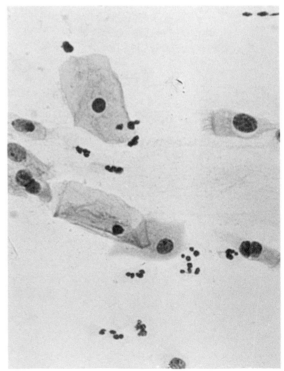

Fig. 16/9 Normal exfoliated cervical cells; at the right edge of the illustration two ciliated endocervical cells can be seen (× 400)

and superficial layers (Fig. **16/8**). The intermediate layer consists of large cells with reticulated nuclei, and vacuoles containing glycogen are found in the cytoplasm. The superficial layer varies in thickness, depending on the oestrogen/progesterone ratio present, and consists of flattened cells with small nuclei. Glycogen is present in the cytoplasm, and a small amount of keratin is produced ('cornified cells'). Desquamation of superficial cells (and some intermediate cells) goes on constantly, and differentiation of new cells proceeds simultaneously by mitotic divisions of basal cells.

The characteristics of the superficial and intermediate cells are best studied by scraping the cervix with a wooden spatula, or a cotton-tipped swabstick, and making a preparation of the smear on a slide. This is then stained by Papanicolaou's stain. The stained preparation is known colloquially as a 'Pap smear'. The principle of the staining is to achieve clear nuclear definition and to define cytoplasmic coloration.

If the epithelium is normal, only superficial and a few intermediate cells appear in the smear (Fig. **16/9**), but markedly abnormal epithelia tend to desquamate more readily and bizarre abnormally-shaped (dyskaryotic) nuclei and cells are seen. This observation led Papanicolaou to suggest that carcinoma might be detected in a preclinical stage by examination of the cytology of exfoliated cervical cells.

THE EPIDEMIOLOGY OF CERVICAL CANCER

Recent studies have shown that in many cases the nuclear dyskaryosis and cellular dysplasia are due to infection with the human papillomavirus (HPV), particularly types 16, 18, and 6. Epidemiological evidence indicates that between 10 and 30 per cent of sexually-active women have been infected by the age of 30, but the infection is clinically obvious in a small proportion.

HPV is sexually transmissible and is the cause of genital warts. In women, the initial infection may be on the vulva or the vagina, spread to the cervix occurring later, or the cervix may be infected from the start. In men, genital warts occur on the penis or other external genitals and may be so small as to be clinically difficult to detect. Studies have shown that about 60 per cent of male partners of women who have HPV infection of the cervix or vagina have evidence of penile infection.

The natural history of HPV infection is still being elucidated. In a 36-month period, infected women may eliminate the virus from the cervix (in 50 per cent); the virus may remain, without causing any further cytological or histological change in 30 per cent; or progression may occur in 20 per cent (3 per cent developing carcinoma *in situ* or invasive cancer of the cervix).

HPV infection of the cervix, particularly with strains 16 and 18 appears to be a major factor in the development of cervical carcinoma, operating with a co-agent.

As the infection at first causes nuclear dyskaryosis and cellular dysplasia, cervical (Pap) smears will identify this early infection.

CERVICAL EXFOLIATIVE CYTOLOGY

In order that the maximum protection against invasive cervical cancer can be offered to women, a cytological and colposcopic service should be made available. It is recommended that it is offered to all sexually active women aged 16 to 60, and to all antenatal patients. So that the full benefit of the service is obtained, it is recommended that the attending doctor examine the patient's breasts, and perform a careful pelvic examination after the cervical smear has been taken. It appears that a single smear will miss about 7 per cent of cases of carcinoma-*in-situ* or early invasive carcinoma, and for this reason it is recommended that a second cervical smear is taken 6 to 12 months after the initial smear. If the two smears are 'negative', smears should be taken thereafter at intervals of 1 to 3 years. After the age of 40 a woman would be advised to visit her doctor annually so that a breast examination may be made and she may be examined vaginally to determine whether ovarian enlargement is present. At this visit the woman may elect to have a cervical smear made, although the cost-benefit of this, over smears taken every 3 years, is not clear.

Technique for taking a cervical smear

A special tray should be available on which are placed the following: a slide, a vaginal speculum, a plastic Ayres spatula and a cotton-wool-tipped swab stick (alternatively a Cervex brush or similar device

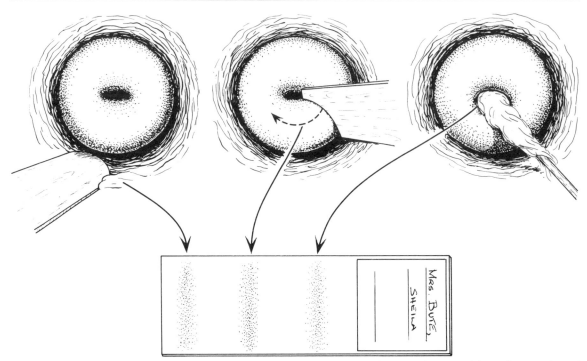

Fig. 16/10 Methods of obtaining cells from the cervix for cytological examination, (1) using a special wooden spatula, and (2) using a cotton-tipped swab stick

can replace the spatula and the swab stick) and spray-on fixative for the smear.

Warm and moisten the speculum in warm tap water and insert it to expose the cervix before doing a bimanual pelvic examination. The tip of the spatula or brush is introduced into the cervical canal and the instrument is rotated through 360 degrees twice. The material from the exocervix and endocervix is smeared on to the slide and fixed. The slide is labelled and sent to a cytological laboratory with the information filled in accurately on the form provided by the laboratory (Fig. **16/10**).

Cytologists have agreed that nuclear abnormalities should form the basis of a cytological diagnosis. They have agreed to report smears as: (1) unsatisfactory, (2) inflammatory or inconclusive, (3) normal, (4) mild dyskaryosis (CIN 1), (5) moderate dyskaryosis (CIN 2), (6) severe dyskaryosis (CIN 3). The diagnosis of 'atypical' cells should no longer be used.

Unsatisfactory smears are those in which a diagnosis cannot be made because of too few cells or incorrect processing of the slide. *Inflammatory or inconclusive smears* (sometimes called borderline smears) are those in which the cells are distorted by the effects of trichomoniasis, candidosis, or herpes simplex virus. Infection by the *human papillomavirus* is included but should receive special mention. In HPV infection the nucleus is often binucleate and the area of cytoplasm surrounding it is translucent (koilocytosis). If trichomoniasis or candidosis is identified treatment should be given. Women showing inflammatory or inconclusive smears should have a repeat smear 4 to 6 months later. Women whose smear shows HPV infection but no dyskaryosis should have the smear repeated in 4 months and if the infection persists should be referred for colposcopy. This also applies to smears showing *mild dyskaryosis*.

If *moderate or severe dyskaryosis* is detected (Fig. **16/11**) a colposcopic examination should be made and punch biopsies taken if indicated.

Over 90 per cent of smears will be reported as normal; 3 to 5 per cent will be unsatisfactory or will show inflammatory changes; 3 to 5 per cent will show HPV infection or mild dyskaryosis, and 1 to 3 per cent will show moderate or severe dyskaryosis.

Colposcopy

The colposcope is a system of lenses which enables a

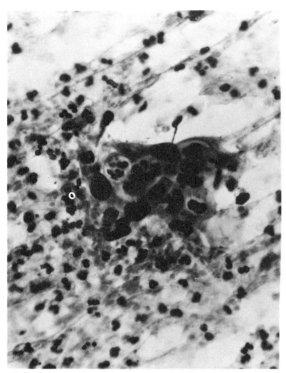

Fig. 16/11 Exfoliated cervical cells showing 'severe dyskary-osis' (× 400)

Grade I	Mild dysplasia	Dysplasia of low degree
Grade II	Moderate dysplasia	
Grade III	Severe dysplasia/	Dysplasia of high degree
	Carcinoma-*in-situ*	

Table 16/1 CIN Classification

An experienced observer can differentiate mild dysplasia, severe dysplasia, and carcinoma with a high degree of accuracy, but confirmation of the probable diagnosis is essential and is made by directed punch biopsy and histological examination.

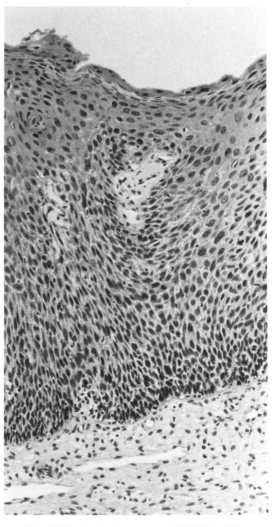

Fig. 16/12 Dysplasia (moderate) CIN II (× 160)

trained observer to examine visually the cervix and upper vagina at a magnification of between × 5 and × 25. Experience has permitted colposcopists to describe the appearance of a normal cervix, particularly the transformation zone, as this is the area where dysplastic changes are most likely to occur.

A normal transformation zone viewed through a colposcope shows a smooth surface, pale in colour. Often there are minute papillary projections, and openings of 'glands' may be seen. Often medial to this is the grape-like appearance of the columnar epithelium which lines the cervical canal.

Dysplasia of varying degrees and carcinoma-*in-situ* lead to alterations in the appearance of the transformation zone, in four specific ways: (1) surface pattern; (2) colour tone and opacity (e.g. 'keratosis'); (3) vascular pattern; and (4) intercapillary distance. The changes which occur are that the surface pattern resembles a mosaic pavement (mosaic effect); there may be evidence of white (keratotic) patches; the blood vessels may appear as punctate dots, and, because of the size of the mosaics, the intercapillary distances are often increased, or bizarre branching vessels may be seen.

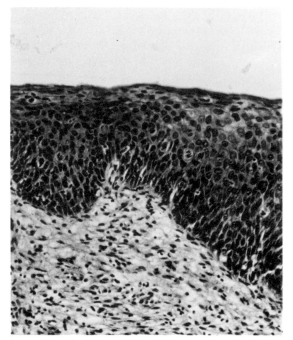

Fig. 16/13 Dysplasia (severe) CIN 3 (× 160)

CERVICAL INTRA-EPITHELIAL NEOPLASIA

The difficulty of making a precise histological diagnosis and the uncertainty of whether the identified lesion will regress, persist, or progress has led to the concept of cervical intra-epithelial neoplasia, which includes all dysplastic cells and cells with dyskaryotic nuclei. Three grades have been described (Table 16/1). The grades can be related to the histological appearance of the tissue.

CERVICAL HISTOLOGY

The cervical tissue obtained by biopsy may show a normal appearance, or may show mild, moderate or severe dysplasia.

Mild dysplasia is characterized by nuclear abnormalities in the basal third of the epithelium. The upper two-thirds is usually well differentiated. The presence of koilocytosis is suggestive of HPV infection. The strain of the virus can be determined by filter-*in-situ* hybridization or HPV DNA analysis.

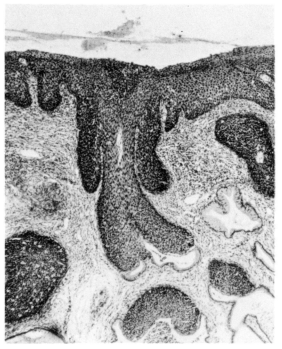

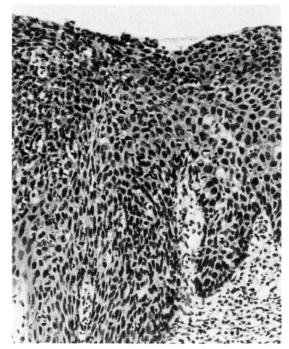

Fig. 16/14 Cervical biopsy from the patient whose cervical smear is shown in Fig. **16/11**. Carcinoma-*in-situ* was found. (A) (× 40) There appears to be invasion of the tissues but in reality the cells have only crept into endocervical crypts. (B) (× 160) The lack of stratification and pleomorphism of the cells is seen

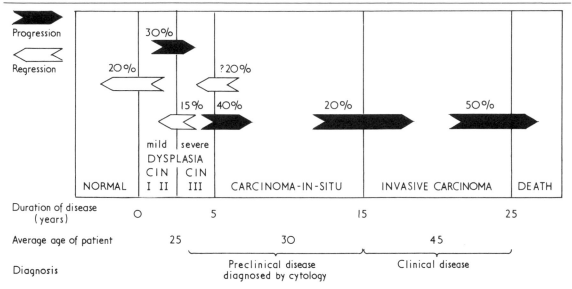

Fig. 16/15 The 'life cycle' of unstable cervical epithelium

Moderate dysplasia (Fig. **16/12**). Some dyskaryotic nuclei are found in the upper layers of the epithelium, abnormal nuclei are more common and reach a higher level in the epithelium than in mild dysplasia.

Severe dysplasia is diagnosed by finding basal cell dysplasia with a high nuclear-cytoplasmic ratio at all levels and only slight stratification of the layers (Fig. **16/13**).

Carcinoma-in-situ is diagnosed histologically when: (1) there is no differentiation as the surface is approached, the entire epithelial thickness being involved, (2) the basal cell layer has lost its pallisade arrangement, (3) the nuclei vary in size and shape and stain deeply, (4) the cytoplasm of each cell is scanty, (5) the cells look crowded (Fig. **16/14**).

THE NATURAL HISTORY OF CIN
(Fig. 16/15)

Nine studies have been made in which patients who

have CIN I have been followed up for at least 3 years. Analysis of the reports shows that between 45 and 60 per cent had regressed to normal, but in some CIN had recurred later. In 20 to 30 per cent the mild dysplasia (CIN I) had persisted, and in 10 to 30 per cent it had progressed to CIN III. If the cervix was infected by HPV (particularly types 16 or 18) progression was more likely to occur.

TREATMENT OF CIN

Treatment of CIN depends on several factors, including the age of the woman and her desire to retain her capacity to reproduce. The use of colposcopy has permitted greater individualization of treatment, and management is now based more on the location and extent of the lesion than on the histological findings.

As mentioned earlier, if CIN I is associated with HPV infection, a further smear should be made in 4

Cytology	Histology		Action
Normal	0.1%	CIN II or III	Repeat in 3y
Inflammatory (excluding HPV)	6%	CIN II or III	Treat. Repeat smear in 6mo
HPV infection	30%	CIN II or III	Repeat in 4mo. If persists, colposcopy
Mild dyskaryosis	50%	CIN II or III	Colposcopy
Moderate dyskaryosis	65%	CIN II or III	Colposcopy
Severe dyskaryosis	85%	CIN II or III	Urgent colposcopy
	5%	cancer	

Table 16/2 Management of abnormal cytological smears

The lesion should be destroyed by laser, cryosurgery or electrocautery. CO_2 laser therapy, under colposcopic control, performed by a trained surgeon is the preferred choice. The treatment is made under local anaesthesia (4ml of 2 per cent lignocaine) and the woman does not require admission to hospital. About 40 per cent of women complain of pain of varying severity for a variable number of days after the procedure (which is similar to that following cautery or cryosurgery), but the vaginal discharge is less and has a less offensive odour. An advantage of laser is that the cervix heals without scarring, which prevents cervical stenosis and makes follow-up Pap smears easier to perform. Cryosurgery can also be performed as an outpatient procedure but may need to be repeated. Electrocautery usually requires admission to hospital and is made under anaesthesia.

Treatment for CIN is followed by psychological as well as physical symptoms. Many women feel depressed and upset, particularly if insensitive health professionals make remarks like 'nuns don't get CIN', or imply that the woman must have been promiscuous.

Follow-up is essential as some lesions recur or are not completely eliminated.

If the abnormal areas on the cervix extend up the cervical canal, and the upper limit cannot be identified by colposcopic inspection, cervical conization (Fig. **16/16**) or hysterectomy is indicated.

Cone biopsy is associated with a 10 per cent chance of postoperative haemorrhage. If the woman subsequently becomes pregnant, she has a three-fold chance the pregnancy will be curtailed and that she will give birth to a low-birth-weight (preterm) baby.

Carcinoma with micro-invasion Stage IA (see p. 182) is treated by hysterectomy with the removal of a vaginal cuff. There is no indication for pelvic lymphadenectomy, and the ovaries should be preserved in premenopausal women.

The knowledge by a woman that she has CIN and that the condition may progress to cervical cancer may cause a considerable disturbance to her relationship with her partner and to her feelings about sexual intercourse. The anxiety and uncertainty should be resolved as far as possible by giving the woman a full explanation about CIN and by giving her the opportunity to ask questions. This requires time and the ability of the health professional to listen to the woman as well as talk to her.

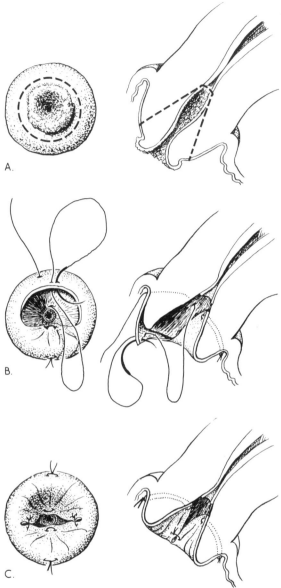

Fig. 16/16 Diagram showing how the raw bed from which the cone has been removed is covered with flaps of cervical epithelium

months and a colposcopy is made. If abnormalities are found treatment by laser, cryosurgery or electrocautery should be made. In the absence of HPV, CIN I may be treated or may be followed with Pap smears at 6-month intervals.

CIN II and III require treatment, after colposcopic inspection has determined the extent of the lesion.

THE PREVENTION OF CERVICAL CANCER

Control of the sexually-transmitted HPV will do much to reduce the incidence of cervical cancer. Preventive measures include: (1) the later onset of sexual intercourse by women, (2) a reduction in the number of sexual partners by men and women, (3) the use of condoms when either partner is uncertain about the sexual behaviour of the other.

Cervical cancer will be controlled if communities can persuade all sexually-active women to have Pap smears taken at one-to-three-year intervals and, if abnormalities are found, to have further investigations performed and treatment offered.

To achieve these objectives will require education, motivation and money.

INVASIVE CARCINOMA OF THE CERVIX

Carcinoma of the cervix is the second most common gynaecological cancer (malignancies of the breast being the most common). Most cases occur in women over the age of 35, and the annual risk of a woman developing cervical cancer is about 1 in 1000 (Table 16/3). As has been noted, the disease is largely preventable by screening, using cervical cytology. By the time cervical cancer is clinically detectable, no matter what treatment is given, one woman in three will be dead within 5 years.

PATHOLOGICAL CONSIDERATIONS

Cervical cancers can conveniently be divided into (1) those which grow outwards (exophytic or fungating types), and (2) those which grow inwards (infiltrating or excavating types). The exophytic type is more common (65 per cent) than the endophytic infiltrating type (35 per cent). In the former, the normal cervix is completely or partially replaced by a friable, granular, necrotic, fungating mass, which surrounds the external os and may extend into the vaginal fornices (Fig. 16/17). The tumour may be ulcerated and usually is associated with a bloody, purulent, offensive discharge. It bleeds easily on slight trauma. The infiltrating type is less obvious, but enlargement of the cervix is common.

Age	Incidence (per 100 000 women)
20–24	1
25–29	15
30–34	25
35–64	45

Table 16/3 The incidence of cervical carcinoma in women who have not been screened regularly

Histology

Two types of cervical carcinoma can be identified: (1) squamous cell carcinoma which develops in the transformation zone of squamous epithelium (Fig. 16/18), and (2) adenocarcinoma, which develops from the endocervical columnar cells. Squamous cell carcinoma accounts for 95 per cent, and the adenocarcinoma for 5 per cent, of all cases. Within the two major classifications, varying degrees of de-differentiation of the cells is found, and the greater the anaplasia, the worse the prognosis. Lymphocytic infiltration surrounds the invading cells, suggesting an immunological response by the host. The greater the lymphocytic infiltration, the better is the prognosis. However, the histological grading is of less value in assessing prognosis than is the clinical staging made under anaesthesia prior to treatment.

SPREAD OF THE TUMOUR BEYOND THE CERVIX

As with any malignant growth, spread of viable tumour cells may be (1) by direct extension, (2) by

	Age			
Organ	30–49	50–59	60–69	All ages
Breast	410	2100	3000	850
Uterus:				
cervix	120	300	450	140
endometrium	60	550	1200	270
Colo-rectum	45	375	1000	95
Ovary	60	230	310	90

Table 16/4 Age specific rates of certain cancers in women (per 100 000). Data derived from Feldman AR, New Eng J Med, 1986; 315, 1394–7; et al.)

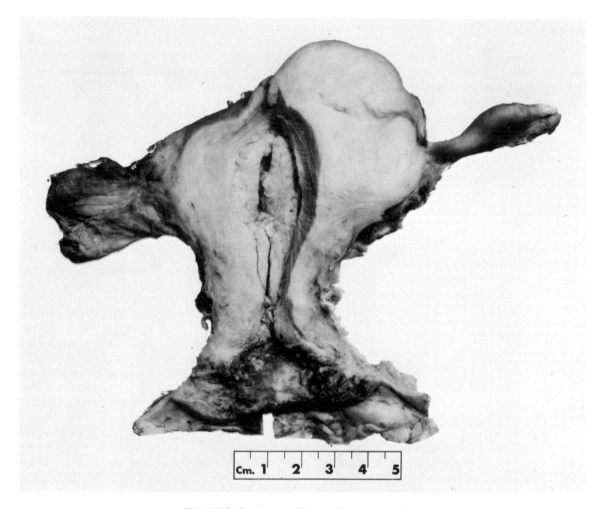

Fig. 16/17 Carcinoma of the cervix – gross specimen

the lymphatics, and (3) by the bloodstream. Carcinoma of the cervix spreads mainly by the first two routes, and haematogenous spread is uncommon except as a terminal event.

Direct spread may be downwards to involve the vagina, or upwards to involve the body of the uterus. Spread in these two directions is usually superficial. The cancer may also spread laterally to involve the parametrium, anteriorly to involve the bladder, or posteriorly to the rectum and cul-de-sac. The parametrial spread is of great importance, as the tumour cells frequently surround and compress the ureter. In all cases of spread, the body resists the invasion and an inflammatory reaction occurs beyond and around the tumour cells. The organ most frequently involved in direct spread is the vagina, followed by the parametrium. Involvement of the corpus uteri and the bladder is infrequent.

Lymphatic spread is of importance because of the rich lymphatic supply of the cervix. Involvement probably occurs early, when small fragments of tumour cells invade the lymphatics, and individual fragments break off as emboli. Most of these are destroyed by the woman's immune processes, but a few may obtain a foothold and grow in lymph nodes as metastases. The nodes most frequently involved are the external iliac nodes (47 per cent of cases with lymph node involvement), followed by the obturator node (20 per cent), the hypogastric nodes (7 per cent), and the paracervical nodes (2 per cent of cases).

Blood vessel spread leads to distant metastases, and is by the veins rather than the arteries.

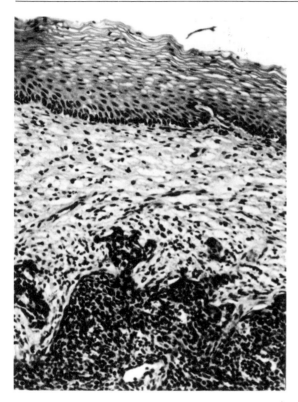

Fig. 16/18 The histological appearances of carcinoma of the cervix. Note that in this section the epithelium is intact and the malignant cells are spreading through the connective tissues of the cervix (× 160)

CAUSE OF DEATH IN CANCER OF THE CERVIX UTERI

About 50 per cent of deaths occur as a result of ureteric compression leading to stasis of urine and pyelonephritis, or to uraemia as the obstruction becomes more marked. In 20 per cent of cases infection, usually pelvic peritonitis, is the cause. In 10 per cent of cases pulmonary complications, mainly due to metastases, and in a further 5 per cent involvement of the intestines (particularly the sigmoid and rectum) is responsible for death.

CLINICAL CLASSIFICATION OF CARCINOMA OF THE CERVIX

As was noted, the clinical classification of carcinoma of the cervix is the most helpful guide to prognosis. The present classification is a modification by the International Federation of Gynaecology and Ob-

stetrics of that suggested by the League of Nations in 1929 (Table **16/5**). Although difficulties occur in accurate 'staging', particularly if the examiner misinterprets the inflammatory reaction as tumour growth, staging has great value for comparing the results of treatment from various clinics.

The higher the stage at the initial classification, the greater is the chance of lymph node involvement and the poorer the prognosis. This is shown in Table **16/6**.

DIAGNOSIS

No specific symptoms characterize carcinoma of the cervix, and frequently there are no symptoms at all, especially in the early stages. It is imperative, therefore, for women to have periodic diagnostic examinations so that cervical malignancy may be detected in the preclinical phase. This requires an intensive effort by each doctor to educate the patients he cares for, in the value of this procedure.

In the later stages, irregular bleeding, particularly postcoitally, or a pink vaginal discharge, particularly after micturition, may be the only indication that a cervical malignancy is present. Indeed, irregular bleeding found in a woman over the age of 35 should be considered due to carcinoma until proved otherwise.

Pain is a late symptom, and is typically of sciatic distribution radiating down the back of the buttock and leg to the knee.

Invasive carcinoma is diagnosed by histological examination of a biopsy of the suspicious area. As the surface of the tumour is often covered with necrotic debris no, or only few, tumour cells are present; for this reason exfoliative cytology may show no malignant cells and cannot be relied upon for diagnosis. The prime place of exfoliative cytology is in the diagnosis of preclinical, pre-invasive carcinoma of the cervix. In this connection, it must be stressed that if the cervical exfoliative cytology is negative and the patient has an unhealthy looking cervix, a further opinion must be sought, and further investigations made, which may include a biopsy of the cervix.

TREATMENT OF CARCINOMA OF THE CERVIX

Study of the literature shows beyond any doubt that the best results of treatment only occur if all patients

Stage 0   Intra-epithelial carcinoma, so-called carcinoma-*in-situ*

Stage I   The carcinoma is strictly confined to the cervix (and extension to the corpus is disregarded)

Stage I(a) Preclinical carcinomas of the cervix, that is, those diagnosed only by microscopy

Stage I(a)1 Minimal microscopically evident stromal invasion

Stage I(a)2 Lesions detected microscopically that can be measured. The upper limit of the measurement should not show a depth of invasion of more than 5mm taken from the base of the epithelium, either surface or glandular, from which it originates, and a second dimension, the horizontal spread, must not exceed 7mm. Larger lesions should be staged as I(b)

Stage I(b) Lesions of greater dimensions than Stage I(a)2 whether seen clinically or not. Preformed space involvement should not alter the staging but should be specifically recorded so as to determine whether it should affect treatment decisions in the future

Stage II   The carcinoma extends beyond the cervix but has not extended onto the pelvic wall. The carcinoma involves the vagina, but not the lower third

Stage II (a) The carcinoma involves the parametrium

Stage II (b) The carcinoma involves the vagina but not the lower third

Stage III   The carcinoma has extended onto the pelvic wall. On rectal examination there is no cancer-free space between the tumour and the pelvic wall. The carcinoma involves the lower third of the vagina

Stage IV   The carcinoma has extended beyond the true pelvis or has involved the mucosa of the bladder or the rectum. However, the presence of bullous oedema is not sufficient evidence to classify a case of Stage IV

Note. It is unavoidable that the personal opinion of the examiner influences his stage of various cases, and this is especially true with those classified as Stage II and Stage III. Therefore, the Cancer Committee recommended that, when reporting results of therapy in carcinoma of the cervix, all cases examined be reported. Also that, in arriving at an opinion of the results achieved at a given institution in Stage II, for instance, the statistics for Stage III be considered simultaneously.

Table 16/5 Clinical stages of carcinoma of the cervix (International Federation of Gynaecology and Obstetrics)

with carcinoma of the cervix are treated in special centres, staffed by radiotherapists, gynaecologists and physicists, and equipped with the most modern apparatus. There is no place for the occasional surgeon or radiotherapist to 'try his hand' at treating cervical carcinoma. A single centre can probably meet the needs of a population of about 3 000 000.

Over the past two decades there has been continuing discussion whether the primary treatment of invasive carcinoma should be surgical or radiotherapeutic. This has now been resolved, and the consensus is that for squamous cell carcinoma Stage I(a), total hysterectomy with an adequate vaginal cuff (or conization, if childbearing capacity is to be preserved) is the appropriate treatment.

For Stages Ib and IIa, there seems to be no advantage of one modality over the other. Those who prefer hysterectomy (with lymphadenectomy) claim

that surgery (1) preserves ovarian and coital function, especially in younger women; (2) enables a more accurate assessment of lymphatic and lymph node spread to be made. If such spread has occurred, they recommend chemotherapy and/or irradiation; and (3) if major complications follow irradiation, they are difficult to treat: surgery avoids this hazard.

Those who prefer radiotherapy, except in special circumstances, claim that the possible residual after-effects are less, and that the 5-year survival is the same as after surgery. They note that after extended hysterectomy (Wertheim hysterectomy), lymphoedema of one or both legs occurs in 10 per cent of women, and about the same proportion have marked bladder dysfunction. In addition between 3 and 20 per cent of women develop lymphocysts in the pelvis.

Radiotherapy may also be followed by complica-

Stage	Lymph node involvement	5-year survival
0	0	100
I(a)	< 1	100
I(b)	15	85
II(a)	25	75
II(b)	35	55
III	55	35
IV	> 65	< 15

Table 16/6 Squamous carcinoma of the cervix – lymph node involvement and survival rates

tions especially when the expertise of the radiotherapeutic team is limited. The immediate complications consist of nausea (radiation sickness), cystitis and moderate diarrhoea during the course of the external radiation. Later complications occur in about 12 per cent of patients, and are mainly due to the internal radiation. They occur on average 6 to 18 months after the initial radiation and consist of 'cystitis' (frequency and dysuria) and proctitis, which is usually mild. In about 1 per cent of cases rectal stenosis, or a rectal fistula, occurs; and in 1 per cent a vesicovaginal fistula develops, mostly when radiation has been used to treat a recurrence. Some degree of vaginal stenosis always develops, but if oestrogen cream is used, and the partner is gentle, coitus is usually satisfactory. In cases where it is painful other techniques of sexual pleasuring can be chosen.

A few centres first give radiotherapy and follow this six weeks later with a radical hysterectomy. Statistics indicate that there is no additional benefit from the combined approach and postoperative disabilities are increased.

In reality, radiotherapy and radical surgery are not in competition in the treatment of carcinoma of the cervix: each has its place and the decision of the most appropriate treatment for the individual patient should be made after discussion between the members of the oncological team. It is unfortunate that few controlled studies defining the place of each therapeutic regimen have been made.

Advanced cervical carcinoma (Stages IIb, III and IV), unfortunately, still occurs in spite of cervical cytological screening. In determining treatment, the wishes of the patient and the 'quality' of her short remaining life must be taken into account. Neither surgery nor radiotherapy provide much hope of cure, and are often followed by marked complications. In some centres these patients are being treated initially with combination chemotherapy. The idea is that chemotherapy will reduce the tumour mass and make it more sensitive to radiation and eliminate distant metastases. Chemotherapy should be followed by radiotherapy to eliminate malignant disease in the pelvis, and possibly surgery.

Chemotherapy is also suggested as the treatment of choice in persistent or recurrent disease, unless the disease is confined to the central pelvis when surgical exenteration may be suggested as an alternative.

Chapter 17

The Endometrium

Abnormal patterns of endometrial growth and the resultant abnormal uterine bleeding have been considered in Chapter 7. In this chapter two benign conditions, which, in certain circumstances, may progress towards a malignant form, will be discussed. The two abnormal growth patterns are endometrial polyps and endometrial hyperplasia. Both result from prolonged unopposed oestrogenic stimulation of the endometrium. The malignant form, endometrial carcinoma, will also be considered.

BENIGN CONDITIONS

ENDOMETRIAL POLYPS

Endometrial polyps are localized overgrowths of endometrial glands and stroma, so that the affected area projects above the surface of the surrounding endometrium in a sessile or pedunculated manner. The change is more common in women above the age of 30, and is most frequently found in peri-menopausal women. There may be no symptoms, especially in older women; or abnormal uterine bleeding may occur, showing as postmenstrual staining or spotting, or as intermenstrual bleeding. When this happens, particularly if the patient is over 35, a careful diagnostic curettage is essential to exclude malignant causes of abnormal uterine bleeding. If the polyps are fleshy and pedunculated, the curettage may fail to remove them; therefore when the condition is suspected, the curette should be supplemented by the use of a narrow polyp forceps. This is inserted into the uterus and advanced to the fundus. The jaws are opened and closed whilst rotating the forceps through 90 degrees. The manoeuvre is repeated several times, and the tissue brought out of the uterus with a curette (Fig. **17/1**).

ENDOMETRIAL HYPERPLASIA

In endometrial hyperplasia there is a generalized overgrowth of the entire endometrium, the glands, the stroma and the capillaries being involved. The condition is found at all ages, but is most common at each end of the reproductive period, and is due to persistent oestrogenic stimulation without the regulating effect of progesterone. The hormonal imbalance may cause myohyperplasia, and consequently the uterus may be uniformly enlarged to some extent, and generally is referred to as being 'bulky'. Endometrial hyperplasia is frequently associated with the clinical entity of dysfunctional uterine bleeding.

Histological findings

In many cases gross inspection of the endometrium merely shows it to be thicker than normal, but occasionally it is polypoidal and profuse. The histological appearance is variable, and different patterns may co-exist in the different areas of the endometrium. The most usual pattern is *cystic hyperplasia*. The

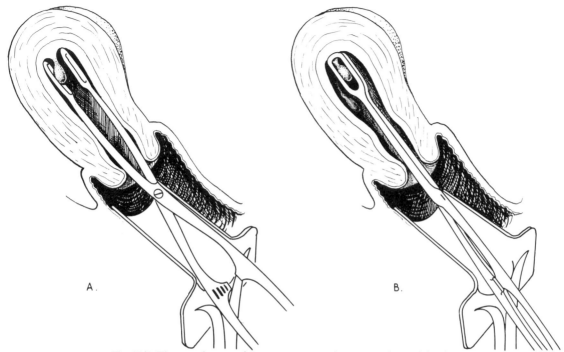

Fig. 17/1 The use of sponge forceps to secure and remove endometrial polyps

endometrial glands show varying degrees of cystic dilatation, some being normal, others greatly distended. The cells lining the glands are tall, columnar and regular in size, with heavily staining nuclei and scanty cytoplasm. There is no evidence of secretory activity. The stroma is compact-looking and cellular, and contains collections of lymphocytes (Fig. **17/2**). A 'burnt-out', inactive form of cystic hyperplasia is found in 10 per cent of postmenopausal women. It is caused by the following sequence of events: in the perimenopausal years an active cystic hyperplasia develops, but later as oestrogen stimulation ceases, cellular activity also ceases, leaving an endometrial hyperplasia which is retrogressive in character. The gland epithelium is inactive and the stroma is fibrotic. Both this form and active cystic hyperplasia are benign.

In a few cases, the glandular epithelium is more active and less well differentiated, so that *atypical (adenomatous) hyperplasia* results. The cells lining the glands show a marked variation in size, shape, polarity and staining. The nuclei are varied in shape and size, and the cytoplasm may be increased in amount. The degree of dysplasia may be such that the pathologist may find it difficult to decide if the condition is benign or malignant.

SYMPTOMS

The patient may complain of menorrhagia or of metrorrhagia; the usual symptoms being irregular, occasionally profuse, bleeding. Short periods of amenorrhoea usually separate episodes of bleeding. The diagnosis is made by curettage.

TREATMENT

Endometrial hyperplasia and polyps

The treatment of endometrial hyperplasia and endometrial polyps depends upon (1) the age of the patient, and (2) the presence, or absence, of other abnormalities, particularly the histological pattern of the curettings. Endometrial hyperplasia found in a young woman should be treated conservatively. Often the curettage made to establish the diagnosis is curative, as the new endometrium regenerates normally; but if the symptoms recur, hormonal therapy using a progestogen is indicated unless the woman is anxious to become pregnant. The choice of progestogen depends on individual preference but norethisterone 5 to 15mg daily from day 15 to 25 of the menstrual cycle for several months is usually curative.

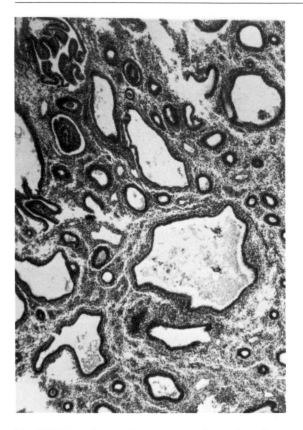

Fig. 17/2 The microscopic appearance of curettings showing cystic hyperplasia

As most patients with endometrial hyperplasia do not ovulate, women desiring to become pregnant should have infertility investigations performed. If anovulation is the main, or only, abnormal finding, treatment with clomiphene should be initiated, as described in Chapter 8. In older women, particularly in the climacteric period, curettage is also curative in many cases, but if menorrhagia recurs, the use of hormones, or resort to hysterectomy, is necessary.

Severe atypical hyperplasia

If the patient has reached the climacteric, or has no desire for procreation, total hysterectomy is the treatment of choice. If the patient wants to retain her reproductive capabilities, or to avoid surgery, the use of progestogens over a period of months is indicated. Several workers have found that atypical endometrial hyperplasia retrogresses, if potent progestogens are administered, and in some cases the endometrium becomes completely atrophic. The use of 17-hydroxyprogesterone caproate, 125mg intramuscularly each week, norethisterone 5 to 15mg, by mouth, daily, or medroxyprogesterone acetate 5mg orally each day, appears satisfactory. The drugs are given continuously for 6 to 12 weeks, when a further curettage is performed. If this shows a normal, or an atrophic endometrium, the patient may be considered cured. If the atypical endometrial hyperplasia persists hysterectomy is indicated.

ENDOMETRIAL CARCINOMA

The most common malignancy of the corpus uteri is adenocarcinoma, which arises from a malignant change in the cells lining the endometrial glands; although sarcoma and choriocarcinoma occasionally develop. Endometrial carcinoma affects 1 in every 1 000 postmenopausal women each year. The peak period of incidence (occurring in 75 per cent of cases) is in the 55 to 65 age group, or 10 years later than the peak age incidence of carcinoma of the cervix; but 25 per cent of cases are diagnosed prior to the menopause.

The type of woman who is likely to develop endometrial carcinoma is very different from the woman who develops cervical carcinoma. She is likely to be postmenopausal, has a 60 per cent chance that the menopause was delayed beyond the age of 50, and that menstruation in the premenopausal years was profuse. She is usually unmarried, or if married is sterile or has had a rather large number of spontaneous abortions. She is likely to be overweight; to have hypertension; and to have an abnormal glucose tolerance, or to be an actual diabetic. One patient in three has coincident uterine myomata.

AETIOLOGY

The profile just delineated suggests that endometrial carcinoma occurs in women with some disturbance of hormone secretion. Postmenopausal women synthesize oestradiol and oestrone from androstenedione by aromatization in their peripheral fat. In conditions of obesity, increased age and hepatic disease, the aromatization rate is increased. Endometrial carcinoma is also increased in women who have raised plasma levels of androstenedione, such as in polycystic ovarian disease and hyperthecosis. These findings suggest that endogenous oestrogens (and administered exogenous oestrogen, if not opposed by progestogen) play a crucial part in the development of endometrial carcinoma. However, there are no differences in the serum levels of oestradiol, oestrone, androstenedione or testosterone in women with endometrial cancer compared with 'control' women of similar age and weight.

The development of malignancy in an area of atypical endometrial hyperplasia has been observed. Active cystic endometrial hyperplasia is a usually benign condition; but in a few instances it develops into atypical hyperplasia, which must be considered potentially malignant. A few cases of atypical hyperplasia de-differentiate further into a severe form of atypical dysplasia and hyperplasia (miscalled adenocarcinoma-*in-situ*), and 10 to 30 per cent of these subsequently, over a period of years, transform into invasive adenocarcinoma of the endometrium. It is impossible to determine if severe atypical dysplasia ever reverts into a less malignant form, as the condition is diagnosed by curettage which also removes all the endometrium, and is usually treated by total hysterectomy, unless the patient is anxious to preserve her reproductive function.

PATHOLOGY

The tumour may develop in any part of the body of the uterus and starts as a localized form, usually in the fundal area, where it forms a sessile or pedunculated growth (Fig. **17/3**). In about 15 per cent of cases it develops in the lower part of the cavity and

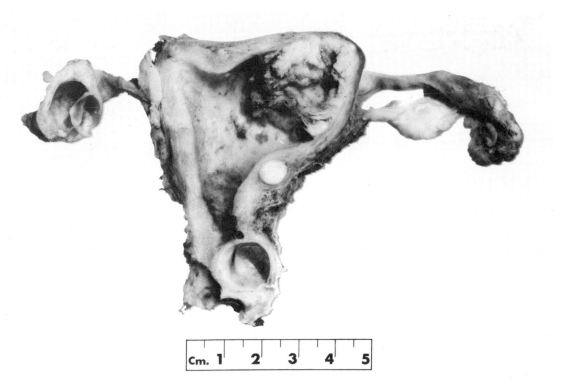

Fig. 17/3 Endometrial carcinoma, localized in the fundal area. Gross specimen. It can be seen that a pyometra and a Nabothian follicle are also present

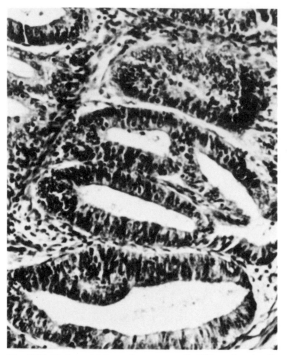

Fig. 17/4 Endometrial carcinoma – well differentiated cells (× 160)

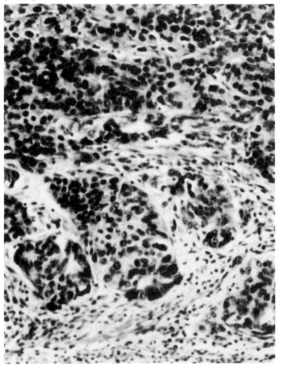

Fig. 17/5 Endometrial carcinoma – poorly differentiated, anaplastic type (× 160)

spreads downwards towards the cervix. The tumour grows slowly, tending to spread over the endometrium to form the diffuse type of malignancy, rather than to invade the myometrium, although this ultimately occurs. Once the cervix is involved, the prognosis is much worse and the patient must be treated as if she had a primary cancer of the cervix.

Endometrial carcinoma shows various histological patterns, and the more undifferentiated the cells, the worse the prognosis. The International Federation of Obstetrics and Gynaecology recommended, in 1970, that a histological grading of endometrial carcinomas be made, based on the overall character of the malignant cells, and the proportion of de-differentiated cells. In Grade 1, the most favourable group prognostically, the tumour is adenomatous and more than 75 per cent of the cells are differentiated (Fig. **17/4**). In Grade 2, the number of differentiated cells is fewer, and partly solid areas are found. In Grade 3, the tumour is mostly solid and the cells are poorly differentiated (Fig. **17/5**).

As the development of endometrial carcinoma is slow, the majority of cases diagnosed fall into Grade 1, and are adenocarcinomas in appearance. In about one-fifth of cases patches of squamous metaplasia occur within the adenoacarcinoma. The tumour is then called an adenoacanthoma (Figs. **17/6** and **17/7**). The prognosis of adenoacanthoma is that of a differentiated adenocarcinoma, not of an anaplastic carcinoma, which is much more sinister. Anaplastic carcinoma accounts for only 5 per cent of all cases, and is diagnosed when histological examination of the tissue shows no glandular pattern in any area. Occasionally the malignant change is found confined to an endometrial polyp but usually by the time symptoms occur, it has spread to involve at least some portion of the endometrium.

Since many of the patients are postmenopausal, atrophy of the cervical canal may have occurred, or the canal may be occluded by growth. Because the carcinoma develops from the epithelium which lines the endometrial glands, it secretes mucin as it grows, and bleeding is likely to occur. If the cervix is occluded, the uterus is unable to expel the secretions, which may become infected causing a pyometra. This alters the prognosis significantly, not only because of the associated infection, but because the increased intra-uterine tension encourages the earlier invasion of the myometrium.

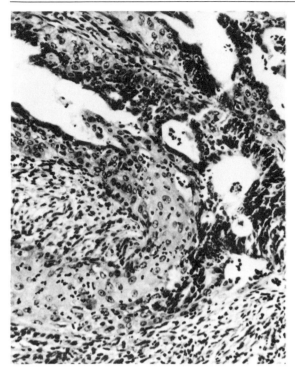

Fig. 17/6 Adenoacanthoma (× 160)

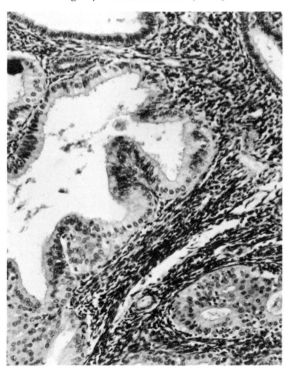

Fig. 17/7 Adenoacanthoma-*in-situ*. The change has occurred in a polypoid endometrium (× 160)

ROUTES OF SPREAD

Although the tumour grows slowly when it is well differentiated, especially in older women, invasion eventually occurs. Most frequently this is confined to the stroma of the endometrium, but may spread in all directions from the initial growth. In time the tumour cells infiltrate the myometrium, and may erode through into the parametrium or the peritoneal cavity. Lymphatic spread tends to be late in onset, but viable cells reach the upper vagina, the tubes and the ovaries via the peri-uterine lymphatics. Metastases develop in the upper vagina in about 2 per cent of cases, and in the ovaries in a further 3 per cent. A more extensive spread via the lymphatic channels occurs in 7 per cent of cases, the regional lymph nodes becoming involved. The actual nodes involved depend on the site of the original tumour. If fundal, the lymphatic channels drain through the broad ligament to the external iliac and common iliac nodes, and, rarely, spread occurs along the round muscle into the superficial femoral nodes (Fig. **17/8**). If the growth involves the cervix, the spread is to the nodes draining the cervical lymphatics, and these channels more readily convey the malignant cells. This is the reason for the worse prognosis when the cervix is involved.

In terminal cases, haematogenous spread occurs, and if the malignant cells are not destroyed, remote secondary deposits of adenocarcinoma arise.

CLINICAL STAGING

In order to obtain some uniformity between clinics so that methods of treatment may be compared, the International Federation of Gynaecology and Obstetrics has recommended a system of clinical staging (Table **17/1**, p. 191).

CLINICAL FEATURES

The only symptom of early endometrial carcinoma is a bloody discharge or irregular bleeding, usually peri- or postmenopausally. The discharge is bloody, watery and offensive, and the bleeding is slight in amount, irregular and recurrent. Pain is a late symptom.

On examination the uterus may be normal in size or enlarged. This depends, to some extent, upon the spread of the tumour, but more upon the associated

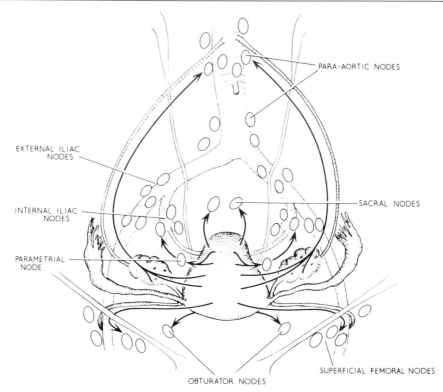

EXTERNAL ILIAC
NODES

INTERNAL ILIAC
NODES

PARAMETRIAL
NODE

PARA-AORTIC NODES

SACRAL NODES

OBTURATOR NODES

SUPERFICIAL FEMORAL NODES

Fig. 17/8 The lymphatic drainage of the uterus

presence of myomata or a pyometra. In most cases the larger the uterus, the worse the prognosis.

DIAGNOSIS

It should be emphasized that *any bleeding, or bloody discharge, appearing in the vagina in a postmenopausal woman must be considered due to carcinoma until disproved.* Although occasionally malignant endometrial cells are found by examining cytologically, a specimen obtained from the pool in the posterior fornix, the method is not very helpful or accurate, and the false negative rate is high. Certain gynaecologists routinely obtain aspiration specimens from the uterine cavity during 'cancer check-ups'; but in general the first sign of endometrial carcinoma is a bloody vaginal discharge in a postmenopausal woman. The diagnosis can only be made by curettage, and because of the worse prognosis and different treatment required if the upper cervical canal is involved, the curettage should be fractional. In this technique, curettings are obtained from the cervical

canal, and the internal cervical os is then dilated so that the curette may enter the uterine cavity. Curettings are next obtained from the lower uterine cavity, then from the upper part and finally a sponge forceps is introduced in case any endometrial polyps have escaped the curette. Each specimen is placed in a separate container and submitted for histopathological examination.

TREATMENT

In the past 5 years a much greater consensus of opinion regarding the treatment of endometrial carcinoma has occurred and areas of controversy have diminished. Few gynaecologists today recommend pre-operative pelvic irradiation, although interest is being expressed in the use of large doses of progestogen (usually either medroxyprogesterone acetate or levonorgestrel) just before and after operation for some weeks. The use of progestogens in this manner is still experimental.

As noted earlier, over 75 per cent of cases of

Stage

IA G123 Tumour limited to endometrium
IB G123 Invasion to < 1/2 myometrium
IC G123 Invasion to > 1/2 myometrium
IIA G123 Endocervical glandular involvement only
IIB G123 Cervical stromal invasion
IIIA G123 Tumour invades serosa and/or adnexa and/or positive peritoneal cytology
IIIB G123 Metastases to pelvic and/or para-aortic lymph nodes
IVA G123 Tumour invasion of bladder and/or bowel mucosa
IVB Distant metastases including intra-abdominal and/or inguinal lymph nodes

Histopathology: degree of differentiation

Cases of carcinoma of the corpus should be grouped with regard to the degree of differentiation of the adenocarcinoma as follows:
G1 5% or less of a non-squamous or non-morular solid growth pattern.
G2 6–50% of a non-squamous or non-morular solid growth pattern.
G3 More than 50% of a non-squamous or non-morular solid growth pattern.

Rules related to staging

(1) Since corpus cancer is now surgically staged, procedures used previously for the differentiation of stages are no longer applicable, such as using dilatation and curettage findings to differentiate between stage I and stage II. (It is appreciated that there may be a small number of patients with corpus cancer who will be treated primarily with radiation therapy. If that is the case, the clinical staging adopted by FIGO in 1971 would still apply but designation of that staging system would be noted.)
(2) Ideally, the thickness of the myometrium should be measured along with the depth of tumour invasion.

Table 17/1 Clinical staging of carcinoma of the corpus uteri (endometrial carcinoma) (International Federation of Gynaecology and Obstetrics)

endometrial carcinoma are Stage I when detected. Stage I cases, graded histologically 1 or 2, are treated by total hysterectomy and bilateral oopho-

rectomy. As lymphatic spread is late, more radical surgery is unnecessary. The ovaries are removed because of the possible oestrogen-dependence of the tumour and because lymphatic spread, if it occurs, involves the ovaries.

The uterus is examined histologically and if myometrial invasion of more than half its thickness has occurred, the prognosis is grave. In such cases postoperative irradiation and/or hormone therapy may increase survival. The irradiation is to the whole pelvis in a dose of 50Gy (5000rads) over 5 weeks. In such cases, and when the histological grade is 3 (irrespective of the degree of myometrial invasion) many gynaecologists also recommend irradiation of the vaginal vault. A total of 40Gy (4000rads) is given 7 to 10 days after operation. This therapy is believed to reduce subsequent vaginal vault recurrences although no randomized trial has been made. An alternative treatment is to administer progestogens postoperatively in large doses for a period of 12 to 24 months. One problem is that the mortality of women with vaginal vault recurrence is high and the recurrence may merely be an obvious sign of wider recurrences in the pelvis. As well as this, vaginal vault irradiation causes vaginal narrowing making coitus uncomfortable, and may be followed by radiation damage to the gut or bladder. At present opinion is divided. One group recommends postoperative vaginal vault irradiation in all Stage I cases; another, in selected cases (as just outlined); whilst a third group avoids postoperative vaginal vault irradiation.

Stage II endometrial carcinoma is treated by radiotherapy, in the manner prescribed for carcinoma of the cervix or by radical hysterectomy and lymphadenectomy.

Following surgery, with or without additional radiation, the rate of recurrence of cancer is about 15 per cent, and is directly proportional to the histological grade of the carcinoma. Surgery is usually of little avail in these cases, nor does intra-abdominal recurrence respond well to irradiation. Obviously, if the carcinoma is staged as Stage III, or Stage IV, surgery is technically impossible, and the prognosis bad. These patients, and those who develop recurrences, may obtain relief of pain and some extension of life from hormone therapy.

Hormone therapy

The biological effect of progesterone and the progestogens is to alter cell metabolism, by altering cell membrane permeability and cytoplasmic enzyme function. The effect of this is to reduce the speed of cell division. About 40 per cent of patients with inoperable endometrial carcinoma, or with recurrence following surgery, show objective improvement if hormone therapy is used. The currently recommended doses are shown in Table **17/2**. It is generally accepted that if there is to be a response, as judged by substantial or complete regression of the tumour, this will occur within 6 to 8 weeks of starting hormone therapy. Treatment should only be continued if improvement is observed.

In some clinics the steroids are used in the period between the diagnostic curettage and hysterectomy by intramuscular injection and direct injection into the uterine muscle. This must be considered experimental at the present time and recent randomized studies show that the use of progestogen does not improve survival.

17-α-hydroxyprogesterone acetate	1000mg daily intramuscularly for 7 days then 500mg × 3 each week. If response in 4 to 8 weeks: 250 to 500mg weekly for life
medroxyprogesterone acetate	500mg intramuscularly twice weekly. If response in 4 to 8 weeks: 1000mg orally each week for 1 year then 500mg orally each week for life
levonorgestrel	20mg twice daily (orally)

Table 17/2 Hormonal treatment of advanced or recurrent endometrial carcinoma

PROGNOSIS

The prognosis for the individual patient depends on (1) the stage of the disease, (2) the histological grade of the tumour, (3) the presence of a pyometra, and (4) the age and health of the woman. The later the stage of the disease and the less differentiated are the cells, the worse is the prognosis. The greater the degree of myometrial penetration, the worse is the prognosis. The older the woman the greater the chance that the disease is more advanced.

In Table **17/3** the mean 5-year survival rate, for each stage, and the preferable mode of treatment is shown.

Stage	Recommended treatment	5-year survival rate
I, G1, 2	Hysterectomy	80 per cent
I, G3	Hysterectomy, post-operative radiation	60 per cent
II	As for carcinoma of the uterine cervix	50 per cent
III	Hormone therapy + megavoltage irradiation of the entire pelvis	30 per cent
IV	Hormone therapy	10 per cent

Table 17/3 The recommended treatment and 5-year survival rate of endometrial cancer related to the stage of the disease

Chapter 18

Benign Enlargements of the Uterus

MYOMA

A myoma is a tumour composed of smooth muscle bundles interspersed with strands of connective tissue. It may arise in any part of the Mullerian duct, but most commonly develops in the myometrium, where several myomata develop simultaneously. It is the commonest tumour encountered in the female, and varies in size from that of a pea to that of a football. It is often, and erroneously, called a 'fibroid'.

INCIDENCE AND AETIOLOGY

The incidence of myomata is difficult to determine, but they probably occur in about 5 per cent of women. The tumours grow slowly and often only become manifest in the 4th decade of life, when the incidence is about 20 per cent. They are more common in nulliparous women or women who have had only one child, and it has been said that 'bad girls get babies, but good girls get myomata'.

The aetiology is obscure, but there is evidence that the growth of the tumour is dependent on oestrogen, as myomata contain more oestrogen receptors than normal uterine muscle, and the majority atrophy after the climacteric.

Many theories of histogenesis have been advanced, and none has been accepted completely. Three main hypotheses exist. Firstly, that the tumour arises from normal mature muscle cells; secondly, that it arises from immature muscle rests in the myometrium; and thirdly, that it originates from embryonal cells found in the walls of uterine blood vessels. Whatever the origin, the tumours begin as minute seedlings which may be single or, more frequently, are scattered through the myometrium. The seedlings grow slowly,

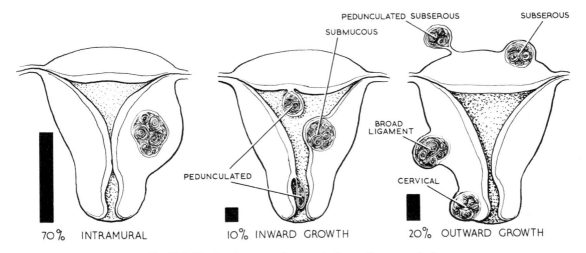

Fig. 18/1 The development of myomata shown diagrammatically

but progressively, and in extreme cases may eventually form a tumour weighing as much as 10kg. If the growth of an ovarian tumour can be measured in months, that of a myoma can be measured in years. Initially all tumours lie within the uterine muscle wall (i.e. they are *intramural*) and in 70 per cent of cases the tumours remain in this situation. Growth may occur inwards, so that the uterine cavity is distorted (*submucous* myoma), or the tumour may become *pedunculated* and lie pendant in the uterine cavity. Inward growth occurs in 10 per cent of cases. In the remaining 20 per cent of cases, the direction of growth is outwards so that the serosal coat of the uterus is distorted, the tumour becoming attached by a broad or narrow base (*subserous* myoma) or becoming *pedunculated* (Fig. **18/1**). If the development is from the lateral uterine wall, the tumour may grow between the two leaves of the broad ligament (a *broad ligament* myoma), whilst if the origin is from muscle remnants in the cervix, a *cervical* myoma will result (Fig. **18/2**).

PATHOLOGY

The gross appearance is variable, but on cut section, the colour is light greyish-white and the tumour pouts above the surrounding myometrium, as the pseudocapsule contracts. The substance of the tumour presents a whorled intertwining appearance (Fig. **18/3**).

The structure of a myoma is one of interlacing bundles of involuntary muscle lying in a network of connective tissue. At the periphery the muscle fibres of the myoma are arranged in concentric layers and the normal myometrial fibres surrounding the tumour tend to be similarly orientated. Between the two concentric muscles layers, a thin layer of areolar tissue is found, which forms a pseudocapsule. It is believed that daughter myomata develop from tumour muscle fibres adjacent to the pseudocapsule. The vascular supply of the tumour enters it after penetrating the pseudocapsule, and usually only one or two large vessels are found, the remainder being inconstant and insignificant. It is clear that the tumour is relatively avascular. On microscopic study, groups and bundles of spindle-shaped cells with elongated nuclei are seen, with the connective tissue elements separating the bundles (Fig. **18/4**).

Since the entire blood supply is derived from the pseudocapsular layer, the growth of the tumour often outstrips its blood supply, and avascular de-

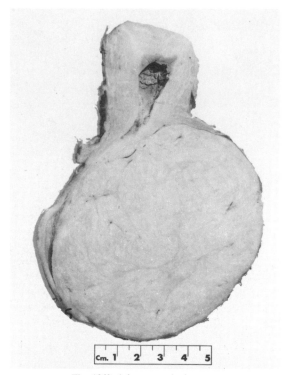

Fig. 18/2 A large cervical myoma

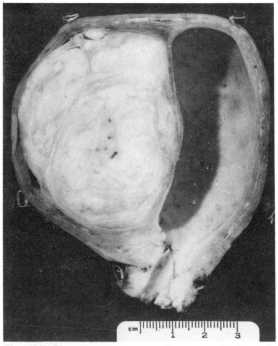

Fig. 18/3 The gross appearance of a myoma is shown in the specimen, which also has a pyometra and a carcinoma of the cervix

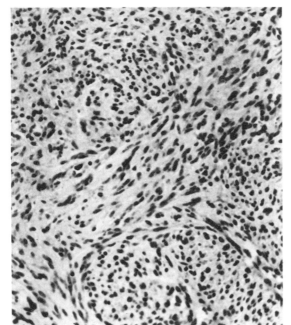

Fig. 18/4 The microscopic appearance of a myoma. The bundles of spindle-shaped muscle cells run in several directions and tend to form a whorl-like pattern (× 160)

generation arises, particularly in the central portion, in about 10 per cent of cases. Initially this is *hyaline* in nature, but if the hyalinization is extensive, liquefaction may occur in the inner part of the hyalinized area, with the development of *cystic degeneration*. In elderly women *calcification* may occur in the hyalinized area – the 'womb stones' of the older writers. *Sarcomatous* change occurs very rarely, the incidence being about 0.2 per cent. Rarely, and usually as a complication of pregnancy, *red degeneration* occurs. This change is probably due to obstruction to the venous return, the back pressure causing rupture of the capillary plexus and extravasation of blood through the tumour, which gives it a red 'raw beef' colour.

Complications may arise because of the position of the myoma. The pedicle of a subserous pedunculated myoma may twist, interrupting initially the venous supply leading to congestion and extravasation of blood, and later as the arterial supply is stopped, to gangrene. Occasionally a large vein on the surface of a subserous myoma ruptures, causing an intraperitoneal haemorrhage. These two complications constitute acute emergencies, but both are uncommon today.

A submucous myoma may become infected at its lower pole; and a pedunculated submucous myoma may be extruded through the cervix and present as an infected necrotic mass, which may be mistaken for a malignant neoplasm.

SYMPTOMS

The symptomology depends to a great degree upon the size and position of the myoma. Most small myomata, and many larger ones, are asymptomatic and are only detected during routine examinations. The effect of large myomata depends on their position in relation to the endometrial cavity – the nearer the cavity, the greater the likelihood of symptoms, usually menstrual disturbances. The myoma itself does not cause the bleeding, which is due to hyperplasia or patchy atrophy of the endometrium overlying the submucous myoma. The duration of the menstrual cycle is not altered, but menorrhagia is usual and is slowly progressive in nature, the bleeding tending to be heavier on the 2nd or 3rd day of the period and often associated with 'flooding', with clots and with pain. This may lead to anaemia.

If the myoma is submucous and pedunculated, a continuous bloody discharge may occur, but the cause should never be ascribed to the myoma until carcinoma has been eliminated, by cervical cytology and diagnostic curettage.

Irrespective of their position in the uterus, large myomata filling the pelvis may cause pressure symptoms. These may be a generalized sensation of pelvic pressure; or may be related to the bladder when frequency and suprapubic discomfort result; or to the rectum when constipation and backache are noted. Despite this, many women have no symptoms until the tumour becomes palpable abdominally.

In other women, symptomless myomata are detected in patients complaining of infertility. However, the myoma should not be considered the cause of the childlessness until all other factors have been eliminated, as many women with myomata succeed in becoming pregnant. Only when the uterine cavity is distorted by the myoma, should the tumour be considered a cause of infertility.

DIAGNOSIS

Examination shows that the uterus is enlarged by a firm, smooth mass, or by masses which markedly distort its shape. The tumour is not tender unless incarcerated in the pelvis, infected or pressing on pelvic nerves. On moving the uterus, the masses move together with it, and not separately unless the myoma is pedunculated.

Enlargement of the uterus due to pregnancy must always be considered, or the surgeon will find to his embarrassment his error at laparotomy. The distinction is not difficult, as amenorrhoea is unusual in association with myomata and in pregnancy an immunological pregnancy test will be positive. Occasionally a solid ovarian tumour may cause difficulty; but the uterus can generally be moved separately from the tumour. If any doubt exists, an ultrasound examination will aid in making the diagnosis, which should be established before surgery.

PREGNANCY COMPLICATED BY MYOMATA

In pregnancy an increase in the size of the myoma usually occurs, due in part to oedema and, in part, to hypertrophy of the muscle fibres. The effect is to cause a softening of the myoma, which may apparently merge into the enlarging uterus. Red degeneration, as already mentioned, may occur in pregnancy, but is rare. The effect of the myoma on the pregnancy is less certain, and at least 75 per cent cause no trouble. If the myoma distorts the uterine cavity, the frequency of abortion and premature labour increases; and malposition or malpresentation of the fetus may occur. If there is a cervical or broad ligament myoma, it may obstruct labour, although in most cases the tumour becomes soft and is lifted out of the pelvis as pregnancy advances. In the third stage of labour, postpartum haemorrhage is a hazard. These matters are discussed more fully in Volume I.

MANAGEMENT

Three possibilities exist, (1) no treatment, (2) hysterectomy, and (3) myomectomy.

No treatment

Small symptomless myomata require no treatment with four exceptions: (1) if the myoma is larger than the size of a 14-week pregnancy, or is growing rapidly, (2) if the myoma distorts the uterine cavity

and the patient is anxious to have a child, (3) if it is situated in the lower part of the uterus and therefore likely to complicate delivery, and (4) if there is any doubt about its nature. In these four cases, operative treatment is recommended. In other cases the patient should be seen annually, when any change in the size of the uterus is determined, and the opportunity can be taken to obtain a cervical smear for cytological examination.

Should the myoma first be detected in a woman who is near the climacteric, hysterectomy is frequently recommended, particularly if the patient complains of menstrual disturbances. However, apart from a careful diagnostic curettage, to exclude other causes of menstrual abnormality such as endometrial polyps, hyperplasia or carcinoma, surgery is usually not essential, as the menstrual irregularity may be coincidental with, and not caused by, the myoma. Provided the curettage excludes endometrial malignancy, and the uterine cavity is not distorted by the myomata, treatment using progestogens is often successful in controlling the menstrual disturbance, and surgery can be avoided.

Hysterectomy

Total hysterectomy is indicated in cases of symptomless myomata, if the uterus is larger than a 14 weeks gestation and the patient is aged 40 or more (or is younger but has no desire for children). Surgery is also indicated when smaller myomata are found, after investigation, to be the cause of menorrhagia, and hormone treatment has failed to control the symptoms. Finally, hysterectomy is the treatment of choice when the myomata are causing pressure symptoms and the patient has completed her family. Before hysterectomy, it is important to undertake preliminary investigations, including cervical exfoliative cytology and diagnostic curettage, to exclude endometrial malignancy.

Since many women erroneously believe that following hysterectomy their sexual urge ceases, that coitus is not possible, and that obesity is usual, the physician must explain that removal of the uterus has no side-effects. Consequently the sexual urge is unaltered, and provided the ovaries are not removed at the same operation, obesity is not due to the surgery but to overeating. Finally, it must be stressed that coitus can take place normally after hysterectomy once the vaginal wound has healed, as the length of the vagina is, if anything, increased. The explanation must be in language which the patient can understand, and should be made well before the date of the operation, so that any other problems which may arise may be discussed and explained.

Myomectomy

Myomectomy is the operation of choice in all women under the age of 40 who require surgery but who wish to preserve their reproductive function. The size and number of the myomata do not prevent myomectomy, although the patient must accept that if the operation proves too dangerous, hysterectomy may be required. Prior to operation, investigations must prove that the husband is fertile, and if at operation occlusion of the oviducts is present, hysterectomy is usually preferable to a difficult myomectomy.

Following myomectomy, about 40 per cent of women who have the opportunity to conceive do so, and this is a measure of the value of the operation. Against this must be set the fact that the myomata recur in 5 per cent of patients, and between 2 and 5 per cent continue to have menorrhagia. The latter symptom can be controlled by the use of progestogens (norethisterone 10mg daily from day 20 to day 25 of the cycle).

If the myoma is submucous and pedunculated, or cervical in site, a vaginal myomectomy may be all that is required.

Because of the increased vascularity of the uterus, myomectomy is unwise in pregnancy or at caesarean section, unless the myoma is subserous or pedunculated, and easily accessible.

GnRH agonist analogue

The parenteral administration of this drug will reduce the size of myomata and will produce amenorrhoea by suppressing oestrogen secretion by the ovaries. Once the drug is withdrawn, the ovaries secrete oestrogen and growth of the myomata begins again. GnRH analogues may have a small place in reducing the size of myomata in young women prior to myomectomy and in premenopausal women who wish to avoid hysterectomy. However, the resulting hypo-oestrogenic state may increase bone loss and predispose the woman to osteoporosis.

MYOHYPERPLASIA

Excessive unopposed oestrogen stimulation in a sensitive individual may cause both endometrial and myometrial hyperplasia, and the condition is often confused with uterine myoma. Its origin is quite different, however, and there is considerable evidence that myohyperplasia has a psychosomatic origin.

Since the endometrium is thickened with hypertrophic glands and hyperplastic stroma, and may be polypoid, menorrhagia is usual. The concurrent hyperplasia of the myometrium enlarges the uterus smoothly, but its size rarely exceeds that of a 10 weeks' pregnancy, and bimanual examination shows it to be soft, almost cystic in nature, and occasionally tender (Fig. **18/5**).

Although frequently subjected to hysterectomy, the condition can be controlled, once examination under anaesthesia and a diagnostic curettage have established the diagnosis, by the use of a 19-nortestosterone progestogen in the second half of the cycle. A convenient regimen is to give norethisterone 10mg daily from the 15th day of the cycle for 10 days, or from the 20th day for 5 days, depending on the severity of the bleeding.

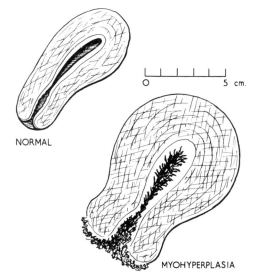

Fig. 18/5 Myohyperplasia

Chapter 19

Endometriosis

The term endometriosis denotes the presence of functioning endometrial tissue in an abnormal location. The development may occur between the muscle fibres of the myometrium (adenomyosis or uterine endometriosis); or in various locations in the pelvic cavity – the ovary and the cul-de-sac being involved most frequently. The lesions have the typical histological appearance of endometrium, and both glands and stroma must be present for histological confirmation of the clinical diagnosis.

AETIOLOGY AND INCIDENCE

The aetiology of the condition remains obscure despite much investigation. The most likely cause is that the uterine lesions are the results of direct extension, or lymphatic transportation of endometrial cells; whilst the extra-uterine lesions result from the retrograde spill of viable endometrial cells through the oviducts. It is probable that most women experience retrograde menstruation at least during some menstruations and the shed endometrial cells are known to be viable. The theory would explain the predominance of the ovary and cul-de-sac as sites of endometriosis. It is also believed that secondary seeding occurs from these primary sites.

The alternative view is that endometriosis results from the development of embryonic cell rests, which have the potential, if stimulated, to differentiate into endometrium and myometrium. The stimulus may be the presence of endometrial cells, leading to imitative metaplasia, or endocrinological factors. Finally, lymphatic or vascular spread of endometrial cells would account for the lesions occasionally found in distant organs.

These theories seek to explain how endometrial cells reach ectopic sites; they do not explain why the endometrial cells grow in the sites. Information on this point comes from epidemiological studies, which show that endometriosis is more common in the higher socio-economic groups, and amongst single women or women who marry late and have few or no children. This information suggests that for the ectopic endometrium to develop, a suitable hormonal climate must be present and the cells must be rhythmically stimulated by oestrogen and progesterone; if the rhythmic stimulation is replaced by a continuous hormone secretion as in pregnancy, the endometriotic sites tend to be attacked by macrophages and fibrosis results.

There is suggestive evidence that immune function is altered in endometriosis and that endometriosis may be an autoimmune disease like SLE. The theory is that there is a deficit in cell-mediated immunity, consequently the viable endometrial cells discharged through the Fallopian tubes are not destroyed but implant.

The incidence of the condition is difficult to determine, particularly as in many instances it is discovered accidentally at laparotomy, but 3 to 7 per cent of women aged 20 to 45 probably have endometriosis.

PATHOLOGY

General

The ectopic endometrium, surrounded by stroma, forms a miniature cyst, which responds to the cyclic secretion of oestrogen and progesterone by proliferating, and by bleeding at the time menstruation occurs in the uterus. The blood and shed cells are trapped in the cyst and distend it, and with each menstruation the collection increases. Between menstruations, absorption of some of the blood serum occurs, so that the remaining contents become thick and dark in colour, producing the 'tarry' or 'chocolate' cyst. Thus there is a slowly progressive growth of the

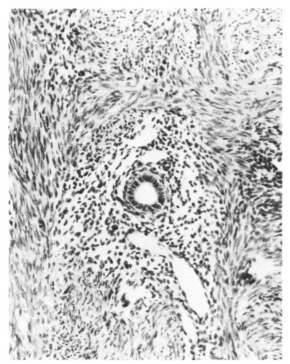 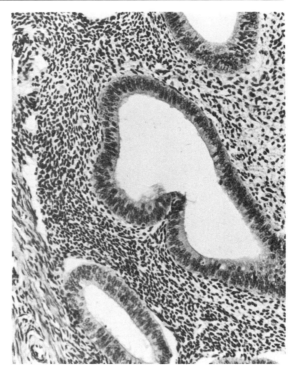

Fig. 19/1 The microscopic appearance of adenomyosis. (A) The endometriotic nodule is lying deep in the myometrium, and both glands and stroma are present (× 160). (B) Another specimen at higher magnification (× 256) clearly showing the glands and the stroma, which is quite dense

endometrial cyst, although the maximum size is rarely larger than that of a large orange. Should the cysts become large, the internal pressure may destroy the endometrial lining, which is replaced by granulation tissue, and the cyst becomes non-functional.

Rupture of even small endometrial cysts is not uncommon, and the inspissated blood is very irritating to the peritoneum, which reacts by forming multiple adhesions. The ectopic endometrium and stromal cells also tend to infiltrate the adjacent tissues, leading to further pelvic adhesions and fixation. In this way ovarian endometriosis may involve the bowel or omentum, and in advanced cases give the impression of a frozen pelvis.

Uterine endometriosis (adenomyosis)

The ectopic cells derive mainly from the basal layer of the endometrium, and infiltrate between the muscle fibres either directly or are carried by the lymphatics. The cells of the basal layer are relatively insensitive to hormonal stimuli, so that the nodules tend to be small, containing little blood, but showing a marked stromal overgrowth (Fig. **19/1**). The pres-

ence of the nodule may also stimulate a proliferative reaction in the myometrium, so that the tumour enlarges and resembles a myoma in appearance. The distinguishing characteristic is that it has no capsule (Fig. **19/2**).

Adenomyosis is a disease of parous women, usually occurring in the later menstrual years, after a long period of infertility. In half of the patients, myomata co-exist, and in 15 per cent extra-uterine endometriosis is found in association.

Extra-uterine endometriosis

The ovary is most frequently involved, and endometriosis may present as small superficial implants (black spots) or as a larger endometrial cyst, which has been described already (Fig. **19/3**). Adhesions to the posterior surface of the broad ligament, to the sigmoid colon and the rectum are common in both forms of the disease (Fig. **19/4**). The peritoneum of the cul-de-sac is the second most common site, and endometriomata may arise either directly from retrograde menstruation, or as a secondary seeding from an ovarian deposit. The lesions in the cul-de-

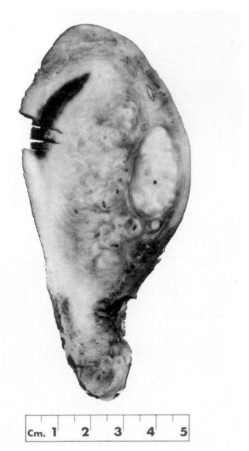

Fig. 19/2 Adenomyosis – gross specimen. The tiny blood cysts can be seen scattered through the myometrium

SYMPTOMS AND SIGNS

It is not easy to describe specific symptoms which are indicative of endometriosis, for at least 25 per cent of patients with the disease have no symptoms, and in a further 25 per cent the disease is found in association with other pelvic conditions. For convenience, the two main forms – uterine endometriosis and extra-uterine endometriosis – are considered separately.

Uterine endometriosis (adenomyosis)

At least one-third of the patients are asymptomatic, and the condition is discovered when a uterus is removed for some other condition and is examined histologically. The principal symptoms are (1) progressively increasing pain, usually found in association with menstruation, and tending to increase in severity during the bleeding episode, and (2) menstrual irregularities, usually either excessive flow or more frequent periods. On vaginal examination, the uterus may be enlarged and feel 'boggy'.

Extra-uterine endometriosis

The symptom complex is often bizarre because of the varying manifestations of the disease. In 60 per cent of cases menstrual irregularities are found, the pattern being premenstrual staining or spotting, menorrhagia, polymenorrhoea or polymenorrhagia, the last two usually signifying ovarian endometriosis. Typically, there is accompanying pain which starts premenstrually, reaches a peak in the last days of menstruation, and subsides slowly after the period, persisting for a varying length of time. This is often referred to as 'acquired dysmenorrhoea'. In other cases, particularly when the cysts are large, constant pain in the lower abdomen and pelvis may be present. About 30 per cent of patients complain of infertility, although the association is due to disturbed ovarian function rather than tubal block, which only occurs in 10 per cent of cases, the tubes in general being patent and functional.

Dyspareunia on deep penetration is often found, should the lesions involve the cul-de-sac, particularly if they fix the uterus in a retroverted position; whilst if the bowel is involved, the patient may complain of pain on defaecation, particularly at the time of menstruation. In a few patients, resorption of the blood causes intermittent pyrexia, especially at the time of menstruation.

sac are usually small, rarely exceeding the size of a pea. They cause puckering of the peritoneum and adhesions to the uterus, often fixing it in retroversion. In 10 per cent of cases, the gut is involved, usually only superficially, but in a few cases marked bowel symptoms occur, characteristically presenting as cramping pains and constipation at the time of menstruation. In a few patients the signs may be suggestive of a bowel malignancy. Since in endometriosis the mucosa of the gut is never involved, the condition can be differentiated by sigmoidoscopy or at laparotomy.

Other sites in the pelvis are reported from time to time, but are relatively uncommon. These include the utero-sacral ligaments, the recto-vaginal septum, the cervix, the round ligament, the bladder and the umbilicus.

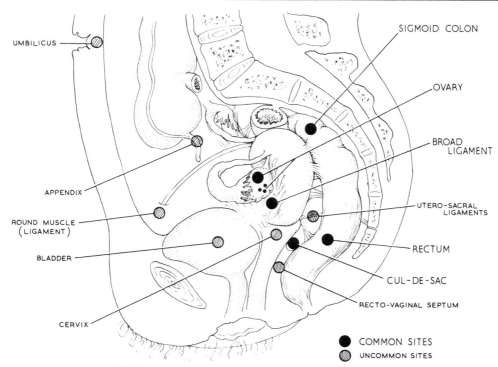

Fig. 19/3 Common and uncommon sites of extra-uterine endometriosis

The signs are also variable. When the lesions are small no abnormality may be felt, whilst larger deposits cause fixed, tender, nodular or cystic swellings. A pelvic examination performed pre-menstrually is valuable, as the lesions are then at their greatest size. At this time tender nodules in the cul-de-sac or enlargement of the ovaries may be detected on bimanual examination. In many cases the symptoms, although persistent, are not diagnostic and endometriosis is only detected when a laparoscopy is performed because of the patient's chronic pelvic pain or deep dyspareunia. Laparoscopy has proved to be of great value in establishing diagnosis of endometriosis. Larger ovarian endometrial cysts are more easily palpable, but may be difficult to differentiate from chronic pelvic infection.

Endometriosis and infertility (see p. 102)

DIFFERENTIAL DIAGNOSIS

Pelvic inflammatory disease

The history of urethritis or acute pelvic infection may be helpful in differentiating the two conditions, for the symptoms are similar. In endometriosis, the pain is maximal towards the end of menstruation, rather than earlier as occurs in chronic salpingo-oophoritis. In difficult cases the pelvis is examined using a laparoscope. This causes the patient minimal disturbance.

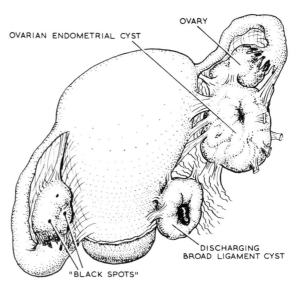

Fig. 19/4 Extra-uterine endometriosis

Ovarian tumours

Ovarian tumours may be impossible to differentiate. They are frequently symptomless, and usually grow to a larger size than do ovarian endometrial cysts.

TREATMENT

Adenomyosis: Unless the disease is associated with extrauterine endometriosis, it is confused with myoma. Adenomyosis does not respond well to hormonal therapy and hysterectomy is required if there are marked symptoms. If the patient has no symptoms, or mild symptoms, no treatment is needed.

Endometriosis: Since endometriosis is a benign condition which is only slowly progressive and is found most frequently in women in the childbearing years, the principle should be to adopt a conservative approach. This is particularly important since the development of potent steroids, which have been shown to cause resolution of many of the lesions. The type of treatment adopted will therefore be determined by the size and extent of the lesions, by the age of the patient and by her desire for childbearing (see Table **19/1** and Fig. **19/5**).

The laparoscope has enabled gynaecologists to 'stage' endometriosis with greater accuracy and to define appropriate treatment (Table **19/1**).

If the woman's main complaint is infertility rather than pain, it may be helpful for her to know the pregnancy rate after treatment. In one series, the pregnancy rate in women whose only reason for infertility was presumed to be endometriosis was: Stage I, 65 to 70 per cent; Stage II, 35 to 45 per cent; Stage III, 25 to 30 per cent.

The lesions of Stage I are clinically indetectable, as are some of those graded as Stage II. These small lesions may either be treated at the time of laparoscopic diagnosis with cautery, or left alone. In like manner, any small periovarian and peritubal adhesions may be divided (which is now usual) or left alone, as the effect of these procedures on improving fertility is not known.

In addition, a complete infertility investigation of the couple should be made before any other surgery is contemplated.

STAGE CHARACTERISTICS	DIAGNOSIS	TREATMENT
I *MINIMAL* AND II *MILD* Small surface nodules with no scarring or peritubal adhesions	Only by laparoscope in investigation of infertility	At most, electrocautery or CO_2 laser to lesions Do not give hormones
III *MODERATE* Small scattered surface lesions with scarring; ovarian endometriomata, <2.5cm, few periovarian or peritubal adhesions; nodules in the cul-de-sac or uterosacral ligaments	Often symptoms but confirmation by laparoscopy needed	Electrocautery or CO_2 laser to lesions Hormones Conservative surgery if hormones fail to relieve symptoms
IV *SEVERE* Ovarian endometriomata >2.5cm; marked adhesions of ovary and/or tubes, cul-de-sac obliteration	Symptoms and signs Laparotomy confirms	Conservative surgery Hormones Hysterectomy and salpingo-oophorectomy
V *VERY SEVERE* Stage III plus involvement of bowel, bladder, ureter etc.	Laparotomy Barium enema IVP	Surgery Hormones, if surgery incomplete

Table 19/1 The management of endometriosis

When the lesions are graded as more advanced, or when pain is present, treatment should be given.

Two main methods of treatment are available. These are the use of hormones and surgery. They should be considered complementary, not competitive. If the endometrial lesions are large, surgery is preferred, particularly if an ovarian tumour is detected.

Hormonal treatment

As a rule, hormonal therapy should not be started until a firm diagnosis of endometriosis has been established. This usually requires laparoscopy or laparotomy (with conservative surgery if necessary). Hormonal therapy produces the greatest successes in extra-uterine endometriosis; by contrast, uterine endometriosis (or adenomyosis) often shows a lesser response, presumably because the basal endometrial cells which form the lesion are less responsive to the sex steroid hormones.

Four regimens of hormonal therapy are currently favoured. The first regimen is the use of an isoxazol derivative, 17-α-ethinyl testosterone, called danazol. The second regimen is to use a gonadotrophin-releasing hormone analogue. The third regimen is to prescribe progestogen-only pills or to give injections of progestogens at intervals. The fourth regimen uses a new-generation progestogen called gestinone. The hormones are those used for oral hormonal contraception. They suppress ovulation and if given continuously also suppress menstruation. In the endometriotic lesion a decidual-like reaction occurs in the stroma and an atrophic reaction occurs in the ectopic endometrial glands – a 'pseudo-pregnancy'. The effect of this is to cause absorption of the decidual-like stroma and subsequent fibrosis which obliterates the lesion.

Hormonal therapy is not a competitor to surgery. The aim in using hormones is to suppress ovarian and endometrial function temporarily, with the minimum of side-effects.

1. *Danazol.* The drug is given in a dose of 200mg 2 to 4 times a day for between 3 and 12 months, depending on the extent of the lesions and on the response. Symptoms are relieved in 2 to 6 weeks and the lesions usually disappear, or are considerably reduced in size, within 3 to 6 months.

The actions of danazol are under dispute. The drug apparently reduces the number of gonadotrophin-releasing hormone receptors in the pituitary and causes a reduction in the level of sex-hormone-binding globulin. A fall in SHBG leads to an increase in unbound (free) testosterone, and a fall in oestradiol. The raised level of free testosterone (T) may be the reason why danazol is effective in curing endometriosis, as androgens inhibit endometrial growth. The inhibition also affects endometriotic areas and the lesions become obliterated by fibrous tissue. The raised T level may account for the side-effects. The drug also may partially suppress FSH and LH release, and act directly on the ovary to reduce steroidogenesis.

During treatment over 70 per cent of women become amenorrhoeic, the remainder becoming severely oligomenorrhoeic. Half of the patients gain more than 3kg in weight, and the same proportion note a decrease in breast size. About 20 per cent develop oily skin or acne and in 10 per cent the voice deepens. In mild endometriosis danazol should not be prescribed as the drug does not improve the pregnancy rate.

2. *GnRH agonist (LH-RH agonist).* The drug is given in a dose of 200μg intranasally twice a day for 3 to 6 months. GnRH agonists render the pituitary gonadotrophs insensitive to stimulation by endogenous GnRH, with resulting suppression of ovarian steroid secretion. Because of this nearly all women experience hot flushes and over 70 per cent become amenorrhoeic. Bone loss of 2 to 4 per cent occurs over a 6-month treatment period. This also occurs when danazol is prescribed.

Both GnRH analogues and danazol given over a 6-month period eliminate or reduce the symptoms in over 75 per cent of women, but only obtain complete remission or marked improvement of the endometrial deposits in about 30 per cent of cases. Following the resumption of ovarian function, after the use of either drug, symptomatic endometriosis may recur. Thus, neither drug treatment nor surgery necessarily cures endometriosis.

3. *Progestogens.* The older treatments of endometriosis using a contraceptive pill containing a high dose of progestogen or a progestogen alone have been superseded by danazol and GnRH analogue. Because they suppressed ovarian function less effectively, they were less successful in treatment. Recently one of the new-generation progestogens, gestinone, has been used but there is, as yet, insufficient information about its value.

Surgical treatment

Small lesions detected at laparoscopy can be treated

by laser or electrocautery under laparoscopic vision. When the lesions are larger, surgery is usually necessary, particularly in cases of extra-uterine endometriosis involving the ovaries. This is because the nature of the ovarian enlargement can only be determined at laparotomy, and occasionally if operation is deferred, the cyst may rupture causing an acute abdominal emergency, or at least the further spread of viable endometrial cells. The extent of the surgical excision must be related to the patient's age, and her desire for children. In regard to the latter, the fertility of the male partner must always be investigated before deciding upon the operative procedure. If surgery is not urgently required, there is evidence that a course of hormone therapy, given over 3 months, will facilitate the surgical dissection. Hormone therapy is also of great value postoperatively if decidual disease is left, as it may well be. In younger women the surgeon's aim should be to remove as much of the endometriotic tissue as possible, whilst conserving ovarian and tubal function. At operation, the surgeon should attempt to dissect out the cysts and then to reconstruct the ovarian tissue (an ovarian cystectomy). He should avoid oophorectomy if at all possible. Should the uterus or tubes be involved in adhesions, these organs should be dissected free. If the uterus is retroverted, or if endometriomata are found in the cul-de-sac, the round ligaments should be plicated to maintain the uterus in an anteverted position, and the nodules of endometriosis in the cul-de-sac should be cauterized.

The situation in older women is different, and a more radical surgical approach is justified. Uterine endometriosis, which fails to respond to a 6-month period of hormonal therapy, or which is encountered in a woman who has no desire for a further pregnancy, is best treated by total hysterectomy with or without oophorectomy, depending on the age of the patient. If the disease is extra-uterine, as much of the endometriosis as can be removed easily is excised, and a total hysterectomy and oophorectomy performed, in the knowledge that with the cessation of ovarian function the remaining lesions will atrophy.

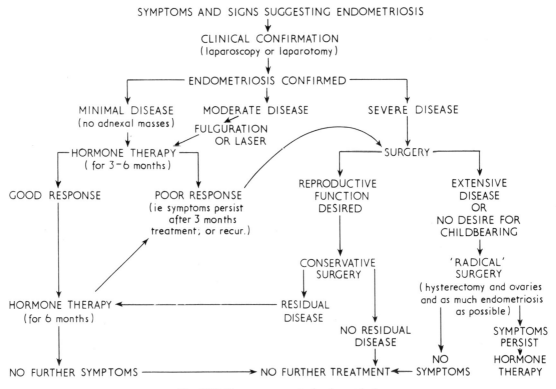

Fig. 19/5 The management of endometriosis

Chapter 20

Trophoblastic Disease

The justification for including a chapter on tropho-blastic neoplasms, which are rarely encountered, is twofold. First, there is increasing evidence that the development of the tumours is due to a failure of the normal materno-ovofetal immunological rela-tions, and secondly, the malignant form of the dis-ease responds dramatically to the use of chemoth-erapeutic agents. Both these matters are of import-ance in sign-posting possible ways to the manage-ment, in the future, of cancerous growths.

Traditionally the benign neoplasm is referred to as 'hydatidiform mole', and the malignant forms as 'invasive mole', 'destructive mole', 'chorio-adenoma destruens' and 'choriocarcinoma'. These terms fail to emphasize the potentially progressive nature of the disease, and the classification shown in Table 20/1 is preferable.

1. *Benign trophoblastic disease* (hydatidiform mole)
2. *Persistent trophoblastic disease* (often malignant)
   Apparently confined to the uterus
   (invasive mole)
   Usually with extra-uterine spread
   (choriocarcinoma)

   Table 20/1 Classification of trophoblastic neoplasms

PATHOLOGICAL DEFINITIONS

Benign trophoblastic tumours

Hydatidiform mole
This is a neoplastic condition characterized by hy-dropic swelling and vesicle formation of the pla-cental villi, paucity or absence of blood vessels within the villus, and is associated with proliferation of trophoblast which is most marked in the placental

bed (Figs. **20/1** and **20/2**). No embryo or fetus is found. A second entity, referred to as partial mole, is characterized by the presence of a fetus, areas of normal villi and patchy areas of cystic villi, some as large as those found in a complete mole, and areas of trophoblastic hyperplasia. Partial moles are rarely followed by malignant change, whilst this event follows a complete mole in 5 to 10 per cent of cases.

Malignant trophoblastic tumours

Invasive mole
This is a term applied when there is penetration of the myometrium by molar tissue with destruction of myometrial fibres, or extension of molar tissue to other organs, the vascular pattern of the original mole always being maintained.

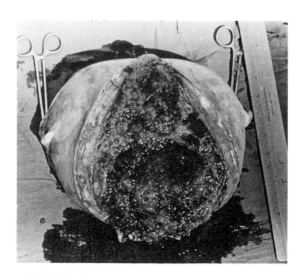

Fig. 20/1 Benign trophoblastic tumour (hydatidiform mole) – gross specimen. Note the grape-like masses

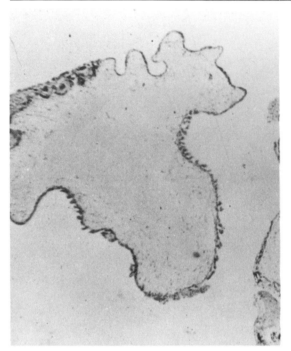

Fig. 20/2 Microphotograph of a benign trophoblastic tumour (hydatidiform mole), showing the distended villi and irregular trophoblastic proliferation

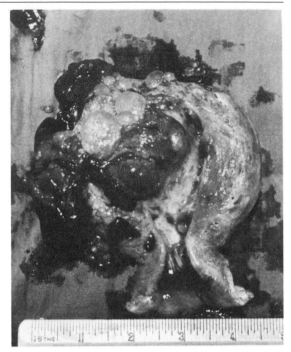

Fig. 20/3(A) Malignant trophoblastic tumour – choriocarcinoma. Gross specimen

Choriocarcinoma

This is a more malignant form in which syncytio- and cytotrophoblast invade the myometrium with marked tissue destruction and haemorrhage, and are usually carried by the systemic bloodstream producing distant metastases. Histologically, the tumour is characterized by sheets of trophoblastic cells, with rarely any vesicle formation (Fig. **20/3**).

AETIOLOGY

Any hypothesis encompassing the aetiology of trophoblastic disease must explain (1) why the disease is four times as frequent in South Asia as in the USA and Europe (the incidence rising from 1:600 pregnancies to 1:2000 pregnancies); (2) why the condition is found more frequently amongst young primigravidae on the one hand, and women aged 35 or more and in women who have borne more than four children on the other; (3) how it is that the malignant form may develop months or years after pregnancy.

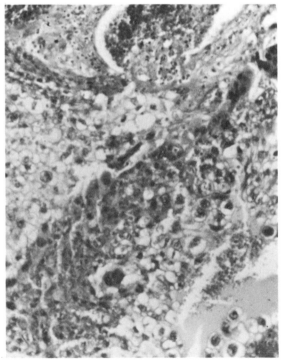

Fig. 20/3(B) Microscopic appearance of choriocarcinoma ($\times 160$)

Cytogenetic and biochemical markers show that over 90 per cent of complete hydatidiform moles are derived entirely from paternal genes. It is believed that the spermatozoon enters an ovum which has lost its nucleus (an empty egg). The haploid sperm duplicates, reconstituting the diploid number of homozygous chromosomes. The haploid sperm must be 23X as sperms with a 23Y complement, on duplication to 46YY are non-viable. About 10 per cent of complete moles result from 2 sperms entering the empty egg, in this case the mole is heterozygous. In contrast, partial moles have a maternal contribution and usually a triploid chromosomal constitution, suggesting dispermy as the probable explanation.

PATHOGENESIS

Trophoblast is unique in that it is an allogenic tissue which normally invades the maternal structures before reaching a state of symbiosis with the host. In human pregnancy this stage is reached, and invasion ceases, between the 80th and 85th day for reasons as yet obscure. In a large number of women, intravascular emboli of trophoblast continue to be shed throughout pregnancy. These appear to do no harm to the woman, and to be destroyed, possibly in the lungs, without invoking an immune response on the part of the host. It has been observed that a coating of 'fibrinoid' covers (from a very early stage) all cytotrophoblastic cells, and syncytiotrophoblast, when exposed to the maternal bloodstream. This fibrinoid layer may inhibit the recognition by the lymphocytes that trophoblast is 'foreign' to the mother, but nevertheless permit the phagocytosis of the embolic trophoblastic tissue.

It has been observed that over one-third of spontaneously expelled abortuses are abnormal, and the placentae of two-thirds of this abnormal group show areas of 'hydatidiform' degeneration (partial moles). The explanation offered is that the trophoblast has continued to absorb nutrients from the decidua and maternal bloodstream, but because of the absent fetal circulation, the nutrients have continued to distend the villi leading to 'hydatidiform' degeneration. This observation offers an explanation for the development of benign trophoblastic tumours, in which all the villi have become distended to give the grape-like appearance of a typical benign trophoblastic tumour (complete mole) (Fig. **20/1**). It is hypothesized that owing to a deficient immunological relationship, the 'aggressiveness' of the trophoblast is excessive and consequently the villi become distended with nutrients. The primitive vasculature within the villi is damaged or defective, and the embryo 'starves', dies and is absorbed, whilst trophoblastic growth continues exuberantly, eventually invading maternal tissue.

The increased trophoblastic activity is also shown by the increased hormonal production mainly by the syncytiotrophoblast. The main hormone produced is chorionic gonadotrophin, but to some extent chorionic thyrotrophin and progesterone production are increased. Since oestrogen steroidogenesis requires enzymes derived from the fetus, the production of this hormone is reduced below the level found in a normal pregnancy of comparable gestation. The effect of high circulating chorionic gonadotrophin levels is to stimulate the development of theca-lutein cysts within the ovary, in about 50 per cent of patients.

BENIGN TROPHOBLASTIC DISEASE

The first sign of trophoblastic disease is uterine bleeding, which in no way differs from that of threatened abortion, except that it tends to occur rather later than is usual for abortion. The bleeding also tends to persist, the colour changing from bright red to dark brown. The bleeding episode may be followed quickly by uterine contractions and the spontaneous expulsion of the grape-like tumour, or may persist until the patient seeks advice. In about 20 per cent of cases, severe vomiting is associated with the bleeding, but this is not diagnostic. Four main diagnostic criteria suggest that the patient has a benign trophoblastic tumour. (1) The uterus is larger than expected from the period of gestation calculated from the date of the last menstrual period. This finding is present in between 60 and 80 per cent of cases. (2) The uterus is 'doughy' in consistency and fetal parts cannot be felt or the fetal heart heard. The absence of fetal heart sounds can be detected by the use of a machine which utilizes the principle of the Doppler sound shift (the Doptone Fetal Heart Detector). Ultrasonic scanning gives a distinct speckled picture on a display system, which has a high diagnostic accuracy, and will also detect theca-lutein cysts (Fig. **20/4**). (3) The serum and urinary gonadotrophin levels are raised. Normally the peak secretion of gonadotrophin is reached between the 60th and 90th day of pregnancy after which it falls. The finding of a high gonadotrophin level in serum or urine after the 100th day of pregnancy is suggestive of tropho-

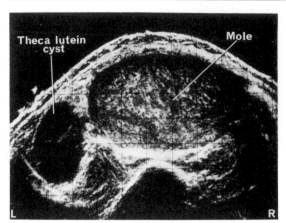

Fig. 20/4 The echogram shows the characteristic vesicular pattern of a hydatidiform mole (by kind permission of Dr W. J. Garrett)

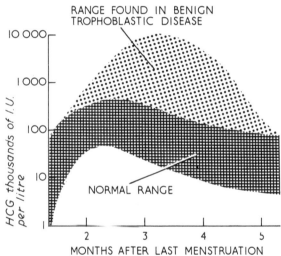

Fig. 20/5 Chorionic gonadotrophin excretion in trophoblastic disease. The normal range is shown shaded; levels found in trophoblastic disease are shown in the stippled area

blastic disease (Fig. **20/5**). (4) Hypertension and/or proteinuria is found in approximately 20 per cent of cases, and the larger the size of the uterus, the greater the likelihood of this occurring. (5) Hyperthyroidism may occur which ceases following treatment of the trophoblastic disease.

Treatment

In about half the cases the patient is admitted in the process of expelling the tumour. Blood loss is fre-

quently heavy, and blood must be obtained for transfusion, should this be needed. If the expulsion is proceeding rapidly, no treatment is required until the greater part has been expelled, when digital evacuation of the remainder is carried out. If the expulsion is delayed, the uterus should be emptied using a suction curette. The alternative is to induce uterine contractions with prostaglandins or an oxytocic infusion, but these methods are associated with a higher risk of intravascular spread of trophoblast. This may lead to persistent trophoblastic disease. Because the myometrium is both thin and vascular, curettage is not performed at the time of molar expulsion, and is delayed for 5 days. An alternative is to perform an ultrasound examination and only curette if the scan reveals trophoblastic tissue in the uterus.

If the tumour is diagnosed prior to its expulsion, two lines of therapy are available, and the choice will depend on the desire of the patient for further children. When the patient has completed her family, irrespective of her age, the best treatment is total hysterectomy with ovarian conservation, as the possibility of malignant development is reduced considerably. Hysterectomy should also be recommended to this type of patient if she has just expelled the tumour vaginally, and should be performed within 5 days of the expulsion. The other method is to evacuate the uterus using a suction curette, having set up a dilute oxytocin infusion before the procedure to ensure myometrial contractions. This method should be chosen if the woman wishes to have a further pregnancy. It is preferable to hysterotomy. Three to five days following the expulsion of the tumour, a careful curettage should be performed to remove any residual trophoblastic tissue.

If theca-lutein cysts are detected they do not require surgical treatment, unless rupture or torsion occurs, as they regress spontaneously over a period of 3–4 months following evacuation of the mole or hysterectomy.

Follow-up is important as the disease persists in between 5 and 10 per cent of women, often developing a malignant form (invasive mole and choriocarcinoma). The period of follow-up should be for 4 to 6 months for women in whom beta HCG is undetectable within 60 days, and 2 years for all other women. Oral contraceptives may be prescribed if the couple desire as there is no evidence that they increase the chance that trophoblastic disease will persist.

PERSISTENT TROPHOBLASTIC DISEASE (MALIGNANT TROPHOBLASTIC DISEASE)

As mentioned, trophoblastic disease persists in between 5 and 10 per cent of women who expel a hydatidiform mole, and in most cases shows malignant characteristics.

Malignancy may also follow an apparently 'normal' abortion and a viable pregnancy. The incidence of malignancy following a benign trophoblastic tumour is 1 in 10; following an abortion 1 in 5000; and following a viable pregnancy 1 in 50 000 cases. This can be stated in a different way: malignant trophoblastic disease is preceded by benign tumour in 70 per cent, by abortion in 20 per cent and by a viable pregnancy in 10 per cent of cases. Because of the relative frequency of malignant change following benign trophoblastic neoplasms the importance of meticulous follow-up of patients expelling a benign trophoblastic tumour is evident. Trophoblastic malignancy following an abortion or a viable pregnancy is much less easy to detect, and

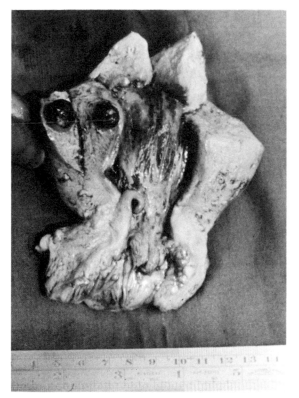

Fig. 20/6 Malignant trophoblastic disease (choriocarcinoma)

most cases are discovered when a patient who was previously pregnant presents with signs of cor pulmonale, or with secondary deposits of tumour in the vagina, the lungs or the brain. Persistent uterine bleeding following an apparently complete abortion, or lasting for more than 8 weeks after confinement, demands curettage and a gonadotrophin estimation in serum or urine. In these cases, the curettings must always be submitted for histopathological examination.

Trophoblastic malignancy following the expulsion of a benign tumour occurs in about 10 per cent of cases, usually within 6 months of the diagnosis of the benign tumour. Two clinical forms occur, (1) malignancy apparently confined to the uterus, and (2) malignancy with extra-uterine spread. These two groups equate fairly closely to the pathological concepts of 'invasive mole' and 'choriocarcinoma', although about 15 per cent of cases of invasive mole show signs of extra-uterine spread, and in approximately the same percentage of cases the choriocarcinoma is confined to the uterus. Malignant trophoblastic tumour is highly lethal, and salvage will only be obtained if it is detected early and treated aggressively (Fig. **20/6**).

Certain women are at greater risk of developing trophoblastic malignancy. Amongst them the risk is 25 per cent, compared with 4 per cent amongst the others.

The high risk group includes those who are:

* Over 40 years of age
* The uterus is 'large for dates' at diagnosis
* The serum beta HCG titre >1000iu/ml before treatment
* Theca-lutein cysts >6cm in size are present.

Patients who have expelled a benign trophoblastic tumour, or who have had a hysterectomy with the mole *in situ*, must be followed up carefully so that malignant change, should it occur, can be detected early. There is evidence that the earlier malignancy is detected and treated, the better is the prognosis.

The woman should be seen at 2-weekly intervals when a vaginal examination is made to evaluate uterine involution (if the uterus has not been removed) and the presence of enlarged ovaries. If bleeding persists, or increases, a further curettage or hysterectomy may be indicated. In general, bleeding should cease within 21 days of the molar evacuation.

The β-subunit of HCG permits the specific

measurement of the hormone and its measurement is essential for the adequate follow-up of all cases of trophoblastic disease. To provide less is inadequate management. The assay is best made in a suitable trophoblastic disease reference centre as the interpretation of the results and the decision when to use chemotherapy is crucial. Although it is customary to increase the level of βHCG in blood plasma, using a radio-immuno-assay, recently a more sensitive βHCG assay has been developed. The test is made on a 24-hour urine specimen as in 24 hours 'the kidney excretes as much HCG as is contained in 1000ml serum'. Recrudescence of trophoblastic activity is detected earlier (by 1–6 weeks) using this assay, which enables chemotherapy to be given earlier and may improve long-term remission. (Fig. **20/7**). The protocol for the follow-up of benign gestational trophoblastic disease, as recommended by the New England Trophoblastic Disease Centre, is shown in Table **20/2**.

1. Radio-immuno-assay of serum βHCG at 7–10-day intervals. If the level falls serially no drug treatment is needed. Complete disappearance of βHCG takes 12 to 14 weeks on average.
2. When βHCG level has been normal for 3 consecutive weeks, test monthly for 6 months.
3. If the assay shows normal βHCG levels for 6 consecutive months, follow-up can be discontinued.
4. During the follow-up period pregnancy should be avoided. Oral contraceptives may be prescribed.
5. If the serum βHCG level plateaus for more than 3 consecutive weeks, or rises, or if metastases are detected, treat with methotrexate or actinomycin D.

Table **20/2** The follow-up of benign trophoblastic disease using a specific radio-immuno-assay

TREATMENT OF PERSISTENT OR MALIGNANT TROPHOBLASTIC DISEASE

As most cases of trophoblastic malignancy follow the expulsion of a benign trophoblastic tumour, the follow-up mentioned in the previous section is mandatory. The failure of the levels of βHCG to fall (over a 3-week period), or a rise in βHCG levels, or the detection of metastases, is an indication for chemotherapy. The choice is between methotrexate 15 to 25mg daily intravenously in divided doses, over 5

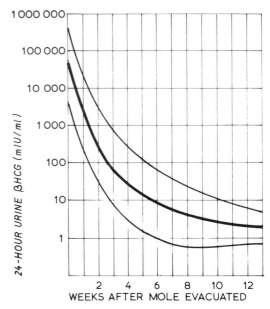

Fig. **20/7** Hormone follow-up of benign trophoblastic disease (mean and 95% confidence limits)

days; or actinomycin D 12μg/kg/day intravenously over 5 days. In certain cases, for example, if the woman is over the age of 40 and has no wish for further children, and the disease is confined to the uterus, total hysterectomy with ovarian conservation may be chosen. The operation should be preceded by methotrexate 20mg daily for 2 days prior to operation and for 3 days after operation. Following surgery, methotrexate is given with folinic acid tissue rescue as shown in Table **20/4**. Response is assessed by measuring the βHCG in serum according to the schedule shown in Table **20/3**.

The adoption of these measures reduces the mortality from non-metastatic malignant trophoblastic disease to less than 5 per cent.

Where the disease has spread beyond the uterus (in other words, a choriocarcinoma is usually present), surgery is only indicated if heavy uterine or vaginal bleeding persists despite chemotherapy. Low dose methotrexate with folinic acid 'tissue rescue' in the schedule shown in Table **20/4** is tried first. If no response is obtained after two consecutive courses as judged by the criteria in Table **20/3**, actinomycin D or etoposide is given for two courses. If this fails to produce a response, multiple chemotherapeutic agents are used.

This method of treatment reduces or eliminates the side-effects of chemotherapy.

1. During treatment the serum levels of the βHCG are assayed each week.
2. Provided that the βHCG level continues to fall after a course of chemotherapy, withhold further courses.
3. When the βHCG level is normal for 3 consecutive weeks, assay each month for 6 months.
4. If the βHCG level remains normal for 12 months, discontinue follow-up. Patients should avoid pregnancy throughout this period.
5. Repeat the course of chemotherapy if the βHCG level plateaus for more than 3 consecutive weeks or rises, or if new metastases are detected.
6. If the βHCG level plateaus after 3 consecutive courses of a chemotherapeutic agent, or if it rises during a course, change to another chemotherapeutic regimen.

Table 20/3 Principles of the management of malignant trophoblastic disease, using a specific βHCG assay

The disadvantage of this therapy is that the chemotherapeutic agents are non-discriminatory, and damage all dividing cells whether normal or malignant. Thus signs of toxicity occur as the cells lining the mouth, the pharynx and the intestinal tract are damaged, and as the maturation of all bone marrow cells is hindered. The toxicity is unpredictable, but the severity of the damage can be reduced if assessment of marrow function (by estimation of red and white cell counts), or liver function and renal function is made prior to instituting therapy. Toxicity varies from course to course, and usually only begins on the 4th day of therapy or after the course has terminated. The main toxic effects are, (1) malaise, (2) stomatitis and pharyngitis, (3) diarrhoea, (4) leucopenia, and (5) alopecia. Apart from the alopecia, which may persist for a prolonged period, toxicity is of short duration, and treatment consists of sedation, analgesic mouth washes or lozenges, and opiates for control of discomfort and diarrhoea. Alopecia causes a considerable psychological upset, but can be hidden by an appropriately styled wig.

A patient undergoing treatment for malignant trophoblastic disease may be discharged from hospital, once toxicity has subsided. She will require readmission for further chemotherapy if the βHCG level rises, or plateaus for 2 consecutive weeks. However, if the βHCG level is zero for 3 consecutive weeks, no further course of chemotherapy is given.

Follow-up is continued with monthly βHCG assays for 12 months.

It will be observed that the administration of the chemotherapeutic agents is based on tumour growth and regression, as evidenced by the level of βHCG in the serum, rather than on the subsidence of systemic toxicity. The use of chemotherapy has reduced the mortality from malignant trophoblastic tumour which has spread beyond the uterus, from 90 per cent to 10 per cent. Such results will only be obtained, however, if all patients with trophoblastic disease are treated in special centres, where careful assessment prior to treatment and meticulous follow-up with sensitive radio-immuno-assays of the βHCG can be conducted.

	Non-metastatic	Metastatic
Initial course		
Methotrexate at 48-hour intervals for 4 doses	1mg/kg IM	1.5mg/kg IM
Folinic acid (citrovorum factor) on alternate days		
24 hours after the injection of methotrexate	0.1mg/kg IM	0.15mg/kg IM

Subsequent courses:
A. If response, that is a fall in the beta HCG level $\pm 20\%$, repeat the regimen
B. Without response, increase methotrexate by 0.5mg/kg and folinic acid by 0.05mg/kg
C. If no response after two consecutive courses change to actinomycin D
D. If no response to actinomycin D after two courses change to three chemotherapeutic drugs used in combination

Laboratory tests
    Full blood count, platelet count, SGOT on day 1 (before starting therapy) days 3, 5, 7, 11, 15, 18, 21

Table 20/4 Chemotherapy in malignant trophoblastic disease

Chapter 21

Uterine Displacements and Uterovaginal Prolapse

Displacements of the uterus and uterovaginal prolapse occupied the minds and the time of most gynaecologists between 1850 and 1950. Many were the disturbances which were considered due to the conditions; many were the operations devised to correct the conditions; many of the operations were not required, and many were failures. The fault lay in the philosophy of the gynaecologists and their failure to appreciate that (1) the uterus is a mobile organ which pivots about an axis at the level of the internal cervical os, (2) the non-adherent retroverted uterus rarely causes symptoms, and (3) even quite marked degrees of uterovaginal prolapse may be symptomless. The pendulum has swung from this anatomical, surgical approach, and a much more rational attitude has come into vogue. Today, the place of surgery is limited, and the extent of the surgical intervention is much more clearly defined.

UTERINE DISPLACEMENTS

The uterus may be displaced in several directions. Upward, forward and lateral displacements of the uterus are of no significance, except as a sign of an underlying disorder which causes the displacement. Backward displacement is caused by a full bladder or by a tumour occupying the vesico-uterine pouch, and is of no significance. Retroversion of the uterus is the term customarily used to include *retroflexion* (in which the long axis of the corpus is bent backwards on the long axis of the cervix), and *retroversion* (in which the long axis of the corpus and cervix are in line, and the whole organ has pivoted backwards in relation to the long axis of the birth canal). The two conditions usually occur together, and for this reason the inexact term *retroversion* is used to encompass them both (Fig. **21/1**).

AETIOLOGY AND INCIDENCE

In infancy the uterus (1) has a cervix much longer proportionally than the corpus, (2) is one-quarter the size of the postpubertal organ, the cervix being larger than the corpus, (3) has a relatively poor vascular supply, and (4) is retroverted. With the onset of ovarian function, the body of the uterus grows rapidly, the blood supply increases, and the adult uterus develops. This (1) has a corpus twice as long as the cervix, (2) has a good vascular and lymphatic supply, (3) is usually anteverted, and (4) since the development of the corpus is so great, is usually anteflexed. But in 20 per cent of women anteversion does not occur, and the uterus remains retroverted.

Acquired retroversion of the uterus is less common, and is due to endometriosis of the uterosacral ligaments or the cul-de-sac; to adhesions formed by pelvic infection pulling the uterus back; or to tumours in the front of the uterus pushing it back. Pregnancy causes a considerable plasticity of the uterine supports, and uterine retroversion is often found in the puerperium. Usually the patient had a retroverted uterus before she became pregnant, but occasionally this is not so. In these cases the uterus spontaneously becomes anteverted once more within 6 months of confinement, and manipulations are not required.

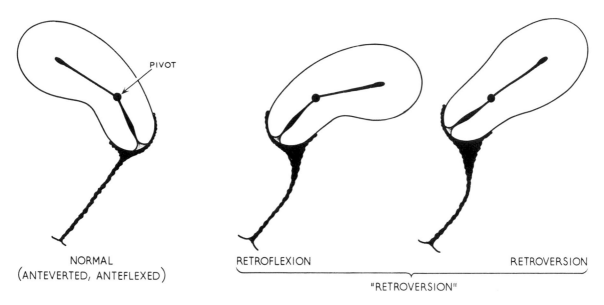

Fig. 21/1 Retroversion and retroflexion of the uterus

SYMPTOMS

Developmental retroversion is symptomless, the uterus being mobile and returning to the retroverted position if anteverted digitally. A few women develop a psychosomatic disorder in which symptoms of pelvic pain and heaviness predominate, and some of these women are alleged to have a bulky, boggy, tender, retroverted uterus. 'Correction' of position of the uterus, if accompanied by sufficient verbal indoctrination of the value of the procedure, has the effect of fixing the patient's mind on a symptom and a 'disease', and sometimes results in a cure. Often it does not.

Despite the belief of some gynaecologists, there is little evidence that uncomplicated uterine retroversion is a cause of infertility or of abortion. However, if no other cause for infertility can be found, anteversion of the uterus and the insertion of a Hodge or ring pessary occasionally results in conception.

When the uterus is fixed in the retroverted position, usually due to endometriosis or to chronic pelvic infection, symptoms are often present. They include dysmenorrhoea, dyspareunia on deep penetration, pelvic pain and low backache.

DIAGNOSIS

Inspection of the cervix through a vaginal speculum will show it to be in the anterior quadrant of the vault and to point forward. A bimanual examination will confirm the position and direction of the cervix, and the uterus can be felt in the cul-de-sac. A rectal examination may help if any difficulty is experienced in outlining the uterus. Often it is difficult to be sure that the uterus is normal, and before diagnosing a complicated retroverted uterus, anteversion of the organ should be attempted. This is done by moving the cervix backwards and pushing the fundus upwards with the intravaginal fingers, whilst the abdominal hand attempts to press behind the fundus and to manipulate it forward on one or other side of the sacral promontory (Fig. **21/2**). Alternatively, a Hodge pessary may be used (Fig. **21/3**).

If the uterus is mobile and of normal shape, one can be reasonably sure that it is not the cause of the symptoms, but if any doubt exists, a pessary test may be applied. The uterus is anteverted, a pessary is inserted, and the patient told that it will hold her uterus in position. If one month later she still complains of the same symptoms, the retroversion was not the cause. If she says that the symptoms are less, the uterus is manipulated backwards and the pessary replaced, the patient being told that her uterus is in

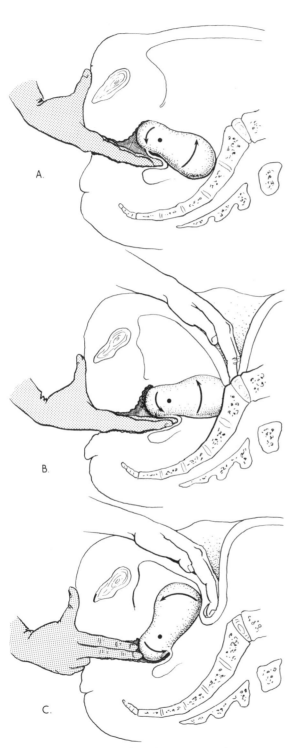

Fig. 21/2 Manipulation of the retroverted uterus

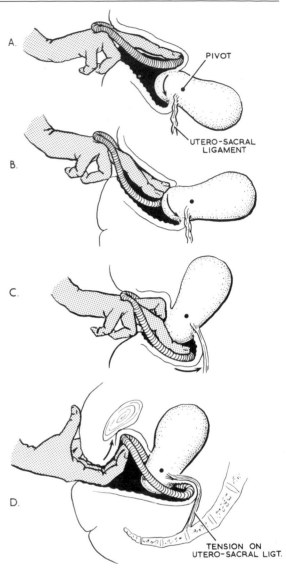

Fig. 21/3 The use of a Hodge pessary to correct the position of a retroverted uterus

the 'normal position'. If after this the symptoms continue to be relieved, the retroversion was not the cause.

TREATMENT

A pessary is required (1) for the pessary test, (2) in pregnancy if a retroverted uterus has not become anteverted spontaneously by the 12th week, and (3) very occasionally in cases of infertility. The Hodge pessary is the most efficient type (Fig. **21/4**). It acts by holding the cervix back in the hollow of the sacrum and putting tension on the posterior fornix and uterosacral ligaments (Fig. **21/3D**).

Operative treatment is contra-indicated, except (1) where the pessary test is positive, indicating that the displacement is *probably* the cause of the symptoms, (2) when the retroverted uterus is 'fixed' and an associated condition, such as endometriosis, is present. In these cases the operation should only be performed if symptoms of pelvic pain and deep dyspareunia are also present. The operation consists of shortening the round ligaments by plicating them with linen thread, or by bringing them out through the internal abdominal ring and suturing one to the other, anterior to the recti abdominis muscles, inside the rectus muscle sheath (Gilliam–Crossen operation).

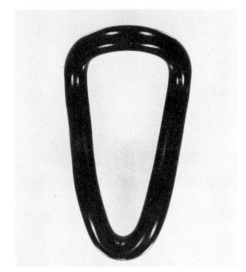

Fig. 21/4 The Hodge pessary

UTEROVAGINAL PROLAPSE

Uterovaginal prolapse implies a descent of the uterus and/or the vagina. A vaginal prolapse may occur independently of any uterine descent, but descent of the uterus always carries some part of the upper vagina with it. It is a form of hernia.

VAGINAL PROLAPSE

Anterior wall – cystocele

The prolapse may involve the upper part of the anterior vaginal wall, and since this is connected to the pubocervical fascia, and thus to the bladder muscular wall, herniation of the bladder, or cystocele, occurs (Fig. **21/5**). Cystocele is fairly common, and often is symptomless, but a large cystocele, particularly of long duration, may cause urethral angulation and hypertrophy of the muscular walls of the bladder, which becomes a thick-walled 'flabby' organ. In such cases symptoms are usual, and the two most commonly met are bladder irritation and the presence of a lump. The bladder irritability is due to the residual urine, which often becomes infected, so that frequency of micturition and dysuria occur. In the later stages, pyelonephritis may result.

Anterior wall – urethrocele

If the vaginal laxity involves the lower part of the anterior vaginal wall, a urethrocele will develop. The urethra is displaced downwards and rotates backwards at its junction with the bladder. The effect of this is that the patient may develop stress incontinence (see p. 247).

Posterior wall – enterocele

The upper vagina and posterior fornix may prolapse, causing an elongation of the conical-shaped cul-de-sac. Since this may contain loops of bowel, it is termed an 'enterocele'. A small enterocele causes no symptoms, but a large one may be associated with deep pelvic discomfort.

Posterior wall – rectocele

Prolapse of the middle vaginal wall brings down with it the rectum, and is called a 'rectocele'. Since the lowest third of the vagina is separated from the rectum by the perineal body, the bulge protrudes from the vulva over this, unless a previous unrepaired laceration has left a deficient perineum. A

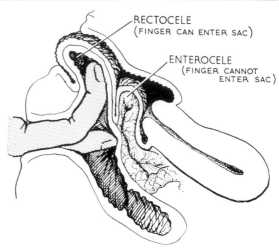

Fig. 21/6 Enterocele and rectocele

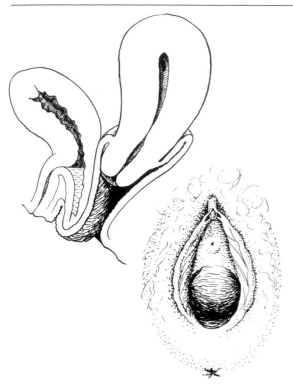

Fig. 21/5 Cystocele

rectocele usually produces no symptoms unless very large, when faeces may enter the sacculated rectum, and defaecation can only be accomplished by digital pressure on the rectocele from the vaginal side. A rectocele may be confused with an enterocele, but this can be resolved easily by inserting a finger into the rectum (Fig. **21/6**). If the finger does not enter the hernial sac and is not palpable per vaginam, the lump is an enterocele.

UTEROVAGINAL PROLAPSE

Descent of the uterus is always accompanied by some descent of the upper vagina, and may be found in association with enterocele, rectocele or cystocele. As the uterus descends, it becomes slightly retroverted, and the cervix elongates.

Three degrees are recognized. First degree prolapse is diagnosed when there is slight descent of the uterus, but the cervix remains within the vagina. Second degree prolapse indicates that the cervix projects beyond the vulva when the patient strains. In third degree prolapse, or complete procidentia, the entire uterus has prolapsed outside the vulva, and most, if not all, of the vagina is everted (Fig. **21/7**).

Once the cervix or the vagina prolapses through the vulva, marked changes in the stratified epithelium occur. In the absence of moisture, the super-

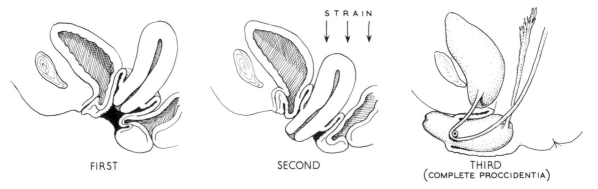

DEGREES OF UTERO-VAGINAL PROLAPSE

Fig. 21/7 Diagram showing degrees of uterine prolapse

ficial epithelial layers become keratinized, thickened and appear whitish. This epithelium is less resistant to trauma and is more sensitive to circulatory disturbances, so that ulceration is not uncommon.

The reason for the elongation of the cervix is not clear, but is probably due to the increased tension placed upon the lymphatics and veins draining the cervix. This causes congestion, hypertrophy and stretching of the connective tissue cells which constitute 90 per cent of the cervix. The congestion can lead to marked cervical oedema, particularly when the uterovaginal prolapse has been present for a long time. A serious complication, particularly when third degree prolapse is present, is that the lower ends of the ureters are carried down, and become kinked and oedematous so that chronic obstruction occurs, leading ultimately to hydroureter and hydronephrosis. It is remarkable how much improvement in the oedema and urinary tract function occurs if the prolapse is reduced, and the vagina packed to maintain the reduction.

AETIOLOGY

Anatomical considerations

The vagina is a hollow muscular tube, the anterior and posterior walls of which are normally in apposition. Fibres of the levator ani muscles pass inwards and downwards from its bony origin on the posterior

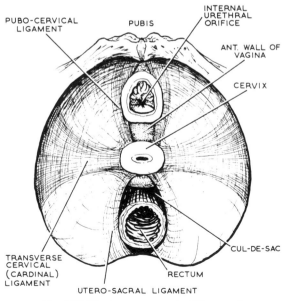

Fig. 21/8 The transverse cervical 'ligament'

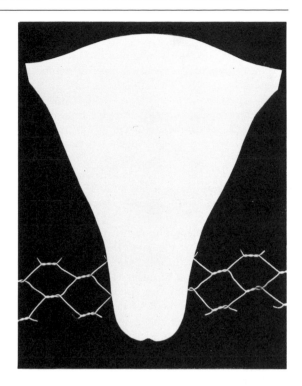

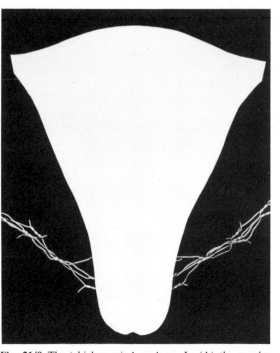

Fig. 21/9 The 'chicken wire' analogy. In (A) the areolar tissue is not stretched; in (B), because of the uterine descent, condensation of the tissue occurs, with the appearance of a ligament

surface of the pubis, to join with the vaginal muscle. In addition, the branches of the uterine artery which supply the vagina add a quantum of muscle tissue. The muscular vagina acts as the inferior support of the uterus.

The cervix projects into the vaginal vault, and above this the supravaginal cervix is surrounded by a felted mass of connective tissue, in which is found smooth muscle and through which pass blood vessels supplying the uterus and bladder. This tissue, which stretches from the fascia covering the internal surface of the levator ani muscles to fuse with the connective and muscle tissue of the supravaginal cervix, is called the 'transverse cervical' or 'cardinal' ligament, although it is not a ligament in the true sense of the word (Fig. **21/8**). Posteriorly on each side a condensation of the tissue forms the uterosacral ligament. The transverse cervical ligaments act as the middle support of the upper cervix and the body of the uterus, and their function has been described in terms of chicken wire. Provided the strain is not too great, they have considerable tensile strength, but if the strain is increased, they stretch, and as they stretch the connective tissue condenses to give the appearance of ligaments (Fig. **21/9**).

The upper supports of the uterus are relatively weak, and operate mostly by maintaining the uterus in an anteverted position. These are the round muscles, usually miscalled the round ligaments.

The uterus therefore has three supports: inferiorly, the muscular vagina; in the middle, and the most important, the transverse cervical ligaments; and superiorly, the round 'ligaments' (Fig. **21/10**).

Functional considerations

The occurrence of prolapse results from the failure of one or more supports just described. The failure may in turn be due to one or more of several factors.

1. *Imperfect development of the supporting tissues.* The infantile uterus is only the size of an olive, and requires little support. With the spurt of growth of the Mullerian duct structures which occurs at puberty, development also occurs in the supports. Should this development be defective, and this applies particularly to the middle supports, prolapse of the uterus may occur. This is the reason for the rare congenital prolapse, and for the observation that uterine prolapse is as likely to follow an easy as a difficult childbirth, the imperfect development of the pelvic tissues permitting a more rapid delivery.

2. *Stretching of the supporting tissues at childbirth.* A more usual cause of prolapse is the stretching of the tissues which make up the genital tract by the passage of the fetus during childbirth. Evolution has endowed man with a large rounded head, which must be forced through the birth canal. The exact mechanism of the damage is unknown, but excessive pressure on the cervix before full dilatation puts a considerable strain on the transverse cervical ligaments, whilst prolongation of the second stage of labour, particularly when the baby is large, may damage the vaginal fibromuscular supports. Finally, undue fundal pressure in attempts to deliver the placenta, will put a marked strain on the transverse cervical ligaments, already strained from the processes of childbirth.

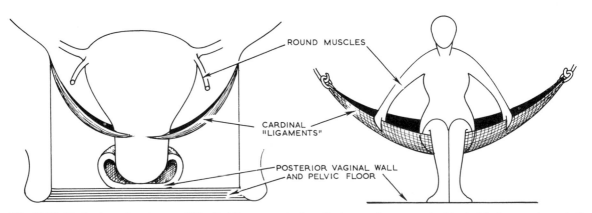

Fig. 21/10 Mechanism of prolapse – if the 'holding apparatus', or the 'supporting apparatus' is stretched, some descent of the uterus, or of the vagina, will occur, particularly if the intra-abdominal pressure is increased

3. *Atrophy of the supporting tissues at the climacteric.* At the climacteric there is a withdrawal of the hormonal support which has persisted since adolescence. Deprived of oestrogen, the musculature and fibrous tissues of the paramesonephric duct atrophy. Prior to this, despite imperfect development, or childbirth damage, there may have been enough tone in the supports to prevent prolapse. But once climacteric atrophy occurs, the prolapse becomes manifest. It is for this reason that symptomatic prolapse is more common after the climacteric.

SYMPTOMS AND SIGNS

The amount of discomfort suffered by patients with uterovaginal prolapse varies considerably, and different types of prolapse are associated with different symptoms; but most are relieved completely if the patient lies down.

The main symptoms are a feeling of 'something falling out', dragging pains in the pelvis, some protrusion at the vulva, and difficulty or discomfort in micturition, or defaecation. Contrary to what has been written, backache is an infrequent symptom of prolapse.

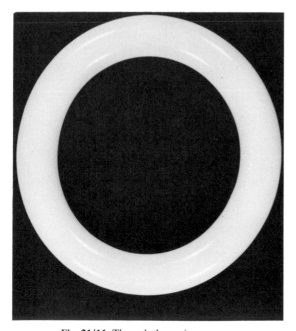

Fig. 21/11 The polythene ring pessary

The type and degree of the prolapse can be determined by observing the vulva when the patient is straining or coughing, and by supplementing this with a vaginal examination. The extent of the prolapse is often revealed more easily if the patient is put in the left lateral position and a Sims' vaginal speculum inserted. The degree of cervical and anterior vaginal wall descent can be more readily appreciated by this technique. Stress incontinence can only be detected if the bladder has not been emptied, and a rectal examination may be required to differentiate a rectocele from an enterocele.

DIFFERENTIAL DIAGNOSIS

Prolapse must be differentiated from the following:

1. Hypertrophy of the cervix with no damage to the uterine supports.
2. Tumours or cysts of the vagina.
3. Tumours or cysts of the uterus, which project through the cervix.
4. Inversion of the uterus.

MANAGEMENT

Preventive

Although inherent developmental defects cannot be prevented, damage and stretching of the tissues can be minimized in childbirth if certain prophylactic measures are undertaken. These include (1) avoidance of pushing by the patient, or of attempts at delivery by the physician, before the full dilatation of the cervix, (2) avoidance of prolongation of the second stage of labour, (3) avoidance of fundal pushing in an attempt to expel the placenta, (4) careful repair, in accurate layers, of all vaginal wall and perineal tears and incisions (colpoperineorrhaphy), (5) early ambulation and pelvic floor exercises in the puerperium.

Active

The treatment of an established symptomatic prolapse, as with other hernias, is basically surgical. However, if no symptoms are present and if assessment shows that there is no chronic urinary infection, no treatment is required, although the patient should be seen and reassessed at annual intervals. The age and marital status of the patient does not alter the principle, although it may modify the surgical procedure adopted. Old women who have complete prolapse should be admitted to hospital prior to surgery and the prolapse reduced, the vagina being packed with gauze impregnated with oestradiol cream. The oestrogen improves the quality of the vaginal tissues, and the reduction of the prolapse permits ulcers to heal, cervical oedema to subside and keratinization to revert. Operation should be delayed for 14 to 21 days to enable this to occur.

The operation required may merely be excision of the redundant vaginal tissue and the repair of the damaged fascia (anterior colporrhaphy or posterior colporrhaphy). If a uterovaginal prolapse is present, these operations are combined with amputation of the cervix and shortening of the transverse cervical ligaments, which are plicated and stitched to the front of the cervical stump (the Manchester operation); or with vaginal hysterectomy and careful approximation of the pedicles of the transverse cervical ligaments, the uterosacral ligaments and the broad ligaments.

Less effective, but valuable in selected patients, is the use of a plastic ring pessary (Fig. **21/11**). Some women refuse operation, some are too debilitated to permit operation, some have a very short life expectancy: these patients benefit considerably if a pessary is used. The size of the pessary chosen is determined by the length of the vagina. It must be large enough to remain in place when the patient strains, but small enough to be rotated in the vagina by the physician. Once in place, the patient should be unaware of its presence. The pessary does not cure the prolapse, but by distending the upper vagina prevents it, and the uterus, from prolapsing. A patient wearing a pessary should be seen every 4 months, when the pessary is removed, the vagina is inspected for tissue damage and the pessary replaced.

Chapter 22

Ectopic Gestation and Non-Infective Diseases of the Oviduct

ECTOPIC GESTATION

Ectopic gestation is the condition when the fertilized ovum fails to reach the uterine cavity and becomes implanted in some part of the oviduct or, rarely, in the ovary. The incidence of ectopic pregnancy has increased in the developed countries from 1 in 250 conceptions to 1 in 150 conceptions and now equals that in the developing countries. The reason for the increase is not clear, but may be due to an increase in pelvic inflammatory disease, or to earlier diagnosis using ultrasound. The latter is suggested as between 15 and 50 per cent of ectopic gestations spontaneously abort or are resorbed. There is no evidence that induced abortions or the use of an IUD as a contraceptive are factors. The right and left tubes are involved with equal frequency, and rarely a tubal pregnancy may occur in both tubes.

AETIOLOGY

Despite many theories, the aetiology of tubal pregnancy remains unknown. Implantation can only occur when the zona pellucida has been partially, or completely shed. This usually takes place in the uterine cavity; but in tubal pregnancy it must occur earlier. This could be because (1) an ovum released

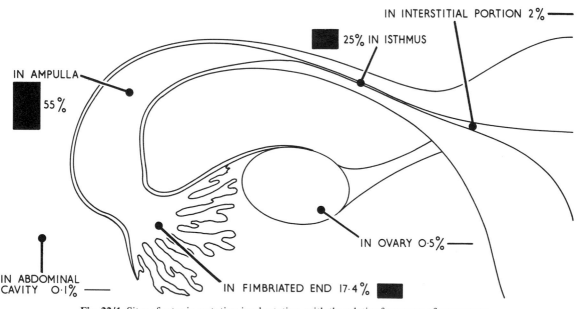

Fig. 22/1 Sites of ectopic gestation implantation, with the relative frequency of occurrence

just prior to menstruation is fertilized and its passage down the tube is delayed by the back-flow of menstrual blood, or (2) the progress of the fertilized ovum down the tube is delayed by mechanical factors such as increased tortuosity, or agglutination of the tubal endothelium caused by previous low-grade infection.

PATHOLOGY

Implantation may occur in the fimbriated end (17 per cent), the ampulla (55 per cent), the isthmus (25 per cent), the interstitial portion (2 per cent), and rarely, the ovary (0.5 per cent), or the abdominal cavity (0.1 per cent) (Fig. **22/1**).

Under the influence of hormones synthesized by the corpus luteum and the invading trophoblast, the uterus enlarges and a decidua is formed. In the tube only a slight decidual reaction occurs with enlargement of the stromal cells of the tube wall, and some hypertrophy of the tubal muscle fibres and blood vessel walls. The further sequence of events depends upon the site of implantation, as the degree the weakened tube can distend before it ruptures varies with the calibre and thickness of the part of the oviduct involved, and the degree of trophoblastic activity.

If the ovum implants in the fimbriated end of ampulla of the tube, the trophoblast initially erodes capillaries supplying the convoluted epithelial-covered folds of mucosa. The resulting haemorrhage is usually slight, but may be sufficient to separate the ovum from its attachment to the mucosa, leading to a tubal abortion. More active trophoblastic invasion maintains the viability of the ovum but causes repeated episodes of haemorrhage from deeper vessels of the tube wall at the implantation site, and some of this blood gravitates from the tube lumen into the peritoneal sac. As the ovum grows the tube becomes progressively distended, and trophoblastic invasion through the muscularis further weakens this layer with more episodes of bleeding. The gradual penetration of the tubal wall finally leads to a small rupture. This is usually sealed at once by blood clot, but repeated episodes cause a peritubal haematoma. If the rupture is larger, part of the ovum is extruded through the rent by the peristalsis of the tube, and bleeding persists which covers the surface of the ovum with clots or gravitates to the pouch of Douglas. In both of these cases a marked local peritoneal reaction occurs and the mass is covered by exudate, adherent omentum and bowel. In time a thick layer of exudate covers the blood in the pouch of Douglas, which is now called a 'pelvic haematocele'. Should the invading trophoblast erode a large vessel at the time of tubal penetration, severe internal haemorrhage into the peritoneal cavity, or between the layers of the broad ligament occurs (a pelvic haematoma) with the sudden collapse of the patient.

If the implantation is in the isthmus, where the mucosa is thinner and the vessels larger, penetration of the muscularis and tubal rupture occurs earlier and internal haemorrhage is usually severe. If the implantation is in the interstitial portion of the oviduct, rupture is often delayed, as the myometrium surrounds the growing conceptus. However, when rupture eventually occurs, it is attended by severe haemorrhage.

OUTCOME FOR THE PREGNANCY

In most cases the pregnancy terminates between the 6th and 10th week in one of several ways.

Tubal abortion

This occurs in 65 per cent of cases and is the usual termination in fimbrial and ampullary implantation. Repeated small haemorrhages from the invaded area of the tubal wall separate the ovum which dies, and is either (1) absorbed completely; (2) aborted completely through the tubal ostium into the peritoneal cavity; (3) aborted incompletely, so that the clot-covered conceptus distends the ostium, or (4) forms a tubal blood mole (Fig. **22/2**).

Tubal rupture

This occurs in 35 per cent of cases, and is more common when the implantation is in the isthmus. Whilst rupture of the ampulla usually occurs between the 6th and 10th week, rupture of the isthmus occurs earlier, frequently at the time of the first missed period. The trophoblast burrows deeply and eventually erodes the serosal coat of the tube, the final break being sudden or gradual. Usually the ovum is extruded through the rent and bleeding continues. If the rupture is on the mesenteric side of the tube, a broad ligament haematoma will form (Fig. **22/3**).

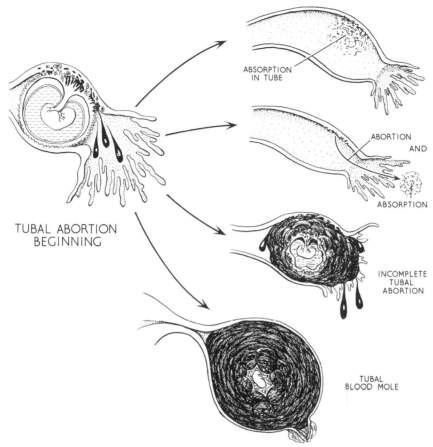

Fig. 22/2 The sequelae of tubal abortion shown diagrammatically

Secondary abdominal pregnancy

Very rarely the extruded ovum continues to grow, as sufficient trophoblast maintains its connection with the tubal epithelium, and later the trophoblast covering the ovisac attaches to abdominal organs. A few of these pregnancies advance to term, and in a very few the fetus dies early and is converted into a lithopaedion.

CLINICAL ASPECTS

The possibility of an ectopic gestation should always be considered in a woman of childbearing age especially if there is a history of acute salpingitis. The history is of greater importance than the physical signs, as these can be equivocal. Usually there is a short period of *amenorrhoea*, although in 20 per cent of cases this may not be present. The *pain* is lower

abdominal in site, but not distinguishable from that of abortion. However, in ruptured ectopic gestation fainting is usual, although this may only be momentary. Vaginal bleeding follows the pain, and may be mistaken for bleeding due to a delayed menstrual period or an abortion. The bleeding is slight, brownish in colour and continuous, and clots are rarely present (Table **22/1**).

	percentage
Abdominal pain	90
Amenorrhoea	80
Vaginal bleeding	70
Adnexal tenderness	80
Abdominal tenderness	80
Adnexal mass	50

Table 22/1 Symptoms and signs in ectopic gestation

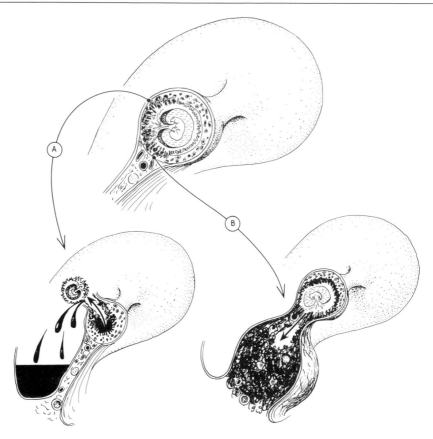

Fig. 22/3 The sequelae of tubal rupture. (A) Intraperitoneal haemorrhage and pelvic haematocele; (B) Broad ligament haematoma

Two clinical patterns occur, and are due to the extent of the damage to the tube wall by the invading trophoblast. The first is subacute, the second acute.

Subacute

After a short period of amenorrhoea, the patient complains of some lower abdominal discomfort, which may be so mild that she considers it normal for pregnancy. Occasionally there is an attack of sharp pain and faintness, due to an episode of intraperitoneal bleeding, and if these symptoms are marked she will seek advice, particularly if the episode is followed by slight vaginal bleeding. Examination may reveal tenderness in the lower abdomen, and vaginal examination may show a tender fornix, or a vague mass, but the signs may be insufficient to make a diagnosis. If the patient is observed, further episodes of pain are likely, and the blood loss per vaginam persists, until acute collapse supervenes (indicating tubal rupture or incomplete tubal abortion), or the symptoms cease (indicating complete abortion with or without pelvic haematocele).

Acute – dramatic

Sudden collapse with little or no warning is more common when the implantation is isthmal, but is not the most frequent type of the acute clinical pattern. It is more usual for the acute rupture to supervene upon the subacute, but the mild symptoms of the latter may have been thought to be normal occurrences in pregnancy and ignored.

As the tube ruptures the patient is seized with a sudden acute lower abdominal pain, sufficiently severe to cause fainting. The associated internal haemorrhage leads to collapse, pallor, a weak rapid pulse, and a falling blood pressure. Usually the condition improves after a short time, as the haemorrhage diminishes or ceases, but abdominal discomfort persists, and pain is felt in the epigastrium or referred to the shoulder. A further episode of haemorrhage and collapse is likely, and continued bleeding can be suspected from increasing pallor and a falling haemoglobin level.

On examination the patient is shocked, the lower abdomen is tender with some fullness and muscle guarding. Vaginal examination, which should only be carried out in hospital, shows extreme tenderness in the fornices and marked tenderness on movement of the cervix from side to side.

DIAGNOSIS

Although in acute cases the presence of internal bleeding is obvious and the diagnosis not in doubt, in subacute cases it can be extraordinarily difficult. Laboratory tests may help, but in most instances are not particularly informative. A radio-immuno-assay for serum levels of βHCG, should be made. A negative result ($<$1ng/ml) indicates that the woman is not pregnant, and ectopic gestation can be excluded. If the βHCG test is positive, a pelvic ultrasound

examination should be made preferably using a transvaginal probe. If this shows an empty uterus (Fig. **22/4**), and particularly if it shows a sac and fetus in the Fallopian tube the diagnosis is certain and a laparotomy should be made. On the other hand if ultrasound shows an intra-uterine pregnancy, a concurrent ectopic pregnancy is extremely unlikely. If the diagnosis remains in doubt a laparoscopy will clear the matter up.

If ultrasound is not available, or is equivocal, the presumptive diagnosis may be confirmed by laparoscopy.

The diagnosis of suspected ectopic gestation is summarized in Table **22/2**.

TREATMENT

Whenever tubal pregnancy is suspected, the patient must be transferred to hospital, *without a vaginal examination*, provided she is not in shock. If she is, this must be treated first by adequate, rapid, blood transfusion if this service is available. If it is not, the patient should be laid flat, morphine or pethidine given to reduce the pain, and an intravenous infusion of saline or a plasma expander given. With

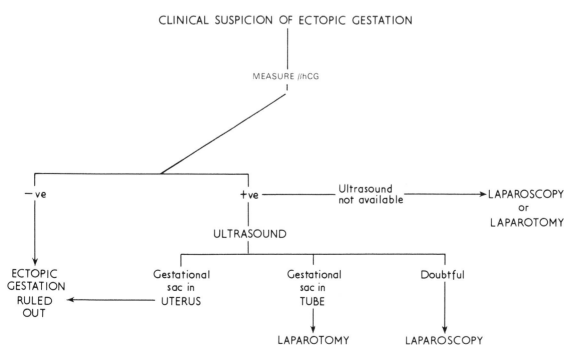

Table 22/2 Algorithm for diagnosis of suspected ectopic gestation

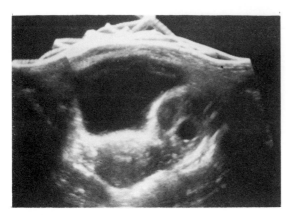 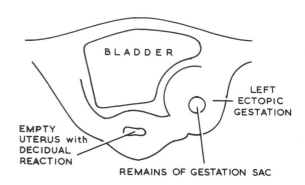

Fig 22/4 Ectopic gestation (ultrasound – transverse scan). Line drawing showing the identification of relevant points

this first aid treatment the patient's condition usually improves sufficiently for her to be taken to hospital.

As soon as the diagnosis of ectopic gestation is made in hospital, laparotomy should be performed *at once*, even if the patient is collapsed. Blood transfusion should be started as soon after admission as possible and continued throughout the operation. When donor blood is not available, auto-transfusion using the blood sucked from the peritoneal cavity can be used. This is collected into bottles containing 200ml sodium citrate per litre and retransfused intravenously.

After opening the abdomen through a sub-umbilical midline incision, the uterus is grasped and brought up into the wound, and the ruptured tube isolated. Before deciding on further treatment, the other tube and ovary should be inspected. Partial salpingectomy, by clamping the tube on each side of the damaged area and excising the wedge, or total salpingectomy is the preferred treatment and can be performed rapidly. If the patient desires further children and the implantation is fimbrial or ampullary, the other tube being absent or damaged, salpingostomy is possible. This will give her a 5 per cent chance of a further pregnancy, and in selected patients may be the operation of choice. If the implantation is interstitial, the damaged cornual area of the uterus must be excised and sutured with haemostatic

sutures. Occasionally the damage to the uterus may necessitate hysterectomy, and the operation may also be required if there is uterine pathology and the patient is able to tolerate the more extensive procedure.

In cases of intraligamentary bleeding, the broad ligament is opened after salpingectomy and the contained blood clot evacuated. Where the bleeding was intraperitoneal, all the free blood and clots should be removed before closing the abdominal wall. This makes for a smoother convalescence and a reduced risk of damage to the remaining tube.

Recent developments using laparoscopic lasers have enabled experienced surgeons to remove the gestation sac from the Fallopian tube and to save the tube in many cases of ectopic gestation.

PROGNOSIS

Only 60 per cent of patients who have had an ectopic gestation become pregnant again. Of the women who do not have a further pregnancy, 75 per cent avoid pregnancy voluntarily, and 25 per cent are involuntarily infertile. The risk of a second ectopic gestation is about 10 per cent, as compared with 0.4 per cent in other women. The chance of delivering a term baby is about 50 per cent. Patients who have previously had an ectopic gestation therefore require additional care during pregnancy.

BENIGN AND MALIGNANT TUMOURS OF THE OVIDUCT

Both benign and malignant tumours of the oviduct are rare; indeed primary carcinoma of the oviduct forms only 0.1 per cent of all genital malignancies. The signs and symptoms of carcinoma of the oviduct are equivocal and the disease is rarely diagnosed before laparoscopy or laparotomy. In premenopausal patients the usual misdiagnosis is chronic salpingitis, and in post-menopausal women, an ovarian tumour. Treatment is surgical, followed by pelvic irradiation. The prognosis is poor.

Chapter 23

The Ovary

OVARIAN TUMOURS

Although details of the embryology of the ovary have been given in Chapter 2, a summary may be helpful. The indifferent gonad develops as an outgrowth of mesenchyme lateral to the root of the primitive mesentery – the intermediate cell mass. The mesenchymal core (which will eventually form the ovarian medulla) is covered by a layer of cells derived from the coelomic epithelium (which will eventually become the ovarian cortex). The epithelial cells penetrate the mesenchymal core in columns, and are subsequently divided into clumps by the mesenchyme. The germ cells, which have been formed in the wall of the hind gut, migrate to, and reach, the gonad by the 35th day. Many are surrounded by a mantle of the epithelial cells to form the primary oocytes, and later as the ensheathing cells secrete fluid, the primary follicles. The remainder are destroyed by proliferation of the medullary (mesenchymal) elements (Fig. **23/1**).

The ovary is therefore made up of (1) epithelial cells derived from the coelomic epithelium, (2) oocytes, which have differentiated from the primitive germ cells, and (3) medullary (mesenchymal) elements. The gonad becomes an ovary because of inductor substances, possibly derived from the oogonia, which stimulate the proliferation of cortical elements at the expense of the male-directed medullary elements. The dominance of the cortical elements is never complete, and this basic bipotentiality is a cause of functional disturbances of the ovary.

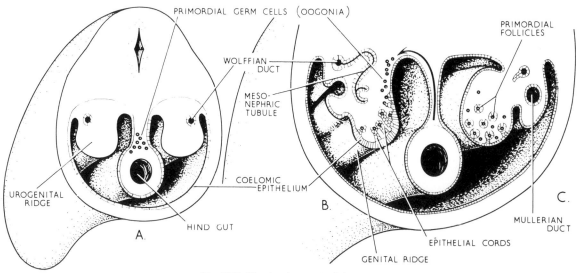

Fig. 23/1 The development of the ovary

PHYSIOLOGY

The tissues which comprise the ovary are particularly dynamic. Each month between puberty and the climacteric, gonadotrophins released by the anterior pituitary gland initiate the growth of up to twenty primary follicles, with the subsequent synthesis of oestrogen by the granulosal cells. Should the regulating 'feedback' of oestrogen to the hypothalamus/pituitary not occur in a proper ratio, or should the pituitary hormonal release be exceptionally marked, one or more of the follicles will enlarge excessively and may persist as a follicular cyst. Similarly, if ovulation occurs and the corpus luteum, formed after the ovum has been discharged, develops abnormally and is maintained for longer than usual by increased release of luteinizing hormone from the anterior pituitary gland, a corpus luteum cyst results. These two types are known as functional cysts of the ovary.

For unknown reasons, growth of the other elements which form the ovary may occur, leading to a variety of ovarian tumours. These may arise from the primitive oocytes (teratoma); from the coelomic epithelium (serous and mucinous cystadenomata); from mesenchymal elements (fibroma, Brenner tumours), from the coelomic epithelium which formed granulosa or theca cells (granulosa-theca tumours); from medullary male-directed cells (androblastoma); or from rests of oogonia which were not destroyed by mesenchymal overgrowth (disgerminoma).

CLINICAL ASPECTS OF OVARIAN TUMOURS IN GENERAL

With the exception of teratomata, and a few of the tumours derived from the sex cell elements in the ovary, ovarian neoplasms are most frequently detected in women aged 35 or more. Ovarian tumours grow slowly, and are usually asymptomatic until they have reached a relatively large size, when the patient, or her physician, may detect an abdominal lump; or when pressure symptoms induce her to seek medical advice. Almost 95 per cent of ovarian tumours are benign, and benign tumours are usually cystic; so that the detection of a solid ovarian tumour (or a cystic tumour containing solid areas) is suggestive of malignancy. The malignancy may be primary, or due to a secondary malignant change in a previously benign tumour. This change tends to occur more frequently after the climacteric than in the reproductive years.

The silent, asymptomatic growth applies equally to benign and malignant ovarian neoplasms, and it is this which makes the latter so lethal. By the time medical advice is sought, the disease is incurable in over 75 per cent of cases. This sinister state of affairs can only be remedied if all women have periodic examinations, including abdominal and bimanual pelvic examinations. If an ovarian tumour is detected at such an examination, further advice must be sought immediately. In general a laparotomy is required.

Benign ovarian tumours never cause pain, unless a complication occurs, and rarely affect menstrual function, unless the tumour is derived from the mesenchymal sex cells. Very large tumours, even if benign, often cause anorexia and abdominal discomfort, and may be associated with cachexia. Malignant tumours are usually accompanied by pain, particularly when the tumour has become adherent to other organs, by ascites and by loss of weight.

DIAGNOSIS

The finding of a painless cystic mass in the cul-de-sac or the presence of an abdominal lump, usually cystic to firm on palpation, is suggestive of an ovarian tumour. Once an ovarian tumour has grown out of the pelvis, it tends to lie centrally, so that it is impossible to be sure from which ovary the tumour has arisen. The distinction, in any case, is of no importance. A large tumour may be confused with ascites, but in the latter the area of dullness on percussion is maximal in the flanks, whilst the ovarian tumour displaces the gut to the flanks and the area of dullness is central, the flanks being resonant on percussion.

An ovarian tumour must be differentiated from all other abdominal tumours, the most usual sources of confusion being (1) pregnancy, (2) obesity, (3) ascites, (4) cystic degeneration in a uterine myoma, (5) pseudocyesis, and (6) a full bladder. The last is an important and embarrassing error, and no medium-sized ovarian tumour should be diagnosed until the physician has made sure that the bladder is empty.

A small ovarian tumour may be easy to diagnose, or may be very difficult, and in some instances the true nature of the swelling is only revealed by ultrasound, or at laparoscopy or laparotomy. The

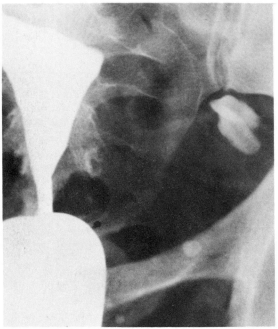

Fig. 23/2 Radiograph of the lower abdomen showing a benign teratoma which contains a tooth

the bladder is empty, (2) remembered that ovarian tumours rarely cause any disturbance in menstrual function, (3) ensured that the patient is not pregnant, and (4) checked by bimanual examination that a cleft separates the tumour and the uterus, and that the uterus moves independently of the tumour.

Additional aids in the form of ultrasound may be required, but should only be utilized after a careful clinical appraisal of the case. A plain radiograph may reveal teeth in a benign teratoma (dermoid cyst) (Fig. **23/2**), whilst ultrasound can identify an ovarian tumour and can distinguish the uterus in the same scan (Fig. **23/3**).

MALIGNANT CHANGE

Malignant change in an ovarian tumour is suggested by the complaints of abdominal pain or tenderness, abdominal swelling and abnormal vaginal bleeding. The pain is of a dull aching nature, and is constant and progressive in severity. Other significant findings are that (1) there has been rapid growth of the tumour, (2) both ovaries are involved (as 75 per cent of malignant tumours are bilateral, compared with 15 per cent of benign tumours), (3) ascites is present, (4) the tumour is fixed, and (5) there are symptoms of involvement of the lower bowel, or a barium enema shows an abnormality. One or more of these signs is suggestive, but not diagnostic, of malignancy, as each of them may occur with benign tumours, and frequently the final diagnosis is only made at laparoscopy and confirmed by the pathologist.

most frequent conditions which may cause confusion are, (1) a pyo- or hydrosalpinx, (2) a broad liagment cyst, (3) a retroverted pregnant uterus, (4) a uterine myoma, (5) pregnancy, either intra-uterine or ectopic, and, finally, (6) a distended bladder.

The confusion can be reduced if before making the diagnosis the physician has (1) made sure that

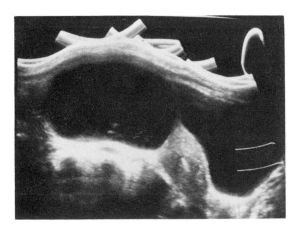

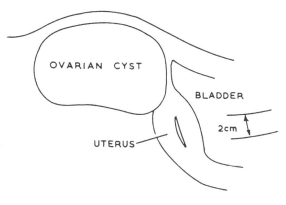

Fig. 23/3 Ovarian cyst (ultrasound–sagittal scan). Line drawing showing the identification of relevant points

COMPLICATIONS OF OVARIAN TUMOURS

Rotation of the tumour

This may take place if the pedicle is long and the tumour relatively small. The amount of rotation varies from a half turn to several turns, and its effect is to reduce or to interrupt the blood supply. Initially the venous return is impeded and the tumour becomes engorged, or else a vein ruptures with severe internal haemorrhage. Later, as the arterial supply is obliterated, gangrene may occur (Fig. **23/4**). The symptoms are marked. The patient complains of severe pain of sudden onset, the tumour increases in size and is acutely tender. If the degree of torsion is less, intermittent pain may be felt and a peritoneal irritation results in the formation of adhesions between the tumour and the peritoneum or omentum.

Haemorrhage into a cyst

This is not uncommon, and usually takes place slowly and in small quantities. Occasionally, particularly during torsion, the haemorrhage may be marked.

Rupture of a cystic tumour

This may occur suddenly after an injury, or be the result of thinning of the cyst's wall following ischaemia resulting from partial torsion, or from malignancy. The symptoms will depend upon the quantity

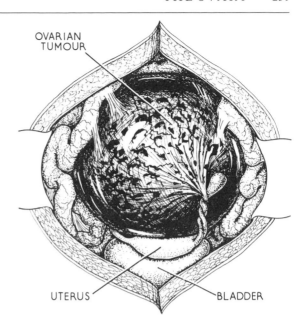

Fig. 23/4 Torsion of an ovarian tumour, in this case a dermoid. The torsion of the pedicle caused thrombosis of the ovarian veins and congestion of the tumour

and quality of the fluid released. Most patients 'feel something has given way', and little else. In the case of a large cyst this is followed by the disappearance of the abdominal swelling and a marked diuresis some 24 hours later. If the cyst contents are irritating, a severe peritoneal reaction may follow.

CLASSIFICATION OF OVARIAN TUMOURS

There is no entirely satisfactory classification of ovarian tumours. This is because of the variety and complexity of potential ovarian new growths, and because the distinction between many of them can only be made by the pathologist. In Table **23/1** a classification is advanced, which emphasizes that certain tumours, mainly cystic, are encountered most frequently, whilst others will be seen only rarely, even by a busy department serving a wide area. Those tumours most commonly encountered will be discussed further.

FUNCTIONAL CYSTS OF THE OVARY

Follicular cysts are enlargements of unruptured Graffian follicles in which the ovum has degenerated and the lining cells of the follicle have continued to secrete fluid. The cyst is usually unilateral, and never grows larger than 5cm diameter. The cells may secrete oestrogen or be relatively quiescent. The symptoms therefore vary. The patient may have a normal menstrual cycle, or it may be shortened, or more commonly lengthened, occasionally with associated

Tumour	Cell origin	Type	Proportional incidence per cent
Benign			
Functional cysts (follicle, corpus luteum)	Normal follicle	Cystic	24
Serous cystadenoma	Coelomic epithelium	Cystic	20
Mucinous cystadenoma	Coelomic epithelium	Cystic	20
Teratoma (dermoid cyst)	Oogonia	Cystic	15
Endometriomata	Ectopic endometrium	Cystic	10
Fibroma (inc. Brenner)	Mesenchyme	Solid	5
Malignant			
Secondary change in serous cystadenoma, occasionally in a mucinous cystadenoma (includes endometrioid carcinoma)		Cystic or semi-solid	5
Rare tumours: Feminizing: granulosa-theca cell Virilizing: androblastoma Neuter: disgerminoma Teratoma (embryoma)		Solid	0.5
Secondary carcinoma: Krukenberg, from stomach Adenocarcinoma, from uterus		Solid	0.5

Table 23/1 A classification of ovarian tumours

menorrhagia. It is unusual for the cyst to persist for more than 3 months. The diagnosis is suggested by the presence of a cyst, less than 5cm in diameter in a young woman. Treatment is to observe the patient, who should be seen each month. Should the cyst enlarge beyond 5cm diameter, or persist for more than 3 months, laparotomy is essential.

Multiple bilateral small follicular cysts, often found in association with obesity, oligomenorrhoea, infertility and hirsutism, constitute polycystic ovarian disease or the Stein–Leventhal syndrome. This is discussed on page 73.

Occasionally a corpus luteum, instead of degenerating when implantation of the ovum fails to occur, persists and forms a *corpus luteum cyst* which continues to secrete oestrogen and progesterone, causing amenorrhoea. In early pregnancy it is not unusual for the corpus luteum to form a cyst which may be mistaken for an ovarian neoplasm. Once again, the tumour never exceeds 5cm in diameter and disappears by the 12th week of pregnancy. Treatment of both forms consists of observation, and surgery is only required if the cyst enlarges or fails to disappear within 3 months of its detection.

Enlargement of the ovaries by theca-lutein cysts is found in trophoblastic disease, and is due to stimulation by the excessive amounts of chorionic gonadotrophin secreted by the tumour. The ovarian condition is overshadowed by the main disease, and surgery is unnecessary as the cysts resolve once the trophoblastic disease is treated.

Iatrogenic enlargement of the ovaries by follicular or theca-lutein cysts may occur following the use of clomiphene or pituitary gonadotrophins for the treatment of amenorrhoea associated with infertility.

It should also be remembered that the ovary is a dynamic organ, undergoing constant changes in size and structure as the hormonal tides wax and wane. Ovarian cystic enlargements are therefore often transient, and the finding of a slightly enlarged organ by a surgeon when operating for another condition is not a reason for sacrificing the ovary.

TRUE OVARIAN NEOPLASMS

The mucinous cystadenoma and the serous cystadenoma account for about 40 per cent of all ovarian neoplasms. Both derive from the multipotential coelomic epithelium. This epithelium forms the Mullerian duct, and can therefore imitate tubal, uterine and cervical epithelium.

Mucinous cystadenoma

The cysts are lined with tall columnar cells, with a basally situated nucleus and an accumulation of mucin within the cytoplasm. They resemble the mucin-secreting cells of the endocervix (Fig. **23/5**). The cells are active and continually secrete mucin into the cyst, so that the wall is kept tense, and the epithelium tends to be compressed to form a flat layer. Occasionally the pressure causes additional strain on a portion of the wall which bulges outwards, and the depression is filled with epithelial cells. If the depression is now occluded at the neck, a daughter secondary cyst is formed (Fig. **23/6**). The tumours, which may grow to an enormous size, therefore tend to be multilocular, but are usually unilateral and only rarely become malignant (Fig. **23/7**). Occasionally, however, the cyst ruptures releasing the mucinous cells, which may transplant and grow upon the omentum and the peritoneum. This

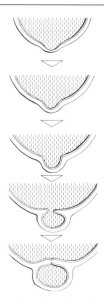

Fig. 23/6 Diagram to show how daughter cysts form in the wall of a mucinous cystadenoma

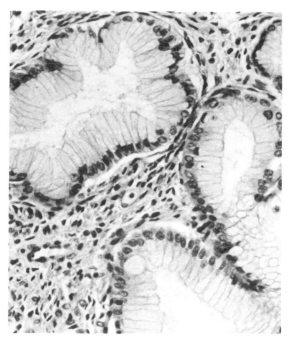

Fig. 23/5 The microscopic appearance of mucinous cystadenoma – note the cells lining the tumour resemble those of the endocervix (× 256)

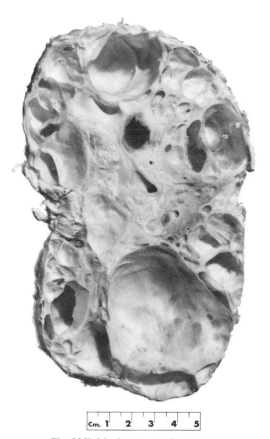

Fig. 23/7 Mucinous cystadenoma

may lead to the continuing accumulation of mucin in the peritoneum, and is called *pseudomyxoma peritonei*. Although biologically malignant, the condition is histologically benign. Mucinous cystadenomata are detected most frequently between the 3rd and 5th decade of life. Treatment is surgical and the type of operation depends upon the age of the patient.

Serous cystadenoma

The cysts, which are most frequently detected in the 3rd or 4th decade of life, are lined with cuboidal epithelium, resembling that of the oviduct (Fig. **23/8**). The cells do not secrete a great deal, consequently there is little intracystic pressure so that the epithelial cells proliferate to form intracystic papillary masses (Fig. **23/9**). In about 15 per cent of cases, the papillary masses grow through the cyst wall to form external papillary projections. Haemorrhage into the cyst is therefore common, and the normally greyish-white of the lobulated cyst is often discoloured in patches. The secretion which fills the cavity is thin and watery, hence the name serous cystadenoma. The tumour, which is unilocular or parvilocular, only grows to a moderate size, and is bilateral in about 30 per cent of cases. Moreover, in contrast to the mucinous cystadenoma, it becomes malignant in about 30 per cent of cases, but usually only in the 5th decade of life or later. Treatment must take into consideration that (1) the tumour is bilateral in one-third of cases, and (2) becomes malignant in one-third of cases. In young women conservative surgery is recommended, but women 40 years or more should be treated by bilateral salpingo-oophorectomy and total hysterectomy.

Teratomata

Benign cystic teratomata or dermoid cysts are relatively common and derive from primordial germ cells, hence they can contain elements of all three layers of the early embryo, but usually the ectodermal layer elements predominate. The cysts contain hair, pultaceous material from sebaceous glands, and often teeth or cartilage derived from mesodermal elements (Fig. **23/10**). The tumour is bilateral in about 10 per cent of cases, and usually between 5 and 10cm in diameter. It often develops a long pedicle, so that torsion is not infrequent.

Teratomata constitute 20 per cent of all ovarian tumours, and may occur at any age, but are most often found between the ages of 20 and 40. Because

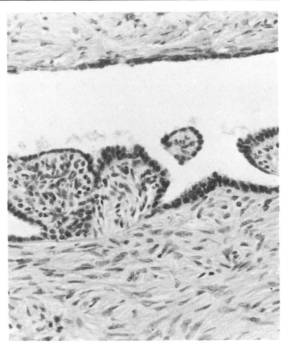

Fig. 23/8 The microscopic appearance of a serous cystadenoma. Note that the cells lining the tumour resemble those of the endosalpinx (× 256)

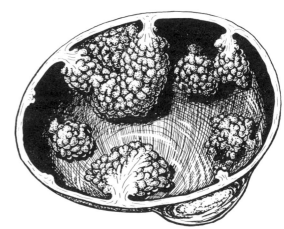

Fig. 23/9 Gross appearance of a serous cystadenoma

they are usually found in a young woman, treatment is to dissect out the cyst and reconstruct the ovary. This operation is termed an ovarian cystectomy.

Endometriomata

These tumours are usually associated with other evidence of endometriosis, which is discussed in Chapter 19. Endometriomata account for about 10

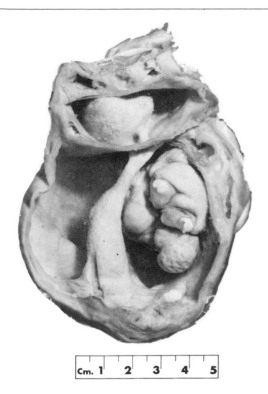

Fig. 23/10 A benign teratoma showing hair, sebaceous material and teeth

per cent of all ovarian tumours. They rarely become malignant and the endometrioid carcinoma found in the ovary has a different origin.

CONNECTIVE TISSUE NEOPLASMS

Fibromata form 5 per cent of ovarian neoplasms, and derive from mesenchymal connective tissue elements. The tumour may be formed of pure connective tissue, or may be found in association with cystadenomata, or with Brenner tumours, which are believed to derive from epithelial elements. Fibromata are usually small, but may grow to a large size, and are bilateral in 10 per cent of cases. An interesting condition associated with fibromata is ascites and hydrothorax (Meig's syndrome). The explanation for the accumulation of fluid is not clear, but clinically it has been found that a simple removal of the tumour is followed by disappearance of the fluid.

RARE TUMOURS

These tumours will rarely be encountered, and are therefore only mentioned briefly. They include the feminizing mesenchymomata (the theca-granulosa cell tumours), which secrete oestrogen and are malignant; the masculinizing mesenchymomata (the androblastoma), which secrete androgen and consequently cause defeminization and later masculinization; and the disgerminoma. The last is very rare and must be considered a malignant neoplasm. It is usually detected in childhood, and is more common in intersex patients. This association is the reason for recommending the prophylactic removal of the gonads just after puberty in patients with testicular feminization.

MALIGNANT OVARIAN TUMOURS

About 6 per cent of ovarian tumours are found to be malignant at surgery, and women who have never had a child are three times as likely to develop the disease compared with multiparous women. In a few instances the tumour, usually a serous cystadenoma, looks benign, but the histology shows it to be malignant. However, most ovarian malignancies have spread beyond the ovary by the time of surgery.

Malignant ovarian tumours have several origins but most derive from the epithelial surface cells of the ovary. Forty per cent arise from malignant change in a serous cystadenoma. Endometrioid carcinoma, which seems to arise primarily in the ovary, and is only rarely preceded by endometriosis, accounts for about 20 per cent of all ovarian malignancies. The histology resembles endometrial adenocarcinoma, which is the reason for the name given to the carcinoma. In about 20 per cent of women who have endometrioid carcinoma, the endometrium is also involved. This may be a simultaneous neoplastic change rather than a uterine metastasis. It is possible that many endometrioid carcinomas arise from malignant change of certain cellular elements in a serous cystadenoma. Malignant change in a mucinous cystadenoma accounts for about 5 per cent of all ovarian carcinomas, and about the same number derive from granulosa cell tumours (Fig. **23/11**).

Metastatic (secondary) ovarian carcinoma, accounts for 10 to 20 per cent of all ovarian malignancies. The tumour usually derives from the stomach or the breast. These tumours, first described by Krukenberg, are thought to occur by 'seeding' of malignant cells or by retrograde lymphatic spread.

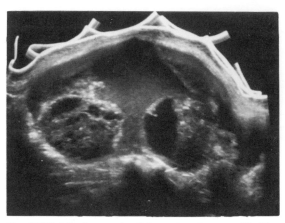

Fig. 23/11 Massive semi-solid ovarian tumour. Bladder (inadequately filled) is on the right. Solid and cystic areas with patchy degeneration in the tumour – cystadenocarcinoma (ultrasound – sagittal scan)

The remaining ovarian malignancies are made up of a variety of neoplasms, including malignant teratomata and disgerminoma.

MANAGEMENT OF OVARIAN TUMOURS

Apparently benign tumours

With the exception of ovarian tumours which are thought to be functional cysts, and which are less than 5cm in diameter, treatment of ovarian tumours is surgical. This is because a tumour cannot be declared benign until it has been seen at laparotomy and has been examined histologically.

The extent of the surgery is determined by the findings at operation and by the age of the patient; but some principles can be stated. (1) In young women an attempt should be made to dissect a benign tumour out of the ovary, and to reconstruct the ovary. This can be performed irrespective of the size of the tumour. The tumour must be examined by a pathologist, and if malignancy is detected, a further operation must be performed to remove the ovary. There is no need to be more radical as this offers no greater chance of survival, and is attended by severe climacteric disturbances. (2) In older women, the entire ovary and tube should be removed; and if the tumour is a serous cystadenoma, the opposite ovary and the uterus should be extirpated should the patient be over the age of 40. (3) Women over the age of 45, who are found to have an ovarian tumour, are best treated by total hysterec-

tomy and bilateral salpingo-oophorectomy. (4) Cysts should not be 'tapped', but whenever possible delivered intact. In this regard it should be remembered that an incision heals from side to side, and not from end to end.

Malignant tumours

Primary ovarian carcinoma accounts for about 20 per cent of all gynaecological cancers, but in more than 70 per cent of cases, the growth has spread beyond the ovaries when first detected. By this time, it is highly lethal, only 10 to 20 per cent of women surviving 5 years.

This high mortality will only be reduced if malignant ovarian tumours are detected earlier in the course of the disease. This in turn may be achieved if women in the vulnerable age group (>50 years) have regular annual bimanual pelvic examinations, to detect ovarian enlargement.

Because most cases of ovarian malignancy are relatively advanced when detected, therapy is best planned by a team consisting of gynaecological surgeon, chemotherapist and radiotherapist, so that the most appropriate regimen of treatment can be devised for the individual woman.

The initial management of malignant ovarian tumours is surgical. As much malignant tissue is removed as is practical without causing severe damage; most of the omentum is excised, the abdomen (including the diaphragm) is explored for the presence of secondary deposits of carcinoma, and a bilateral salpingo-oophorectomy and total hysterectomy is performed, if feasible. When the malignancy is not confined to the ovaries, a decision has to be made whether or not to give adjuvant therapy. Unless the tumour is a disgerminoma, chemotherapy, using cytotoxic drugs, gives a better survival rate than does radiotherapy.

Chemotherapy in the treatment of advanced ovarian malignancy is palliative, not curative, but may improve the quality of life of the woman and enable her to live longer.

The most effective type of chemotherapy has not been established. Courses of combinations of several chemotherapeutic agents (e.g. cyclophosphamide, hexamethyl-melamine, doxorubicin and cisplatin) may be used initially, or after courses of a single alkylating agent has failed to produce a response. The response is evaluated by a reduction in size of the residual tumour masses. Combination chemotherapeutic agents are associated with severe side-effects. Some 60 to 80 per cent of patients have moderate or severe nausea and vomiting during treatment; severe hair loss occurs in 45 to 65 per cent, peripheral neurotoxicity in 5 to 35 per cent and renal toxicity in 15 to 60 per cent.

Because of the severity of the side-effects, the patient must be fully informed of the benefits, the distressing side-effects and the chances of remission, so that she can make an informed choice whether to accept or reject the physician's advice.

Megavoltage radiotherapy may be valuable as an adjunct to surgery in certain malignant tumours, particularly disgerminoma. The dose is 65-95Gy (6500-9500 rads) distributed over the pelvis. The response, however, is unpredictable.

OVARIAN TUMOURS COMPLICATING PREGNANCY

About one pregnancy in 1500 is complicated by an ovarian tumour, usually a serous cystadenoma or a benign teratoma. The treatment of ovarian tumours is surgical, an ovarian cystectomy being the preferred operation. However, if the tumour is less than 5cm in diameter and detected prior to the 12th week of pregnancy, it may merely be a cystic corpus luteum, and consequently operation should be delayed until the 12th week when the patient is re-examined. Should the cyst be the same size or have increased in size at this time, laparotomy should be performed between the 12th and 18th week. If the tumour is first detected after the 28th week, technical difficulties may make it necessary to delay surgical intervention until the early puerperium, but each patient must be given individual consideration. These problems are discussed further in Chapter 33 of Volume I.

OVARIAN RETENTION AFTER HYSTERECTOMY

The sudden ablation of the ovaries invariably leads to severe climacteric symptoms in the premenopausal woman, and even in the postmenopausal woman may deprive her of a valuable source of oestrogen precursors. It should therefore be stated clearly that a normal ovary should never be extirpated in a woman under the age of 45.

Several arguments have been advanced recommending the bilateral removal of normal ovaries in women aged 45 or more who require hysterectomy. These are (1) the ovaries atrophy after hysterectomy, (2) ovarian steroidal function is ceasing at this age, and (3) malignancy may subsequently develop in the conserved ovary. These arguments do not stand up to critical scrutiny, as (1) ovarian atrophy does not occur after hysterectomy provided an adequate blood supply has been maintained, (2) ovarian steroidogenesis continues postmenopausally in at least 25 per cent of women, and a natural reduction in activity is preferable to a sudden surgical castration, (3) the risk of an ovarian malignancy developing in an ovary retained after hysterectomy is less than 1 in 1500 cases.

From this, it follows that provided no uterine malignancy is present and the ovaries are clinically normal, they should not be removed when hysterectomy is performed on the perimenopausal woman.

UTERINE RETENTION AFTER BILATERAL OVARIECTOMY

There is no reason for retaining the uterus when a bilateral ovariectomy has been performed, unless technical difficulties make hysterectomy hazardous. Indeed, the retention of the now useless uterus may be dangerous, as it may become the site for pelvic inflammatory disease or for cancer.

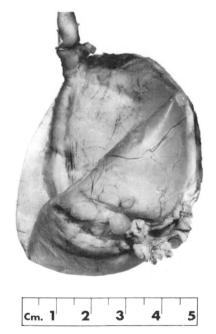

Fig. 23/12 A broad ligament cyst, note how the oviduct curves over the surface of the cyst

TUMOURS OF THE PAROVARIUM AND BROAD LIGAMENT

The parovarium and broad ligament contains vestigial structures derived from the mesonephric duct, and small cystic tumours may arise anywhere along the line of the duct by distension of one or more of the remnants. The cysts are thin-walled and contain clear fluid. More frequently a remnant in the parovarium becomes cystic, and as it grows separates the ovary from the Fallopian tube, which becomes stretched over its surface (Fig. **23/12**).

The treatment is to dissect out the cyst and to restore the tissues to their normal anatomical relationships. Ovariectomy should be avoided.

Chapter 24

Accidents and Injuries

The effects of trauma to the tissues of the genital tract occurring during childbirth are dealt with in Volume I and will not be mentioned here, except in so far as inadequate treatment at that time may leave residual defects. Nor will rupture of the uterus be discussed, for this is usually an accident occurring during pregnancy or in labour. However, it should be mentioned that occasionally perforation of the uterus, by a sound or by a curette, occurs during curettage. Contrary to what might be expected, this accident has few sequelae. The main dangers are haemorrhage, and the introduction of infection; but the former is unusual as the uterine muscle is contractile, and the latter is uncommon unless the indication for curettage was to evacuate infected products of conception from the uterus, or to procure an abortion.

When the accident occurs, the operation should be abandoned, and antibiotics given, but laparotomy is unnecessary unless (1) evidence of internal haemorrhage appears, or external haemorrhage persists, (2) the gut prolapses through the tear in the uterus, or (3) the lesion is one of endometrial cancer or pyometra. In these circumstances laparotomy is essential, and the uterus is repaired or removed according to the findings at operation.

VULVA AND VAGINA

Trauma to the vulvovaginal area may follow accidents, coitus or childbirth. Accidental injury is rare, as the external genitalia are in a well-protected situation, and such injuries as occur are due to direct violence from kicks, to falling astride some object, or to injuries from coitus. Injuries to the external genitalia are treated on the same general principles as injuries in other locations: (1) the haemorrhage should be stopped, (2) the injured parts should be reunited to obtain the best restoration of function, and (3) infection should be prevented.

Coital injuries

As has been noted, the hymen is generally torn during a first coition, but bleeding is slight and ceases spontaneously. Occasionally a larger vessel is torn which requires attention. Pressure on the bleeding point is usually sufficient to control the haemorrhage, but occasionally a suture is required. Rough coitus, particularly rape, may cause vaginal injuries to a pre-pubertal child and to an aged woman, as the tissues are not able to distend so readily as during sexual maturity. Such injury is unusual in the reproductive era. The vaginal wall may be torn or the vaginal vault damaged. Treatment is to repair the rent, under anaesthesia and in a good light.

Accidental injuries

Cuts and lacerations are unusual, and when found suggest that a criminal abortion has been attempted. The usual injury is a haematoma, which may be small or large, and is due to damage to one or more of the many venous plexuses in the vulva (Fig. **24/1**). A haematoma may also follow inadequate haemostasis during suture of incisions and tears, or following rupture of a vein during childbirth. The haematoma usually increases in size rapidly, and presents as a tender purple-coloured swelling, unless a deeper vein has been ruptured, when it may produce a hard indurated area in the position of Bartholin's gland. In these cases, a vaginal examination will show that a mass displaces the vaginal wall medially. The patient complains of severe pain; and shock, which is out of proportion to the blood lost, is often present. Treatment is to replace the blood lost, and then to incise the tumour and evacuate the clots.

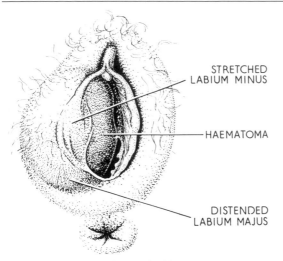

STRETCHED
LABIUM MINUS

HAEMATOMA

DISTENDED
LABIUM MAJUS

Fig. 24/1 A large vulval haematoma

The resultant cavity is obliterated by haemostatic sutures, and any obvious spurting vessels secured. Pressure packs are then placed in the vagina and on the vulva, and the patient given analgesics and antibiotics. Only if it is impossible to obtain haemostasis should the cavity be packed, as convalescence is stormy and prolonged following this method of treatment.

INJURIES RESULTING FROM CHILDBIRTH

Defective perineum

Uterovaginal prolapse is considered in Chapter 21, but lesser damage at childbirth, or inadequate suturing of perineal tears may leave the patient with a defective perineum. The skin of the perineum may be intact, but the muscles of the perineum are widely separated so that the vulva gapes (Fig. **24/2**). The condition is usually symptomless, but occasionally the patient complains that water enters the vagina when bathing; or that vaginal flatus occurs; or that coitus is less satisfactory to both partners than before childbirth. A few women complain of a feeling of 'weakness in the vagina'.

Perineal deficiency should be sought at the postnatal visit, and pelvic floor exercises prescribed if it is found. These consist of tightening the pubococcygeal muscles, and can best be described as trying to 'make the anus touch the chin'. The physician should make sure that the patient is using the correct muscles by getting her to contract the levators whilst

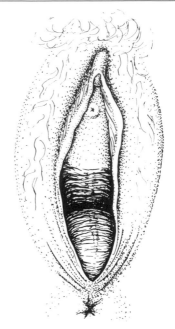

Fig. 24/2 Marked perineal deficiency

he keeps two fingers in her vagina. Once learned, the exercises should be performed 100 times or more a day. Only if the anatomical defect is marked, or if no improvement occurs after the exercises have been practised consistently, or if symptoms are marked, should surgery be contemplated. The operation is a posterior colpoperineorrhaphy, and care should be taken to ensure that overcorrection is not made, and the lax vaginal introitus replaced by a tight introitus and a high perineum which produces dyspareunia.

Complete perineal tear

This is the most severe form of perineal injury produced at childbirth, the skin, muscles and anal sphincter being torn (Fig. **24/3**). The main complaint is incontinence of faeces, but in lesser degrees of damage, control is obtained if the patient avoids loose stools. Treatment is surgical, which may be performed (1) immediately after the injury, (2) as a secondary suture if the initial repair breaks down and infection has been eliminated, (3) 4 to 6 months after delivery, or (4) when the condition is detected at a later date.

VAGINAL ACCIDENTS AND INJURIES

Injury, or infection, of the vagina can result from foreign bodies in the vagina. The foreign body may

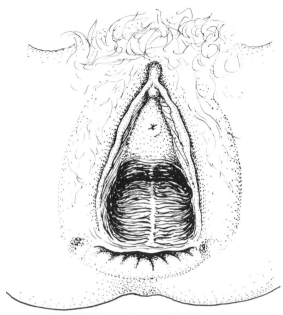

Fig. 24/3 A complete or third degree tear

be a forgotten vaginal tampon, or some object introduced to produce an abortion or for experimental reasons. In old women, a supportive pessary may be introduced to control a uterovaginal prolapse and then forgotten. Over the months, or years, it becomes encrusted and abrades, or even perforates, the vaginal walls. Once the foreign body is removed, the vagina heals rapidly, although cleansing douches (administered by a nurse) may occasionally be helpful in controlling the smell, and in old women an oestrogen vaginal cream will speed up the healing process.

Vaginal burns

This injury is uncommon, and may follow the use of an abnormally hot douche; the accidental burning by a physician using a cautery; or the deliberate introduction of a caustic agent, such as rock salt or potassium permanganate crystals, to procure an abortion, or in some Asian lands, to tighten the puerperal vagina and render coitus more satisfying to the male. The results can be the opposite, a rigid stenosed vagina occurring, and apareunia resulting.

THE CERVIX AND CORPUS UTERI

Childbirth, or excessively rigid, roughly performed

dilatation of the cervix by a physician can lead to a lacerated cervix (Fig. **24/4**). The laceration usually runs from one or other side of the external os, and may lead, in a few patients, to an incompetent cervix and recurrent abortion or to the birth of a preterm baby between the 20th and 29th week of pregnancy. Treatment is surgical.

Cervical stenosis may result from excessive zeal in cauterizing the cervix or from conization. Treatment is to dilate the cervix, and this may have to be repeated. Occasionally excessively forcible curettage removes all the endometrium, and adhesions form between the uterine walls. The adhesions become fibrous, forming synechiae, and amenorrhoea results (Asherman's syndrome). Treatment is largely unsuccessful in restoring either menstruation or fertility.

GENITAL TRACT FISTULAE

Genital tract fistulae may occur between the vagina or the uterus and any adjacent organ, but the most frequently encountered fistulae are between the bladder and vagina (vesicovaginal fistula) or the rectum and vagina (rectovaginal fistula) (Fig. **24/5**). Other types may occur, but are rare, and occasionally multiple fistulae may be found in the same woman. The fistula may be tiny, or a large area of tissue may be deficient.

In the developing countries about 85 per cent of fistulae follow an obstructed labour, and 15 per cent surgery or radiation for gynaecological conditions. In the developed countries, the reverse applies. Obstetrical and surgical fistulae arise either immediately due to direct trauma, or 5 to 14 days after delivery or operation when the traumatized, ischaemic tissue

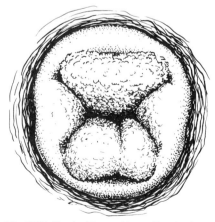

Fig. 24/4 Cervical laceration, stellate in shape

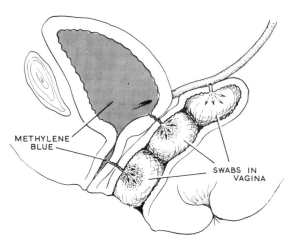

METHYLENE
BLUE

SWABS IN
VAGINA

Fig. 24/5 Vesicovaginal fistula

sloughs. Fistulae following irradiation rarely appear until one or more years after treatment.

The patient complains of incontinence of urine or of faeces. In cases of vesicovaginal fistulae, urinary incontinence is continuous night and day, and the patient does not need to void. If the fistula is large, the defect can be seen, but pinpoint fistulae may require special tests for diagnosis. One such test is to place three cottonwool swabs in the vagina, one above the other, and to run methylene blue dye into the bladder. If only the lowest swab stains, the fistula is urethral; if the middle swab stains, it is vesical; if no swab stains, but the uppermost swab is wet, the fistula is ureteric.

Rectovaginal fistulae may be obvious or extremely difficult to identify, and proctoscopy or the introduction of dyes may be required.

The treatment of all fistulae, except small fistulae which have formed recently following childbirth or operation, is surgical. Some recently formed vesicovaginal fistulae will heal if the bladder is drained continuously for 21 to 28 days; and some rectovaginal fistulae will heal if a low residue diet is given for the same period. Most fistulae require operation. The principles involved are: (1) the fibrosed edges of the fistulous tract must be excised so that well-vascularized viable tissue may be brought into apposition. (2) The apposition must be effected without tension on the apposed edges. (2) The tissues must not be placed under tension for at least 3 weeks (this principle implies constant bladder drainage in cases of vesicovaginal fistulae). (4) The best results are obtained if fistulae are treated in special units, where experience in the operative technique and, more important, the meticulous postoperative management of the case can be offered.

Chapter 25

The Urinary Tract and its Relationship to Gynaecology

The close connection between the vagina and the bladder, and the shortness of the female urethra, subject the female urinary tract to hazards avoided by the male. Since many complaints in women relate to disturbances in micturition, the anatomy of the lower urinary tract and the mechanics of voiding urine are first discussed.

ANATOMY

The urethral meatus lies in the anterior part of the vestibule, and the urethra runs upward and backward for 4cm to join the bladder base at an angle. It is intimately connected with the anterior vaginal wall, and a series of small crypts open into its posterior surface in the lowest third. These crypts are known as Skene's tubules and lie between the lateral urethral wall and the vagina. They are homologues of the male prostate, and may become the site of chronic infection.

The bladder is a muscular organ with a considerable capacity for distension. The base is relatively flat, lies parallel with the axis of the vagina, and contains the internal urinary meatus and the orifices of the ureters (Fig. **25/1**). The triangular area between these three openings constitutes the trigone. The dome, or fundus, of the bladder varies in shape and position depending upon the degree of distension. It is lined by transitional epithelium, and external to this is the muscular layer. The involuntary muscle which forms the bladder can be divided into two parts, that forming the fundus, which is poorly supplied by autonomic nerves, and that forming the base (the detrusor muscle), which is richly supplied by autonomic nerves. The female urethra is a muscular tube, composed of two muscle layers. It is about 4cm long. The inner layer of muscle is longitudinal and is a direct continuation of the inner longitudinal layer of the detrusor muscle. It is embedded in dense collagen. The outer layer, which is a continuation of the outer layer of the detrusor muscle, is composed of semicircular fibres which never form a complete ring around the urethra. They loop around the urethra, at various degrees of obliquity, turning back to reach the bladder. Collectively they form a thick muscle layer, which encircles the urethra, to form a 'sphincter'.

Elastic tissue, collagen fibres and fascial attachments are intermingled with the involuntary semicircular fibres of the urethral muscle, and with the striated, voluntary fibres surrounding the mid-third of the urethra. This complex combination gives the urethra an 'inherent tone', or intra-urethral pressure, which is greatest at the mid-third of its length and which is important in maintaining urinary continence.

The voluntary muscle surrounding the mid-third of the urethra is part of the levator ani muscle (the puborectalis muscle), and its contraction cuts off micturition voluntarily. It also contracts to prevent urine leakage in response to the stress of coughing, bearing down, sneezing or heavy lifting. It therefore acts as an external sphincter.

The external sphincter is under the control of the pudendal nerve; whilst the involuntary musculature is mainly under the autonomic control of the parasympathetic (cholinergic) nerves.

How does the urethra resist sudden increases in abdominal pressure? It is now known that as well as contraction of the voluntary external sphincter, the raised abdominal pressure is transmitted not only to the bladder but also to the proximal urethra, thus increasing the intra-urethral pressure as well as the intravesical pressure. This concept is important in understanding 'stress incontinence'.

The ureters pass from the renal pelves, behind the peritoneum, lying on the psoas muscle, to enter the

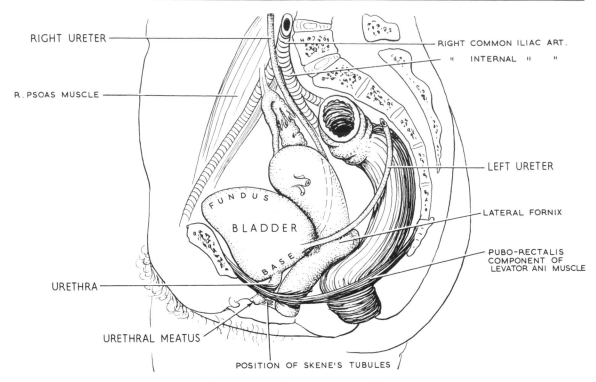

Fig. 25/1 The relations of the urinary tract within the pelvis

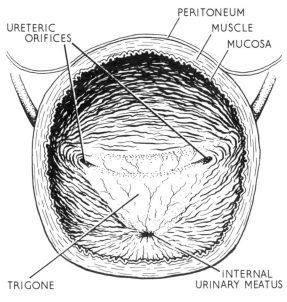

Fig. 25/2 The trigone of the bladder

true pelvis anterior to the sacro-iliac joint. They are separated from the joint by the ligaments of the joint, the psoas muscle and the common iliac vessels, and enter the pelvis in front of the common iliac artery at its bifurcation into the external and internal branches. Inside the true pelvis each ureter turns downward and runs on the medial side of the internal iliac artery. In the parametrium, as it courses forward to the bladder, it is crossed by the uterine artery, and lies 1cm lateral to the supravaginal cervix and 1cm above the lateral fornix. It passes obliquely through the bladder wall on the posterior aspect of its base, and the ureteric orifices mark the posterior points of the trigone of the bladder (Fig. **25/2**). The ureter is lined with transitional epithelium, and the main coats of its wall consist of involuntary muscle which constantly moves as peristaltic waves pass along it. The obliquity with which the ureter enters the bladder acts as a valve preventing reflux of urine when the bladder is full.

MECHANICS OF MICTURITION

The bladder fills as urine trickles down the ureters. To accommodate the urine, the walls of the bladder distend. The organ can accommodate 250 to 350ml of urine without any increase in the resting intravesical pressure, which remains below 10cm of water. Once the bladder contains more than this amount of urine, the intravesical pressure rises and stretch-receptors in the muscular wall are stimulated. In the infant a reflex arc is initiated, which leads to contraction of the detrusor muscle of the bladder and an increase in the intravesical pressure. If this pressure exceeds the intra-urethral pressure, voiding occurs. The adult has learned to inhibit detrusor contractions by higher centre control so that micturition is regulated.

Continence is maintained by the 'inherent tone' of the urethra, and by the muscles which envelop the urethrovesical junction and the proximal urethra. These muscle fibres are continuations of the detrusor muscle. They surround the bladder base in a circular manner and the proximal urethra in a spiral fashion. Their tone maintains a 'flat' bladder base and creates an intra-urethral resting pressure, which normally exceeds that of the bladder by 7 to 10cm of water.

Owing to the distribution of the muscle fibres at the urethrovesical junction, the urethra enters the bladder almost at right angles (as a stalk enters an apple), and this angle is called the 'urethrovesical angle' (Fig. 25/3A). Although the detrusor and its proximal urethral extension is a single muscle, paradoxically owing to the spiral arrangement of the fibres around the urethra, when the detrusor is relaxed, the proximal urethral muscle is contracted, and the urethral walls are kept in apposition. Conversely, when the detrusor muscle contracts, its extension around the proximal urethra relaxes and urine passes into the urethra.

The portion of the urethra between the layers of the urogenital diaphragm is surrounded by the external sphincter, which is under voluntary control, and the whole urethra is supported by a fibromuscular layer derived from the pubococcygeus portion of the levator ani muscle. These muscles act as a second line of defence against incontinence.

VOLUNTARY MICTURITION

The discomfort of the distended bladder induces a relaxation of the pubococcygeal muscle tone and a reduction of the urethral support. This relaxation does not affect the external sphincter of the urethra, which remains closed. Almost immediately the detrusor muscle contracts, drawing the urethra downward and backward, obliterating the urethrovesical angle and changing the shape of the bladder base to that of an inverted cone. This brings the urethra into line with the bladder trigone. A further effect of the detrusor contraction is to raise the intravesical pressure to 40cm of water. Simultaneously a reciprocal relaxation of the proximal urethra occurs, probably due to a reflex, with a considerable fall in the intraurethral pressure, which falls below the intravesical pressure. When this occurs, urine is forced into the proximal urethra, which adopts a 'funnel'

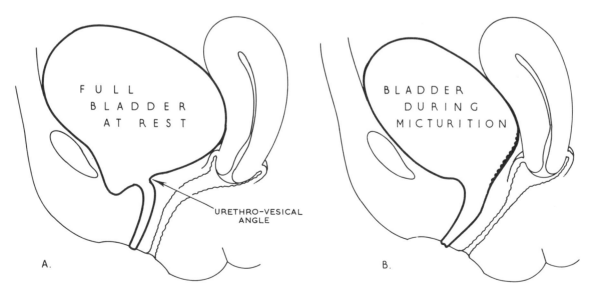

Fig. 25/3 Tracing from radiographs of the bladder and urethra. (A) At rest; (B) During micturition

or pear shape (Fig. **25/3B**). Abdominal muscle activity doubles the intravesical pressure and urine is forced along the urethra. The external sphincter is relaxed voluntarily and urine is voided until the bladder is empty. When this occurs, the detrusor is no longer stimulated and relaxes, and the proximal urethra contracts from the distal end to the urethrovesical junction, 'milking' back a few drops of urine into the bladder. The bladder base becomes 'flat' and the posterior urethrovesical angle is restored. Finally the external sphincter closes.

URINARY INCONTINENCE – INVOLUNTARY VOIDING

In women two main and two subsidiary forms of involuntary voiding or urinary incontinence occur. The two main forms are (1) urge incontinence and (2) stress incontinence, and the two subsidiary forms are (3) reflex incontinence and (4) overflow incontinence. *Urge incontinence* is an involuntary loss of urine associated with a strong desire to void usually due to uninhibited detrusor contractions. *Genuine stress incontinence* (*urethral sphincter incontinence*) is an involuntary loss of urine when the intravesical pressure exceeds the intra-urethral pressure in the absence of detrusor activity. *Reflex incontinence* is an involuntary loss of urine due to abnormal reflex activity in the spinal cord in the absence of the sensation usually associated with a desire to micturate. *Overflow incontinence* occurs when the intra-

vesical pressure exceeds the intra-urethral pressure because of excessive bladder distension, but detrusor activity is absent. The first two forms of incontinence will be considered further. Stress incontinence is the more frequent, but must be carefully distinguished from 'urge incontinence' as surgery is contra-indicated in the latter.

DIAGNOSIS

Before either of the two main types of incontinence are diagnosed, asymptomatic urinary tract infection must be excluded, as it may produce symptoms and signs of incontinence. General medical conditions such as early Parkinsonism, multiple sclerosis and diabetic neuropathy must also be excluded. The patient should be asked if she is taking tricyclic drugs or lithium as they may cause symptoms of urge incontinence. Local bladder causes of urinary incontinence, such as a bladder stone or a pelvic tumour pressing on the bladder should also be excluded. The social inconvenience caused by the incontinence should be evaluated and the symptoms analysed. In between 60 and 75 per cent of incontinent women, consideration of these matters will lead to a diagnosis. In the remainder urodynamic tests are required to determine whether the patient has urethral sphincter incontinence or urge incontinence. A simple test is the 'flow-bridge' test. A special plastic catheter, calibrated at 0.5cm intervals is introduced into a full bladder, and the urinary flow is

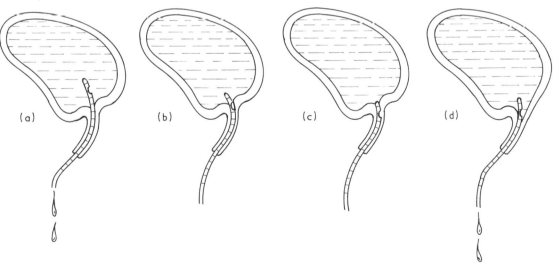

Fig. 25/4 The fluid bridge flow test: (a) the catheter is passed into the bladder; (b) locating the bladder neck; (c) selecting the test position; (d) the bladder neck opens as the patient coughs

observed. The catheter is slowly withdrawn until the flow ceases. This locates the vesico-urethral junction (the bladder neck). The catheter is now withdrawn a further 0.5cm and the patient, who now stands up, is asked to cough. If urine flows, the bladder neck is incontinent to that point, and the test is positive. The catheter can be withdrawn at 0.5cm intervals to see how far the urethra opens when the patient coughs (Fig. **25/4**). If doubt regarding the cause of the incontinence persists after these tests, urodynamic testing in special centres is required.

Urge incontinence (the 'unstable bladder')

In this condition the detrusor muscle of the bladder contracts (or can be made to contract) involuntarily. Over the age of 35 about 1 woman in 10 has the problem. Two categories of unstable bladder are described. In the first, *sensory urgency* (hypersensitive bladder), the woman micturates, not because of involuntary detrusor activity but because it hurts if she does not empty her bladder. This means that the woman micturates frequently and if she also has cystitis may experience painful micturition. In the second category, *motor urgency* (detrusor instability), the urge to micturate before the bladder is full, occurs at variable intervals when variable amounts of urine are voided. This may be accompanied by urinary frequency and by urge incontinence, especially if the woman is unable to reach a toilet, or at night when bed wetting may occur. Pain on micturition is not usually a feature.

Treatment is rather unsatisfactory. Bladder drill may help. In this the woman tries to increase the interval between micturating, no matter how difficult she finds it. Women who try bladder drill need considerable support and help, preferably from a trained person, or the outcome is poor.

In some cases drugs may help. As detrusor muscle contraction is under cholinergic control, anticholinergic drugs may reduce the incontinence. Current practice suggests that oxybutynin (which also has a local anaesthetic effect) in a dose of 5 to 10mg 4 times a day may be of benefit. Some side-effects may occur, and if these are severe, dicyclomine 30mg 4 times a day may be substituted. If these measures fail, some urologists inject the paravesical nerve plexuses with phenol or perform an augmentation ileocystoplasty. These extreme methods should not be undertaken without counselling and discussion with the patient.

A variety of the unstable bladder is so-called *urethro-trigonitis*. This condition is frequently diagnosed in patients complaining of urgency, by finding hyperaemia of the mucosa of the bladder base without any evidence of bacteriuria. In the past, treatment has been directed to eliminate a non-existent infection; and urethral dilatation, cautery of the internal urethral meatus and trigone, and bladder washouts have had a vogue. As the condition is psychosomatic, these measures depended upon a placebo effect for their variable success. Treatment should be that for urge incontinence.

Urethral sphincter incontinence (genuine stress incontinence)

In urethral sphincter incontinence the involuntary loss of urine occurs when the intravesical pressure exceeds the intra-urethral pressure in the absence of detrusor activity. Clinically, the woman complains that a small amount of urine escapes when she coughs, laughs, or jumps. The urine can escape when the bladder is full or when it is apparently empty after voiding. The condition is fairly common, but relatively unimportant in most cases, and it is only when severe that it causes distress.

In stress incontinence the main defect is that the normal closure mechanism of the urethrovesical junction is inadequate, the bladder base is funnelled not flat, and the posterior urethrovesical angle is diminished or lost. As well, the descent of the urethrovesical junction prevents the proximal urethra from receiving the benefits of raised intra-abdominal pressure when stress occurs (Fig. **25/5**).

The effect of these changes is to bring the upper urethra and trigone into alignment, a situation found in the normal woman in the early stages of micturition, so that relatively small increases in intravesical pressure permit urine to enter the upper urethra, from whence it is voided. The urethral supports are not usually damaged, and if the woman has a warning of an increase in vesical pressure, she can control the loss by contracting the levator ani muscles.

The aetiology of stress incontinence is due to (1) defective development of the vesical and urethral muscles, or (2) to damage to the bladder neck supports at childbirth. Although often associated with vaginal prolapse, it is not a symptom of prolapse, and minor degrees of damage may cause stress incontinence without any evidence of prolapse. The condition is aggravated in pregnancy, as the muscles of the bladder and proximal urethra relax under the

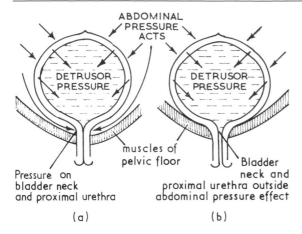

Fig. 25/5 The effect of the position of the bladder neck on stress incontinence. In (a) the urethrovesical junction is normally situated. An increase in abdominal pressure acts *equally* on the detrusor pressure and on the bladder neck pressure, so that the pressure gradient is maintained and a positive 'closure' pressure is present. In (b) the urethrovesical junction is *outside* the effects of abdominal pressure as the junction is below the pelvic floor. An increase in abdominal pressure is transmitted only to the detrusor pressure, which exceeds momentarily the intra-urethral pressure. The positive closure pressure is lost and the patient passes a small amount of urine

influence of progesterone.

Treatment is directed to restore the function of the muscles of the urethrovesical junction, and to strengthen the supports of the urethra. The latter are only a second line of defence, but if the stress incontinence is mild, may be sufficient to control the symptom. Pelvic floor exercises to strengthen the pelvic muscles are often helpful. The exercises should be taught to the woman by an experienced physiotherapist. Once learned the woman should continue to do the exercises hourly during the day for at least 3 months. A study from Britain showed that using this regimen, over two-thirds of women had improvement or complete relief of the symptoms. The severity of the incontinence or the age of the woman did not alter the success rate. If physiotherapy is unsuccessful, surgery should be offered if the symptoms are distressing to the woman. However, post-menopausal women should use vaginal oestrogen cream daily for 6 weeks before surgery as the treatment suits some women. The objective of surgery is first to elevate the bladder neck so that it lies within the abdominal pressure zone (Fig. **25/5**). This increases the closing pressure of the urethra. Second, to support the vesicourethral junction to prevent it 'funnelling', in other words

opening in response to a raised intravesical pressure.

These objectives can be accomplished by the vaginal or the abdominal approach. The vaginal operation consists of exposing the urethrovesical junction, and proximal urethra, and providing support by plicating the pubocervical fascia and muscle fibres beneath them. The abdominal approach indirectly does the same thing by placing sutures in the paravaginal fascia and into the iliopectineal ligament on the same side. When the sutures (usually 3 or 4 on each side) are tied, the proximal urethra and the urethrovesical junction are lifted to lie close to the posterior surface of the symphysis pubis (Burch operation) (Fig. **25/6**). Long-term follow-up suggests that none of the available surgical techniques is better than any other and that after 6 years only 75 per cent of women will be continent.

A recent suggestion may simplify treatment in some cases of bladder neck weakness. An injection of Teflon paste is made into the peri-urethral tissues at the junction of the bladder neck and the urethra. Preliminary results indicate that this simple procedure may be as successful in producing a cure as more complex surgical operations.

URINARY TRACT INFECTION

The short urethra and its intimate relationship with the vagina considerably increases the risk of a

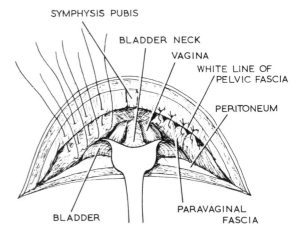

Fig. 25/6 Modified colposuspension (retropubic approach). Sutures are placed between the paravaginal fascia and the ileopectineal ligaments. These sutures elevate the bladder neck. The sutures on the right have been tied, those on the left are ready to be tied. During exertion the intra-abdominal pressure rises and compresses the urethra against the symphysis pubis, thus controlling the incontinence

woman developing urinary tract infection. The lower urethra, the vulva and the lower vagina are colonized by bacteria early in life, but the bacteria are non-pathogenic. However, once coitus occurs, the irritation of the urethra by the movement of the penis in the vagina encourages bacteria to ascend and to colonize the bladder, so that between 3 and 8 per cent of non-virgins have an asymptomatic bacteriuria (more than 100 000 organisms per millilitre of urine). Provided the bladder is emptied regularly and completely, the condition is without consequence, but should stasis occur, as in pregnancy, bacterial growth may lead to renal tract infection. Initially this is confined to the bladder, when it is termed cystitis, but the further multiplication of bacteria in the urine, and their ascent, either along the peri-ureteric lymphatics or along the ureter itself by reflux of infected urine, inevitably leads to pyelonephritis. In older women, particularly those who have a cystocele, stasis of urine and distortion of the anatomy of the ureteric orifices occur and are conducive to renal tract infection.

In most cases of acute urinary tract infection (UTI) only the lower urinary tract is infected (cystitis and the urethral syndrome); in a few the upper urinary tract is also infected (pyelonephritis). In the latter case parenchymal tissue infection is usual. In a proportion of cases pyelonephritis is sub-clinical, smouldering quietly with occasional exacerbations.

The symptoms of UTI are dysuria, frequency and urgency of micturition, and it has been estimated that about 20 per cent of women may complain of an episode of dysuria each year. Occasionally haematuria occurs. In a few cases, the symptoms of UTI may be mimicked by urinary incontinence and psychosomatic conditions. Acute pyelonephritis is associated with pyrexia, loin pain and rigors, but sub-clinical pyelonephritis is not uncommon.

A patient who presents with dysuria (with or without other urinary tract symptoms), requires investigation.

1. The presence or absence of an irritating vaginal discharge should be looked for, and if present, vaginal swabs should be taken.
2. A history of sexual contact with a new partner or a partner who has had a urethral discharge, or if the symptoms have had a gradual rather than an abrupt onset, suggests possible gonorrhoeal or chlamydial infection. A mucopurulent cervical discharge adds support to this diagnosis.

3. A previous history of UTI or symptoms of more than 10 days duration, may indicate sub-clinical pyelonephritis.
4. A midstream specimen of urine is obtained and examined for pus cells. The presence of 8 leucocytes per high power field in a centrifuged sediment indicates UTI. If pyuria is detected and the history suggests an upper UTI, a colony count of the urine should be made. Even if the count is less than 100 000 bacteria per ml treatment should be given.
5. A midstream specimen of urine is sent to a laboratory for culture. A count of 100 000 bacteria per ml indicates UTI, probably upper UTI.

Aetiology: In over 80 per cent of cases *E. coli* is the infecting organism ; in 15 per cent *Klebsiella, Proteus mirabilis* or *Staphylococcus saprophyticus* is found.

Treatment: Most cases of lower urinary tract infection are treated by a single dose of amoxycillin (3g), trimethoprim 600mg or co-trimoxazole (2 double strength tablets). This treatment is as effective as the earlier 7–10 day courses. The urine should be re-examined 2 to 7 days after treatment and, if bacteria are present, upper UTI is diagnosed.

If chlamydial infection is diagnosed or thought to be the cause of the dysuria, a 10-day course of doxycycline 100mg twice daily or tetracycline 500mg four times daily should be prescribed.

Upper UTI is diagnosed (1) by the presence of a colony count of > 100 000 organisms per ml, (2) failure of the single-dose regimen to effect cure, and (3) if the symptoms of loin pain, nausea, and pyrexia (including rigors) are present. In the first two instances the infection is sub-clinical. Treatment for sub-clinical pyelonephritis is to give a standard 7-day course of an appropriate antibiotic.

Clinically diagnosed pyelonephritis requires aggressive treatment, using an appropriate antibiotic regimen. In infections with few symptoms, amoxycillin (or ampicillin) 500mg 4 times a day, or co-trimoxazole 2 tablets twice daily are given for 7 days. If the patient is severely ill, hospital admission is arranged and amoxycillin or ampicillin is given parenterally. Lack of response within 48 hours demands a critical review.

THE URETHRAL SYNDROME

In this form of lower UTI, the woman complains of dysuria, frequency and pain, which usually occurs within 12 to 36 hours of sexual intercourse. The symptoms last for 1 to 4 days and recur when sexual intercourse is resumed, although not after each episode. The relation of the symptoms to intercourse gave the condition its old name of 'honeymoon cystitis'.

The severity of the symptoms and their anticipated recurrence may cause considerable problems in the relationship, and marked sexual frustration. The cause of the urethral syndrome is unknown but may be due to an increased adherence of bacteria to receptors in the urethral epithelium.

Although the urethral syndrome is usually related to sexual activity, in a few women it occurs at other times.

A specimen of urine should be examined for pyuria, which is usually present, and if appropriate a urine culture should be made. In the past many urologists have claimed that the urethral syndrome was caused by trigonitis, which they diagnosed at cystoscopy. The diagnosis was based on the red granular appearance of the trigone and, if a biopsy was taken, on a report of squamous metaplasia. These conditions are found in women with no urinary tract problems and the concept of trigonitis should be abandoned, as should treatment by cauterizing the supposed condition. Most women who have the urethral syndrome can be cured relatively simply. Immediately before sexual intercourse (or just after) the woman drinks 3 to 4 glasses of water and about 20 minutes later empties her bladder completely. Should this not relieve the symptoms (or she is not sexually active) she should be prescribed trimeth-oprim 100mg, or nitrofurantoin 50mg each day indefinitely.

URETHRAL TUMOURS

Prolapse of the lower urethra

This condition occurs most frequently in old age, and may be acute or chronic. In the acute form the whole circumference of the lower urethra suddenly everts and becomes engorged as the venous return is impeded. The patient complains of severe dysuria, pain and frequency. The immediate treatment is to reduce the prolapse and to insert a large catheter; later a surgical correction of the prolapse is required. In the chronic form, the atrophy of the vulval and urethral tissues after the climacteric causes the external meatus to gape, and permits some part of the posterior urethral wall to prolapse (Fig. **25/7**). It appears as a small red tumour, and is usually symptomless. However, if infection occurs, the tumour becomes larger and dull red in colour, and the patient complains of severe dysuria. The condition is sometimes called a 'granulomatous caruncle'.

TREATMENT

Unless symptoms are present, no treatment is required. Symptoms should be treated by local applications of chlorohexidine cream, and oestrogen cream in postmenopausal women. If the symptoms persist, the prolapsed area should be excised and the urethral meatus tightened.

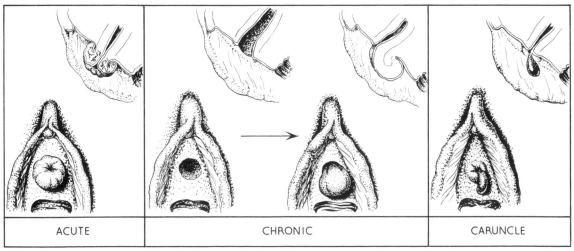

| ACUTE | CHRONIC | CARUNCLE |

Fig. 25/7 Urethral prolapse and urethral caruncle

Urethral diverticulum

This is a relatively rare condition, causing non-specific complaints, the most frequent being urgency, frequency and 'recurrent urinary tract infection'. In about half of patients a palpable, tender, suburethral mass is found. Diagnosis is confirmed by cysto-urethroscopy or by a voiding cystogram. Treatment is to excise the diverticulum, close the aperture in the urethra, using a transvaginal approach.

Urethral caruncle

This is a pedunculated polyp, which arises from the posterior margin of the urethral meatus. It is highly vascular and dull red in colour. It is extremely tender to touch, and the patient complains of pain, dysuria and dyspareunia. Treatment is surgical, the caruncle and its bed being excised and cauterized.

Chapter 26

The Breast in Gynaecology

The breasts develop from an ectodermal swelling in the thoracic region of the embryo. Initially this ridge extends the entire length of the ventral surface of the fetus, from the fore limb bud to the hind limb bud, but it rapidly atrophies and only the thoracic portion remains by the 12th week of intra-uterine life. During the 20th week solid cords of cells grow down in the tissues beneath the ectodermal swelling, and between the 30th and 36th week these become canalized to form the lactiferous ducts. At this time the original ectodermal swelling sheds its surface central cells, which creates an epithelial pit. This becomes everted at about the 38th week to form the nipple.

In the newborn infant, the breast consists of a nipple and a system of 15 to 25 lactiferous ducts, the growth of which has been exaggerated to some extent by maternal oestrogen. Within 2 to 3 weeks of birth, involutional changes occur and thereafter the breast is quiescent until 2 or 3 years prior to the menarche. At this time, under the influence of increasing oestrogen secretion, its development begins. Initially this is in the area around the nipple, and consists of growth of the duct system, a discoid mass forming beneath the areola. Later the ducts proliferate through the breast area, and divide into smaller ducts and primitive acini. At the same time fat is deposited around the duct systems, so that the pubertal breast becomes prominent and round. Following puberty development proceeds more rapidly, and when the influence of progesterone is added to that of oestrogen, the development of the acini increases considerably.

THE ADULT BREAST

The adult breast is of variable size, the size bearing no relationship to the function of lactation. It is divided into 15 to 25 lobes, separated from each other by fibrous septa radiating from the nipple. Each lobe has its own duct system which terminates in a dilated area (the lactiferous sinus) within the nipple, and then opens onto its surface as a punctate orifice. The lobes divide into lobules, each of which contains from 10 to 100 acini grouped round a collecting duct. The number of the lobes and acini varies between individuals, but are most numerous in young adulthood. After the menopause the numbers decrease, so that in old age each lobule has only 3 or 4 acini. The collecting duct from each lobule joins with others, and these link with the main duct draining the lobe. Traced backward from the nipple, the duct system resembles a tree, the acini forming the leaves, the ducts the branches, and the main duct the trunk. Both the ducts and acini are surrounded and supported by fatty and fibrous tissues (Fig. **26/1**). The acini, when not secreting milk, are lined by two layers of epithelium. External to this is a network of myo-epithelial cells, contraction of which empties the alveolus. A mesh of fine capillaries mingles with the myo-epithelial cells, and the lactiferous ducts are also well supplied, so that the entire breast is very vascular.

The adult breast undergoes a cyclic change which is dependent upon the cyclic release of the female sex hormones. In the proliferative phase of the menstrual cycle some development of the ducts occurs, but the maximal activity is in the luteal phase, when increased epithelial activity occurs in the ducts and acini, both of which hypertrophy to a variable extent. At the same time engorgement of the vascular system and transudation of fluid into the breast tissues occurs, so that the breasts become heavier. In an exaggerated form this may lead to premenstrual breast tenderness and discomfort. The use of oestrogen-progestogen combinations for ovulation suppression may exaggerate these symptoms in susceptible women.

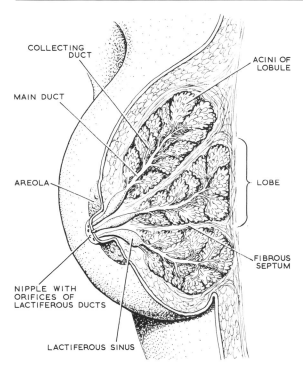

COLLECTING DUCT

MAIN DUCT

AREOLA

NIPPLE WITH ORIFICES OF LACTIFEROUS DUCTS

LACTIFEROUS SINUS

ACINI OF LOBULE

LOBE

FIBROUS SEPTUM

Fig. 26/1 The anatomy of the breast, showing the acini and collecting ducts of the lobes

EXAMINATION OF THE BREAST

This has been described in detail in Chapter 1.

DISORDERS OF THE MAMMARY GLAND

Small breasts

In Western cultures a considerable emphasis is placed upon mammary size and shape as a potent sexual symbol. Eastern cultures place less emphasis upon the erotic nature of the breast, and the organ is considered more as a means of survival for the race, than as an erogenous zone. Because of the symbolism of a well-developed breast in Western society, many young adults whose breasts are small seek advice. Absent breast development may be due to a failure of oestrogenic production (as in ovarian agenesis) or its cessation (as after castration), or may be due to intrinsic defects in the gland itself. The last is not amenable to treatment, but considerable mammary development can be obtained in the former conditions by the use of oral, parenteral or locally applied oestrogen. However, to maintain the size of the breast, oestrogen must be continued indefinitely. In cases where menstrual function is normal, it is clear that adequate quantities of endogenous oestrogen is being secreted, and it is illogical and futile to administer additional exogenous oestrogen in the hope of increasing breast size. In such patients the small size of the breast is due to lack of fat deposition rather than lack of duct formation. Apart from dietary advice, treatment is not particularly satisfactory. If the condition is causing the woman marked psychological distress, augmentation mammaplasty using a silicone prosthesis may be advocated.

Increased size

The size of the breasts tends to increase as the woman enters the late reproductive era (from aged 30 to 45), and particularly if she has been pregnant. Most of this enlargement is due to increased fat deposition. Associated with the increased size is a tendency for the breasts to become more pendulous, due to stretching of the fibrous tissue septa, which in Western (but not African) cultures, is considered unattractive. Unfortunately exercises are of little value, and if the condition is unacceptable to the patient, reduction mammaplasty may be considered. Unfortunately the reduction effected may not persist and the breast size may increase after a time interval. This must be taken into account and discussed with the woman prior to surgery.

Asymmetry

As is normal with paired organs, the size of the breasts is rarely identical, one having more gland tissue than the other. Inequality in breast size is not uncommon during adolescence, the breasts usually becoming equal in size as the girl reaches late adolescence. Occasionally the inequality persists and this may cause marked psychological disturbances, as the girl feels 'abnormal'. The use of oestrogens (especially in the form of oral hormonal contraceptives) may help, but in cases of extreme distress mammaplasty may be indicated.

Asymmetry may occur in adulthood and again in marked cases plastic surgery may be sought, preferably to reduce the size of the larger breast, but once again its effect may be only temporary.

Accessory breasts

Theoretically a breast, or at least a nipple, may develop anywhere along the site of the ectodermal ridge, rudiments of which may persist along a line extending from the axilla to the pubic spine. The commonest site for breast tissue is as a 'tail' extending into the axilla; but accessory nipples may be found anywhere along the 'nipple line'. No treatment is required.

Inverted nipples

These are due to a developmental error, the epithelial pit failing to evert under the stimulation of oestrogen in the last weeks of intra-uterine life. The condition requires no treatment until the patient becomes pregnant, when digital manipulation by stretching the tissues surrounding the inverted nipple, or the periodic use of a negative pressure pump, is useful. If the condition is detected in pregnancy and the patient wishes to breast-feed her baby, she should wear a Waller plastic nipple shield beneath her brassière.

LACTATION AND ITS PROBLEMS

These are discussed in Volume I as they are mainly obstetric problems, apart from the suppression of lactation required during weaning. The management of this is considered further in Chapter 30.

DISEASES OF THE BREAST

Benign mammary dysplasia

The increase in the development of the ducts and acini which normally occurs during the luteal phase of each cycle, and which diminishes during menstruation, may be exaggerated in some women, so that the duct system increases in size, the breasts become tender, and are coarsely nodular on palpation. Benign mammary dysplasia is characterized by exceedingly variable pathological findings, but there is generally a hyperplasia of both glandular (epithelial) and fibrous elements. These alterations may be diffuse or localized affecting only one lobe, or even only part of a lobe. In most cases the upper outer quadrant of the breast is most affected.

Women with mild mammary dysplasia complain of painful, tender heavy breasts in the week to ten days before menstruation. The pain may be severe and the condition disabling. Benign mammary dysplasia is the most common cause of breast pain in women during their reproductive years. Although stress may play a part in the aetiology of the condition, in many cases there is an imbalance in the oestradiol progesterone ratio, with a relative decrease in progesterone; or the breasts are especially sensitive to the effects of prolactin.

In the past the condition was called 'chronic mastitis' (which it is not), fibrocystic disease of the breast, fibroadenosis or mazoplasia. These epithets should now be abandoned, in favour of benign mammary dysplasia or benign breast disease. Long-term studies show that benign breast disease does not increase a woman's risk of developing breast cancer.

The development of mammography has enabled physicians to be more precise in diagnosing benign breast disease. It is usual to describe two types: (1) a diffuse form and (2) a localized form.

Diffuse mammary dysplasia

This form is mainly found in women aged between 30 and 50. The symptoms vary from mild discomfort through marked tenderness, to severe pain and are intermittent in intensity and duration. The condition may be present throughout the cycle, but is worse premenstrually. Examination may show that both breasts are affected, but usually one is more involved, especially in the upper and outer quadrant. Palpation reveals a coarsely nodular area of increased thickness, resembling ill-defined lumps which merge into normal tissue, and these signs are most obvious in the premenstrual phase of the cycle. The patient often has a considerable anxiety that the condition may be a 'breast cancer', and treatment should start with a full and careful discussion of the disorder, and an explanation that it is an exaggerated, persisting form of a normal cyclical change. Some of the women complaining of breast pain have associated psychosomatic disorders (such as deep pelvic discomfort) so that it is important to discuss the problem with the patient.

Most patients will obtain a reasonable amount of relief by wearing a well fitting brassière day and night. Some women benefit by the use of diuretics (in the belief that fluid is retained in the breast) or tranquillizers.

Women who have marked mammary dysplasia and have severe breast pain require additional therapy. A recent report indicates that dietary fat may play a part in relieving the swelling and pain. A diet should be chosen which reduces the daily intake of fat to about 20 per cent of total energy intake (from about 37 per cent in most Western diets) and increases the carbohydrate consumption to about 60 per cent of energy intake (from about 45 per cent in the average diet). On this diet the symptoms were relieved in over 60 per cent of the women studied. If the woman does not choose to change her diet three other approaches are suggested. The first is to prescribe dydrogesterone 10mg twice daily from day 12 to 26 of the menstrual cycle to correct any postulated progesterone deficiency. This therapy produces a cure rate of about 60 per cent. The second approach is to prescribe danazol 200mg twice daily, from day 12 to 26 of the cycle. Danazol, which is an antigonadotrophic drug, reduces the FSH and LH stimulus to the ovary with a resulting reduction in the secretion of oestradiol and progesterone.

The third approach is to prescribe the prolactin antagonist, bromocriptine, daily throughout the menstrual cycle in a dose varying between 2.5 and 5mg daily.

Local mammary dysplasia
This form is found at all ages from 25 to 50, and in the perimenopausal patient, especially, single large cysts are occasionally detected. In general there are few, if any, symptoms, and the patient seeks help because she has noticed a lump in her breast and is fearful that it may be cancerous. The physician must exclude this by careful palpation, by mammography or thermography, or by biopsy if any doubt remains. Apart from this, no treatment beyond reassurance is required.

Duct ecstasia ('periductal mastitis')

Duct ecstasia is the second most common cause of breast pain. The pain occurs at all times during the menstrual cycle, and may be worse in cold weather. Its site is localized to an area below the areola or to the inner quadrants of the breasts. Mammography may identify characteristic flame-shaped shadows. Treatment is to excise the affected wedge-shaped area and the subareolar duct system.

Breast pain, other causes

Some women complain of breast pain, which is, in reality, due to pain over an enlarged costochondral junction. The pain is localized, chronic and bears no relationship to the premenstruum. Radiology shows no abnormality, and a mammogram shows a normal breast. The condition is called 'the Tietze syndrome' and no effective treatment is available.

Trauma, usually localized at the site of a previous injury or surgical incision (for biopsy or to treat a breast abscess) is another cause of breast pain.

Fibroadenoma

These are benign encapsulated tumours, which are found most frequently in women in their twenties. The tumours are symptomless, and are generally discovered by accident or at self-examination. Palpation of the breast reveals a firm tumour with a smooth surface, which is very mobile and may be found in any quadrant of the breast. Treatment is simple excision,

Age:	> 30	30 to 50	40 to 50
Clinical findings	Discrete, firm mobile, painless lump	Breast lumpy, especially in pre-menstruum, tender. Later, discrete, tender. Cystic masses may occur which appear and disappear. Still later, a 'blue-domed cyst'.	Serous or bloody discharge from nipple
Name(s):	Fibro-adenoma Benign	Benign mammary dysplasia (Mazoplasia)	Intraductal papilloma (rare)

Table 26/1 Benign tumours of the breast

with a wedge of surrounding normal breast tissue, as the capsule tends to be adherent (see Table **26/1**).

Benign breast disease and cancer

What is the relationship between benign breast disorders and carcinoma? Studies indicate that neither mammary dysplasia nor fibroadenoma predispose to breast carcinoma.

This observation is important as about 1 woman in every 5 develops benign breast disease, usually mammary dysplasia, during the reproductive years. It is important to reassure these women that they are at no greater risk of developing breast cancer than other women. The preventive measures which they should take, particularly breast self-examination and annual breast check-ups are no different from those recommended to all women.

INFECTIONS

Acute mastitis

In a lactating patient breast abscess is the most common inflammatory condition. The infection reaches the breast parenchyma from the nipple, and is more frequent if the nipple is 'cracked' or abraded by forceful sucking. The diagnosis is easy, and treatment is by the administration of antibiotics, and incision if pus formation is marked. The condition is discussed more fully in Volume I.

Periductal mastitis

This is the most frequent breast infection in a non-lactating patient, and is usually unilateral and associated with an inverted nipple. The infective agent is usually *Staphylococcus aureus*. Generally the onset is subacute, and the condition is characterized by tenderness, inflammation and induration in a wedge-shaped zone beneath the areola. Treatment, initially, is conservative, antibiotics being administered. Incisions should be avoided unless definite pus formation occurs.

ECZEMA OF THE AREOLA AND NIPPLE

This condition is occasionally encountered, and is usually bilateral, which identifies it from Paget's disease of the nipple which is unilateral. However, in

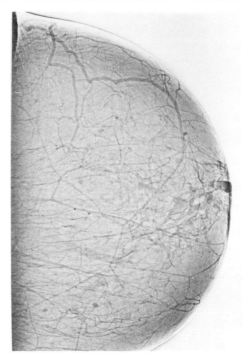

Fig. 26/2 A mammogram of a normal breast

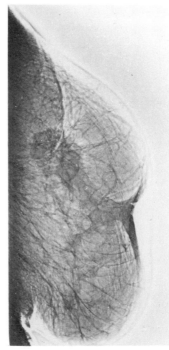

Fig. 26/3 A mammogram of a breast containing an advanced carcinoma. Note the retracted nipple and skin thickening

doubtful cases biopsy is essential. The treatment of eczema is the topical application of an ointment containing corticosteroids (for example, Betnovate or Synalar).

CANCER OF THE BREAST

Cancer of the breast is the commonest malignancy in the female, the incidence being three times that of carcinoma of the cervix. It has been estimated that 1 woman in 16 will develop the malignancy. Only by detecting the disease in the earliest stages can cure be expected. Many health authorities recommend intensive educational programmes to teach women over the age of 35 breast self-examination (BSE), although the value of this procedure in detecting early breast cancer is doubtful. Other authorities recommend that women over the age of 35 have their breasts examined by a doctor each year. The value of this procedure in detecting early breast cancer has not been established.

Mammography has been shown in studies from Sweden, the Netherlands and the USA to be a superior screening method to BSE or annual breast examination. Women between the ages of 40 and 50 should have a mammogram made to give base-line information about the glandular structure of the breasts. From the age of 50 a woman should have an annual mammogram (Fig. **26/2** and Fig. **26/3**). Mammography is currently the only way in which breast cancer can be detected at an early stage. Unfortunately, by the time most breast cancers are detected at present, the 5-year survival rate is less than 50 per cent.

The aetiology of breast cancer remains obscure, despite much research. Childbearing before the age of 30 seems to be protective; and, possibly, Western diets, rich in fat and unrefined carbohydrate, may be provocative by altering the bowel flora and leading to the ingestion of oestrogenic-type hormones.

The treatment of breast cancer is in the hands of the general surgeon. The knowledge that in 60 to 70 per cent of operable early breast carcinoma, the disease has already disseminated widely has led to new procedures. These procedures attempt to strike a balance between mutilation and adequate local control. If the tumour is <3cm in diameter excisional biopsy ('lumpectomy'), axillary lymphadenectomy and radiation is resulting in the same tumour-free survival, when compared with modified radical mastectomy and, because the woman keeps her breast, is attended by considerably less psychological trauma. Larger tumours are treated by modified radical mastectomy and, if the patient wishes, by breast reconstruction about 3 months later. If the axillary lymph nodes are positive for carcinoma, adjuvant chemotherapy improves survival, at least in premenopausal women; an alternative is to use tamoxifen. Tamoxifen is an antioestrogen which occupies oestrogen receptors, blocking the effects of oestrogen, and may have a cytotoxic effect on tumour cells. Tamoxifen is also used in advanced breast carcinoma.

The second major change is the realization that breast cancer affects women in two ways. The first is the knowledge that she has cancer; the second is that the loss of a breast affects her femininity, her body image and her self-esteem. For these reasons counselling before and after operation is important. The role of an informed lay counsellor who has herself undergone mastectomy may be crucial in the rehabilitation process after operation.

Chapter 27

Paediatric Gynaecology

Gynaecological conditions which require diagnosis and treatment may occur at any age, although they are relatively uncommon in infancy and childhood. The main neonatal problem is the identification of intersexuality; whilst in childhood, vaginal infection, ovarian tumours and precocious puberty can cause diagnostic and therapeutic problems.

EXAMINATION OF THE NEONATE

Congenital anomalies occur in 2 or 3 per 100 infants, and should always be sought by careful examination of the neonate, at birth by the obstetrician, and before discharge from hospital by the paediatrician. Particular attention should be paid to the child if any ambiguity of the external genitalia is found, or if a small penis or hypospadias is present and no testes can be palpated in the scrotum at repeated examinations, as the anomalies may indicate that the child is an intersex (pseudohermaphrodite).

FEMALE INTERSEX

The majority of neonates with ambiguous genitalia are female intersex, but three other intersex forms may be encountered. The differentiation of these types is discussed in Chapter 3, and in this chapter only female intersex is considered further. Three forms of female intersex occur: (1) congenital adrenal hyperplasia, (2) drug-induced virilism and (3) adrenal tumour. The last two types are uncommon. Female intersex should be investigated by (1) buccal smear for the presence of Barr bodies, (2) karyotype (using marrow aspirate), (3) hormone assays of 17-OH progesterone and androgens (including precursors) and (4) serum electrolyte levels.

CONGENITAL ADRENAL HYPERPLASIA (adrenogenital syndrome)

The condition (affecting 1 in 10 000 neonates) is due to a group of enzyme defects which prevent the synthesis of cortisone from progesterone. Since cortisone is not produced, the hypothalamus-pituitary is not subjected to a negative 'feedback' and considerable quantities of corticotrophin are released, which stimulate the adrenal gland to undergo hyperplasia and to produce increasing amounts of androgens. The androgens cause masculinization of the external genitalia, but do not interfere with the differentiation of the Mullerian duct structures. This means that the oviducts, uterus and upper vagina are normally formed, but the external genitalia appear masculine to a greater or lesser extent (Fig. **27/1**).

Three forms of congenital adrenal hyperplasia exist due to three related enzymatic defects. (1) The most common, which is found in 87 per cent of cases, is C-21-hydroxylase deficiency. In three-quarters of the cases, the deficiency is characterized by uncomplicated virilism; but in one-quarter the enzyme defect is more severe, so that aldosterone production is lost and the virilism is accompanied by a salt-losing syndrome. (2) C-11-beta-hydroxylase defect occurs in 8 per cent of cases, and is associated with hypertension and hyperpigmentation. (3) The remaining defect, 3-beta-ol-dehydrogenase deficiency occurs in 5 per cent of cases, and is very severe. It is associated with adrenal deficiency and sodium loss.

As all cases are genetically determined, there is a likelihood that other siblings may be affected. The diagnosis is made, therefore, by studying the family history, by determining the nuclear sex from a buccal smear, and by estimating the levels of plasma 17-hydroxy progesterone and androgens. Because the salt-losing variety of the adrenogenital syndrome is rapidly lethal, serum electrolytes should be esti-

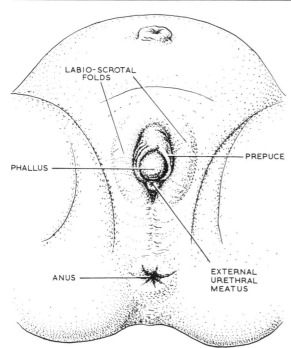

Fig. 27/1 Ambiguous external genitalia due to the adrenogenital syndrome

mated immediately in all neonates with ambiguous genitalia.

The diagnosis is confirmed if the 17-hydroxy progesterone level exceeds 200ng/dl. Plasma pregnanetriol levels are also raised (above 5µg/100ml).

Treatment must be instituted quickly or death will supervene. Cortisone or one of its derivatives is given in order to suppress ACTH activity and provide circulating cortisol. Initially a high dose is given, and this is later reduced. If treatment is started sufficiently early, the patient can live a full life. Surgical correction of the genital malformations should be undertaken before the child goes to school, but it is unwise to operate in the first year of life. With corticosteroid supplementation these children survive and their secondary sexual characteristics develop normally. However the menarche tends to be delayed and the girl tends to be shorter than her peers.

DRUG-INDUCED VIRILISM

This condition may occur when the mother has received progestogens in early pregnancy. A history

will provide information of iatrogenic therapy and a buccal smear is positive for Barr bodies.

Unlike congenital adrenal hyperplasia, no further masculinization occurs after birth. In most cases the degree of virilization is slight, minimal enlargement of the clitoris and minimal, or no, fusion of the scroto-labial folds occurring. These infants require no surgery unless the clitoris is greatly enlarged, when partial clitoral amputation may be required.

FUSION OF THE LABIA MINORA

This condition may occur as a minor form of masculinization following maternal ingestion of androgens, or may be acquired, when it is encountered in the toddler stage. Treatment is to separate the fused labia digitally, and to apply oestrogen cream for 2 to 3 weeks to enable epithelial growth to occur.

THE GENITAL CRISIS

The female fetus *in utero* receives, via the placenta, a considerable quantity of oestrogens. Although most are immediately converted into the relatively inactive form, oestriol, sufficient remains in the circulation to thicken and stratify the fetal vaginal epithelium. In some cases, owing to a tissue sensitivity, the uterus also responds, the endometrium is stimulated, and the breasts react to maternal oestrogen and progesterone by developing the alveolar and duct systems. Following birth, the maternal hormonal support is withdrawn and in a few infants uterine 'withdrawal bleeding' occurs. The amount is small and settles within a few days. This is known as '*the genital crisis*'. Similarly, withdrawal of the hormonal suppression of growth hormone or of prolactin, leads in a few female infants to increase in the size of the breasts (*gynaecomastia*) and to the secretion of a watery milk. No treatment is required as the condition is self-limiting.

VULVOVAGINITIS

As noted, the neonate acquires an appreciable amount of oestrogen and progesterone transplacentally and from the syncytial cells of the placenta. These hormones are of sufficient quantity to cause variable, but distinct, physiological and cytological alterations, until they are finally degraded over a period of 7 to 14 days. The effect upon the vagina is to increase the number of layers of the epithelium, the cells of which synthesize glycogen, and consequently there is an increase in vaginal acidity. However, once the sex hormones are metabolized and excreted, the superficial and intermediate vaginal cell layers are exfoliated and only a few layers of parabasal epithelial cells remain, until growth is stimulated once again by the endogenous secretion of oestrogen which occurs at puberty.

The vagina becomes colonized within the first 24 hours of life by various cocci and by lactobacilli, and as the acidity falls with the withdrawal of the sex hormones, invasion by staphylococci, streptococci, diphtheroids and colon bacillus occurs. Only occasionally, however, do they become pathogenic. When they do, or when more virulent organisms are introduced, they multiply readily in the alkaline environment of the prepubertal vagina. The vulva is usually involved in the inflammation, so the term *vulvovaginitis* is preferable to vaginitis.

A classification of vulvovaginitis is shown in Table 27/1.

			Percentage
1. Non-specific			60
2. Specific			
(a) Bacterial: *E. coli*	12		
N. gonorrhoea	2	20	
Other	6		
(b) Fungal (*Candida*)			10
(c) Protozoal (trichomonad)			5
(d) Foreign body			5
(e) Helminthic/viral			1

Table 27/1 Vulvovaginitis: causes

Investigation

It should be remembered that the vulva and introitus in infants and young girls is normally red in colour, and this must not be confused with the rubor of infection. The vulva should be inspected, and the groins palpated for lymphadenopathy. The anal area should be inspected and a smear taken for pin and threadworms. The urine should be examined for protein and sugar. A smear for bacteriological examination should be taken from the vagina. To exclude the presence of a foreign body introduced into the vagina by the child, many gynaecologists insist in passing a vaginoscope, and there is merit in this investigation provided the proper instrument is available. Alternatively, a rectal examination should be made to detect a foreign body in the vagina.

In a few cases the examination of the vaginal exfoliative cytology is helpful. A lateral wall vaginal smear, placed immediately in 95% ethyl alcohol for 15 minutes and stained with Papanicolaou or Shorr's stain, gives some indication of the hormonal state of the child. In the neonate, a predominantly intermediate or superficial cell population is found; but this changes rapidly and for the next 9 or 10 years the smear shows only parabasal cells. With the steroidogenesis which occurs during the 2 or 3 years preceding menstruation, intermediate cells progressively replace the parabasal cells. The quantity of hormonal secretion varies, so that varying patterns of vaginal exfoliative cytology are found.

Treatment

As a diagnosis is made in only 40 per cent of cases, general principles apply. These are (1) general cleanliness, using only a mild soap or none at all, (2) careful drying and powdering after vulval washing, (3) avoidance of nylon panties, and (4) the wearing of cotton panties day and night.

With these measures over 75 per cent of cases will be cured within 2 weeks, and no other treatment should be given initially unless a specific cause has been isolated. If the condition persists after 2 weeks, the local application of oestrogen cream twice daily will usually result in a cure. When a specific cause is found, specific therapy is given. Trichomoniasis is treated by oral metronidazole; fungus infection by the local application of fungicides; gonococcal vaginitis by penicillin (25 000 units per kg daily for 4 days); helminths by the oral administration of piperazine or viprynium.

In non-specific vaginitis which fails to respond to general hygienic measures, slim vaginal pessaries containing 9-aminoacridine HCL may be used nightly for 14 nights provided they can be inserted into the vagina painlessly.

OVARIAN TUMOURS IN CHILDREN

Ovarian tumours are rare in childhood, and this group forms no more than 2 per cent of all cases

| | Non-neoplastic | Neoplastic | |
| | | Benign | Malignant |
	%	%	%
Functional cysts	25		
Germ cell tumours			
Teratoma		33	
Disgerminoma			8
Embryonal carcinoma			4
Other			2
Sex cord tumours			
Granulosa cell			3
Androblastoma			2
Fibroma		3	
Other		1	2
Epithelial tumours			
Serous cystadenoma		8	
Mucinous cystadenoma		5	
Cystadenocarcinoma			2
Other			2
	25	50	25

Table 27/2 Ovarian tumours in childhood (from literature 1940–79:1200 reported cases). Figures are given as percentages

seen. If present, there is a 25 per cent chance that the tumour is malignant (Table **27/2**). The symptoms are abdominal distension, usually of short duration, and pain in the case of malignant tumours. Examination shows a mass in the lower abdomen. Treatment is surgical; benign tumours should be treated by ovarian cystectomy if possible, and malignant tumours by oophorectomy. Radiation therapy may be given in cases of disgerminoma, and, perhaps, granulosa cell tumours, when extension beyond the ovary has occurred.

OTHER GENITAL TRACT TUMOURS

Carcinoma is extremely rare in prepubertal children, and the prognosis poor. Sarcoma botryoides, although only affecting children, is infrequently encountered, and is very lethal. The most common symptom is a bloodstained vaginal discharge. Inspection will reveal a haemorrhagic tumorous mass. Treatment is unsatisfactory, and recently it has been suggested that chemotherapy (vinblastine) may help and may be followed by exenteration in some cases. However, the mutilation is so great that the principle:

'Thou shalt not kill, but needst not strive
Officiously to keep alive . . .'

may apply.

Bleeding per vaginam

Bleeding per vaginam is an alarming symptom in a young child. In babies the sign is usually due to a lesion of the genital tract; in older children the sign is usually due to precocious puberty, when other signs of sexual development are often but not always, present. Investigation to exclude vaginitis, a foreign body in the vagina, an ovarian tumour and genital tract malignancy is mandatory before the diagnosis of precocious menstruation and/or puberty is made.

PRECOCIOUS PUBERTY

Precocious puberty indicates that sexual maturation has occurred before the age of 9. It may be due to (1) a constitutional factor in which activation of the hypothalamus-pituitary-gonadal axis occurs without any other lesion, (2) a hormone-producing tumour, usually a granulosa or theca cell tumour of the ovary, (3) a central nervous system lesion or (4) an adrenal tumour.

The condition is relatively uncommon, but when it occurs the normal sequence of pubertal changes are apparent – first the breasts develop, then pubic and axillary hair appear, and finally menstrual bleeding occurs. The latter may be preceded by a bloody vaginal discharge for some weeks. The child is usually relatively tall for her age, but her skeletal maturation is advanced relative to her age so that skeletal growth tends to cease early. This means that the girl will be shorter than her peers by the age of 16.

Investigation of a young girl showing signs of precocious puberty should be thorough, and constitutional precocious puberty only diagnosed by exclusion.

The following investigations should be made to exclude organic causes. (1) full history and physical examination, (2) bone age studies, (3) x-ray of skull, or CAT scan to exclude a brain (pituitary) neoplasm, (4) CAT scan or ultrasonography to exclude an adrenal or ovarian neoplasm. If the scan shows that the uterus has a cross-sectional area greater than 4 cm² and/or an ovary with a volume greater than 3 cm³, the diagnosis is confirmed. In certain cases the following are needed; (5) hormone assays, plasma FSH and LH; plasma oestradiol 17 beta and a plasma testosterone assay may be needed, to exclude an adrenal tumour, (6) a pelvic examination, under anaesthesia, to exclude a functioning ovarian tumour, (7) if any doubt persists, laparoscopic examination of the pelvis.

Treatment in the case of an intracranial tumour or a functioning ovarian tumour is surgical. Constitutional precocious puberty usually requires no treatment, apart from careful explanation to the mother that the condition is not 'abnormal'. However, if the physical appearance of the girl is causing psychosocial problems, drugs may be offered. Medroxyprogesterone acetate will inhibit menstruation but has no effect on breast development or on skeletal maturation (i.e. height). If the bone-age studies show that the bone age is 11 or less, cyproterone acetate (70 to 150mg/m²/day) will suppress signs of sexual maturation and growth, but may suppress adrenal function. The most effective drug for the treatment of constitutional precocious puberty is a synthetic superactive GnRH analogue. It is given daily by subcutaneous injection, by nasal insufflation, or by giving a depot preparation each month until the girl reaches the normal age range of puberty. The GnRH analogue 'blocks' the GnRH receptors so that they become refractory to endogenous GnRH. The effect of this is to reverse the pubertal changes. The breasts diminish in size, menstruation ceases and acne clears.

TALL GIRLS

Some girls in the prepubertal years are considered to be excessively tall by their parents. The height of the child depends to some extent on the stature of the parents and this must be taken into account. For children aged less than 9 there are reliable charts devised by Professor Tanner against which the child's stature can be compared. Excessive height may be due to excessive growth hormone production, and to certain other rare conditions, but is usually constitutional when the girl is normal apart from her height.

If the height of the girl is causing her psychological problems, and her skeletal bone age is less than 13, treatment with oestrogens may be effective in reducing the girl's final height by producing premature epiphyseal closure, although oestrogens are usually not prescribed unless the girl's height exceeds 180cm.

Before prescribing oestrogens, the girl should be aware that she will bleed vaginally at monthly intervals. Ethinyl oestradiol 50–100μg (or its equivalent see p. 282) is given for 25 days each month, and norethisterone 1 to 2.5mg is given daily from day 15 to 25. After 5 days rest, during which withdrawal bleeding may occur, the regimen is repeated. Recently bromocriptine 5mg daily (which suppresses growth hormone synthesis) has been suggested. This regimen avoids the side effects of the sex steroids. After 3 months, the height is measured to determine if the growth velocity has diminished. Side-effects may occur and the girl may choose not to have medical treatment, but to wait until her final height is reached and then seek surgery to shorten the length of the femur and/or tibia and fibula.

Chapter 28

Adolescence and Puberty

The period between childhood and maturity is adolescence, which biologically extends between the ages of 10 and 19. During this period the most important event is the onset of menstruation, or the menarche, which marks puberty, and which occurs at any time between the ages of 10 and 16, although the median age in the developed nations is 12.8 years. Prior to this, between the ages of 5 and 8, an increase in adrenal androgen production occurs in both sexes. The reason for this androgen secretion and its relationship (if any) to the events which result in puberty is obscure at present.

SOMATIC CHANGES

The somatic changes characterizing female adolescence begin some years before puberty, but are most marked in the 2 years preceding the menarche. They are due in part to the increasing amounts of pituitary hormones produced, but mainly to oestrogen secreted by the ovary and the adrenal cortex. These organs, in their turn, are stimulated by the awakening hypothalamus/pituitary complex. Perhaps the most marked somatic change is the prepubertal spurt of growth occasioned by the secretion of human growth hormone (HGH) and of adrenal androgens. It starts between 3 and 4 years before the menarche and is maximal in the first 2 years (Fig. **28/1**). Physical growth slows down as the menarche approaches, because HGH secretion diminishes as oestrogen secretion increases, due to a 'feedback' mechanism. In the absence of oestrogenic feedback, hypersecretion of HGH produces symmetrical overgrowth of the whole body, including the long bones. This leads to a tall, thin girl with poor breast

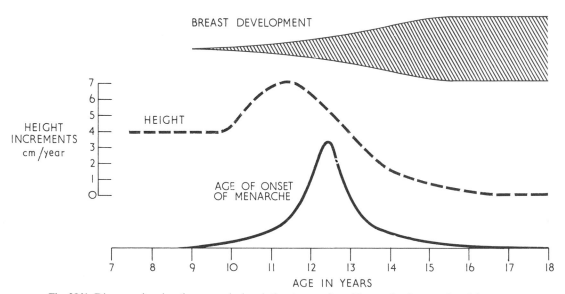

Fig. 28/1 Diagram showing the menarche in relation to growth and breast development in adolescence

development, the so-called eunuchoid or hypogonadal type. Oestrogen secretion is therefore of the greatest importance for normal female development. The secretion of oestrogen largely depends on ovarian stimulation by pituitary gonadotrophic hormones.

Shortly after the HGH surge, which occurs at about the age of 8, the hypothalamus begins to secrete the gonadotrophic releasing hormone (GnRH), in an episodic pulsed manner. Prior to this time there is evidence that GnRH is secreted but at low levels and with a low but steady release (and if pulses occur they have low amplitude). The high amplitude pulsed episodic release of GnRH occurs during sleep initially, but after an interval of $1\frac{1}{2}$ to $3\frac{1}{2}$ years, it occurs during the day as well, at about 2-hourly intervals. The pulses of GnRH induce a release of FSH and LH.

The effect of these changes is to lead to a rapid rise in circulating FSH between the age of 9 and 11, and an inconstant rise in LH. As puberty approaches, the FSH bursts increase in amplitude and the FSH level continues to rise, reaching a plateau when the girl reaches the age of about 14 when it approximates to adult levels (Fig. **28/2**).

The LH bursts continue, becoming more pronounced as puberty is reached when a rise to adult levels occurs.

The age of menarche has been reduced by 2 to 3 years in European nations in the past 100 years. The reason for this and for the stimulus to the awakening activity of the hypothalamus-pituitary is not understood. It may be related to the need for a minimum height and weight ratio (more accurately a fat:lean ratio) to be reached before menstruation starts. Children today are better nourished than they were in the past, and increased body fat may be a factor in the earlier age of the menarche. One hypothesis is that as the body fat increases, androgen is more easily aromatized to oestrogen. The higher circulating levels of oestrogen lead to a 'positive' oestrogen feedback with surges in FSH and LH.

In summary, the menarche is associated with a rapid rise in LH secretion on a previous relatively high level of FSH. After the menarche FSH and LH levels reach those of normal menstruating women.

The raised levels of FSH and LH stimulate the ovarian follicles with the result that oestrogen is secreted by the ovary and blood levels rise. Up to the age of 7 oestrogenic secretion is maintained at a very low level. Between the ages of 7 and 9 a gradually rising secretion occurs, and this rise increases more steeply between the ages of 9 and 11. After the age of 11, a rapid acceleration of oestrogen secretion occurs. This culminates in the menarche and cyclical oestrogenic secretion throughout the reproductive era.

The effect of the increased secretion of oestrogen is (1) to stimulate the growth of the breast ducts and the subareolar button, and produce enlargement of the areolae, (2) to cause deposition of fat in breasts, on hips and lead to a rounding of the figure, (3) to induce growth of oviducts, uterus and vagina, (4) to induce growth of the external genitalia and stimulate activity of the sebaceous glands in the area, (5) to lead to proliferation of the vaginal mucosa, with deposition of glycogen and exfoliation of the superficial and intermediate cells. The glycogen in the exfoliated cells is acted upon by Döderlein's bacilli, with the production of lactic acid, and increased vaginal secretions results.

The time of appearance of these sexual characteristics is shown in Table **28/1**.

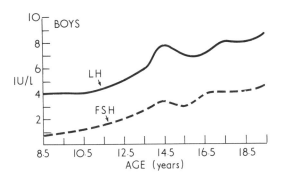

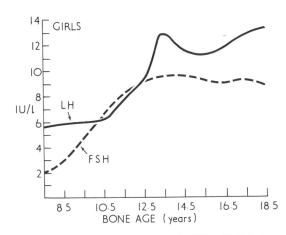

Fig. 28/2 Pubertal changes in level of FSH and LH in boys and girls. (Derived from Aptar, D. *et al. Acta Paediatric. Scand.* 1978, **67**, 417.)

Age	Characteristics
9 to 10	Growth of bony pelvis begins Fat deposition initiates beginnings of female contour Budding of nipples
10 to 11	Budding of breasts Appearance of pubic hair (androgens are responsible for pubic and axillary hair)
11 to 13	Growth of internal and external genitalia Glycogen content of vagina increases; the height of the epithelium increases with change in cell type, and the pH is lowered. Occasionally a vaginal discharge is noted.
12 to 14	Pigmentation of nipples Growth and rounding breasts
13 to 15	Axillary hair appears Menarche occurs (mean 13 years, range 9 to 16) Pubic hair increases in amount Acne present in 60 per cent of adolescents
16 to 18	Cessation of skeletal growth

Table 28/1 Time of appearance of sexual characteristics in Australian girls

PSYCHOLOGICAL CHANGES

The tremendous somatic changes are matched by equally disturbing psychological changes, which occur in adolescents of all races, but which may be modified by different cultural patterns. During these years each facet of the girl's growth affects others, and her task of adjustment can be helped or hindered by parental attitudes. At this time she begins to realize the force of new, ill-understood heterosexual inclinations and attractions; to demand a loosening of parental ties; to question previously accepted dogma. Because of these conflicts, her emotional moods, altered by the tides of hormonal secretions, tend to be volatile, and, often, to be little understood by parents who may have forgotten their own adolescence.

ADOLESCENT AMENORRHOEA

The onset of menstruation is influenced to some extent by racial, but more particularly by nutritional,

factors. In general, the mean age of the menarche is 13, with a normal bell curve distribution of 9 to 16.

In about 1 per cent of girls the menarche is delayed beyond the age of 16. This may be constitutional, but is as likely to have an organic cause. It is therefore difficult to differentiate it from primary amenorrhoea, which implies the failure of menstruation to occur, and the final diagnosis can only be made after a full investigation has revealed that the reproductive and endocrine systems are intact and may be expected to function in the future. Primary amenorrhoea in this age group may also be difficult to differentiate from secondary amenorrhoea (absence of spontaneous bleeding for an interval of at least 1 year) as some girls fail to discriminate between spontaneous and hormonally induced bleeding. However, with the exception of congenital and genetic abnormalities, the causes are similar, as can be seen in Tables **28/2** and **28/3**.

	Percentage of cases
Gonadal dysgenesis (inc. Turner's syndrome)	45
Congenital absence of uterus or vagina	15
Low body weight (inc. anorexia nervosa)	10
Congenital adrenal virilism	5
Testicular feminization	5
Other (inc. hypothyroidism 4 per cent; systemic disease, 4 per cent)	15
No cause (i.e. constitutional delayed menarche)	5

Table 28/2 Primary amenorrhoea

	Percentage of cases
Physiological – pregnancy	25
Psychological – depression, dieting anorexia nervosa, exercise	25
Pathological	
Pituitary/hypothalamic dysfunction	25
Other endocrine: thyroid, adrenal	5
Ovarian: polycystic disease, etc.	10
Endometrial disease	1
Systemic disease	9

Table 28/3 Secondary amenorrhoea in unmarried adolescents

Investigation

Provided that the girl is not excessively short in

height and that her breasts are developing, investigation is not required until after her 16th birthday, but she (and her mother) have the right to an explanation and to be counselled. If she has no, or poor, breast development, and is short, gonadal dysgenesis is a possibility. In this case, investigations are required.

The investigation of delayed menstruation comprises three mandatory and seven selective measures. It is mandatory to obtain a full and carefully analysed history, to perform a careful general physical examination, and to perform a pelvic examination (under anaesthesia if necessary). Although the latter will cause stretching, or rupture, of the hymen, it is an essential step in the investigation of the patient.

The elective investigations are determined to some extent by the findings during the mandatory phase of the investigation. One or more of the following will be required, (1) x-ray of skull, (2) nuclear sex chromatin, (3) hormone assays (gonadotrophin, oestrogen, 17-ketosteroid), (4) vaginal cytology, (5) cervical mucus examination, (6) karyotyping of cell nuclei grown in tissue culture, (7) laparoscopy.

For example, an amenorrhoeic girl who at the age of 16 years has no breast development and a eunuchoid appearance, is likely to have hypogonadism; whilst a girl of similar age with well-developed secondary sexual characteristics and normal genital organs probably has a constitutional delayed menarche. These two types can be distinguished by hormone assays and vaginal cytology. More details of methods of investigation and treatment are given in Chapter 8.

INTERSEX AT PUBERTY

The majority of cases of intersex are diagnosed at birth, but three forms may not be recognized before puberty. These are:

1. Attenuated congenital adrenal hyperplasia, leading to postpubertal virilism.
2. Gonadal dysgenesis in girls of normal stature.
3. Testicular feminization.

The investigations of these cases are those outlined for the diagnosis of intersex in infancy, and the problem is discussed in Chapter 3.

IRREGULAR MENSTRUATION IN ADOLESCENCE

The periods following the menarche are usually anovulatory and frequently irregular in rhythm and flow, often showing irregular bleeding patterns, such as oligomenorrhoea, polymenorrhoea or menorrhagia. The rhythm becomes regular within one or two years, but the flow may remain variable for rather longer before the individual's menstrual pattern is established. In many cases the cause of the irregularity in menstrual rhythm and flow is a failure of the awakening ovary to respond consistently to gonadotrophic stimulation, so that oestrogen secretion is variable, and the positive feedback of oestrogen necessary to initiate the LH surge fails to occur, anovulation resulting. Thus a variety of endometrial histological patterns may be found. In other cases, the hypothalamus, affected by emotional influences, fails to release sufficient gonadotrophin releasing hormone to stimulate the pituitary adequately. The influence of emotions and behavioural patterns upon hormonal secretion is considerable during

the period of adolescent instability, and is frequently manifested in menstrual disturbances. The adolescent is therefore entitled to a reasoned explanation of what the doctor proposes to do, and how the therapy will help. Sympathy, understanding and explanation are as important as drugs.

INVESTIGATIONS

The investigations required can conveniently be listed:

1. History of illness in the past.
2. History of the menstrual pattern.
3. General examination, seeking blood dyscrasias (which occur in 10 to 20 per cent of young women who have menorrhagia) and hypothyroidism (which is uncommon, comprising less than 5 per cent of cases).

4. Rectal examination, or
5. Vaginal examination and/or vaginoscopy.
6. Examination under anaesthesia and, if needed, cervical smears and diagnostic curettage.

The number of investigations required will depend on the individual case, but the first four are mandatory, the last two only being required if the patient has irregular staining or does not respond to medical treatment.

PATTERNS OF DISORDERED MENSTRUATION

The main patterns of menstrual disorder may be discerned. There are (1) oligomenorrhoea, and (2) dysfunctional uterine bleeding.

Oligomenorrhoea

This is defined as normal menstrual loss occurring at intervals exceeding 42 days and is more frequent during adolescence than during the fertile years, but may persist as the normal menstrual pattern of the individual. In most cases the condition is of no clinical significance, and ovulation will be found to occur in most cycles. However, if oligomenorrhoea develops in a young woman who previously had normal periods, it may presage the development of amenorrhoea in a few cases (5 per cent) or occasionally dysfunctional uterine bleeding (3 per cent).

Treatment is rarely required on medical grounds, but may be needed for psychological reasons if adequate explanation of the normality of the condition does not suffice. In this event, the cyclic use of sex steroids will usually provoke bleeding. The condition is discussed further in Chapter 8.

Dysfunctional uterine bleeding

This is defined as profuse, prolonged or frequent bleeding in the absence of genital pathology or systemic disease. It occurs with a greater frequency in adolescent girls than later in the reproductive years. The physiological cause is a failure of the positive oestrogen feedback, so that the LH surge is inhibited or is inadequate to provoke ovulation. The interval between episodes of bleeding, which are usually anovulatory, lasts from 14 days to several months. The heavy bleeding may follow a period of amenorrhoea

and last 2 to 4 weeks; or bleeding may be completely irregular. The endometrial histological pattern is variable, but because of the anovulatory nature of the disorder, most will show a proliferative pattern, secretory patterns are unusual and hyperplastic patterns rare.

Probably the most common aetiological precursors of acquired adolescent dysfunctional bleeding are psychogenic factors. These may be provoked by excessive exercise, dieting, domestic strife with parents, boyfriend problems or peer group pressures.

Management

The adolescent girl must be examined to exclude general disease and a vaginal examination is indicated, especially in sexually active girls, to exclude pregnancy complications and local disease. A blood count is required and blood coagulation studies may be indicated, especially if there is other clinical evidence of blood dyscrasias. The absence of other causes of bleeding establishes the diagnosis of dysfunctional uterine bleeding. If the bleeding has been sufficiently heavy to produce anaemia, curettage may be required, but most bleeding episodes can be managed using hormones. Most bleeding episodes can be 'medically curetted' by giving an oral progestogen (norethisterone 10mg every 6 hours) until bleeding ceases, and then reducing the dose to 5 to 10mg daily for as long as the physician wishes. Thereafter the hormone can be given cyclically from day 5 to 25, or preferably from day 15 to 25, for a period of 3 to 4 months. Alternatively, hydroxyprogesterone caproate 250mg can be injected every 28 days on the 25th day of the cycle. With this regimen the majority of adolescents return to a normal pattern of menstruation. Another choice is to prescribe a combined oestrogen/progestogen tablet from day 5 to 25, although logically this is less reasonable if the girl is secreting oestrogen in adequate quantities.

Prostaglandin antagonists (fenamates and naproxen) are currently under investigation for the treatment of menorrhagia (dysfunctional uterine bleeding) in adolescents. The drugs have the advantage that they need not be taken before the onset of bleeding.

Dysfunctional uterine bleeding ceases with this treatment in most cases, but in 5 per cent of women the pattern tends to persist or to recur. A proportion of these women develop endometrial cystic glandular hyperplasia, which requires repeated episodes of hormonal therapy. In later years, they tend to be infertile, or, if they succeed in becoming pregnant, have a higher than normal chance of abortion and fetal loss.

DYSMENORRHOEA

Although, in general, dysmenorrhoea of a spasmodic nature only occurs in ovulatory cycles, some earlier anovulatory cycles occurring soon after puberty may be painful. In these cases the pain is due to the passage of clots, or the shedding of a hyperplastic endometrium. However, the distinction between dysmenorrhoea following ovulatory and anovulatory cycles is unimportant, and the diagnosis of the type of cycle is seldom necessary for treatment.

The pattern of the pain is that it is cramping in character, and is felt in the lower abdomen, occasionally radiating down the inner surface of the thighs. The pain usually starts during the 24 hours before the onset of menstruation, and may last for the first 24 to 36 hours of bleeding, although it is rarely severe for longer than 12 hours. In severe cases vomiting or diarrhoea may accompany the dysmenorrhoea. Spasmodic dysmenorrhoea is experienced by between 60 and 75 per cent of women, with a peak incidence between the ages of 15 and 25. It decreases in incidence with age and usually ceases after childbirth. In 75 per cent of the affected women, the menstrual cramps are mild or moderate, and in 25 per cent they are severe and incapacitating. The severity of the pain may be influenced by cultural attitudes, particularly those of the child's mother and older sisters. Thus adolescents in 'primitive races' are said to suffer less severe pain than those in more sophisticated Western societies. Within a single community the incidence of dysmenorrhoea is higher in the higher social classes. In adolescents associated premenstrual symptoms are unusual, and the nausea, irritability and 'bloating' noticed by their older sisters is uncommon.

The aetiology of spasmodic (or primary) dysmenorrhoea has been clarified recently. Following ovulation, progesterone transforms the endometrium into the secretory state. Prostaglandins are synthesized in the secretory endometrium, and are released when the premenstrual fall in oestradiol and progesterone is followed by constriction of the spiral arteries of the endometrium. The excessive release of prostaglandins by the endometrium or a raised sensitivity to prostaglandins ($F_{2\alpha}$ and E_2) by the myometrium, leads to uterine myometrial hypercontractility and ischaemia ('uterine angina') with resulting crampy pains. Prostaglandin $F_{2\alpha}$ may cause contractions of the gut musculature with resulting nausea and vomiting. In addition, vasopressin may be involved in dysmenorrhoea. Vasopressin increases prostaglandin synthesis but also increases myometrial activity directly. This may account for the failure of antiprostaglandins to relieve all cases of dysmenorrhoea.

INVESTIGATIONS

A careful history followed by a rectal or vaginal examination and an assessment of the girl's and her mother's attitude to sexual matters is all that is needed. The last should be obtained from each without the other being present.

TREATMENT

The variety of drugs and treatments given in the past (pelvic exercises, sitz baths, cold showers, pelvic diathermy, salt-reducing and other diets) indicates that their effect was largely that of a placebo. Since there is little fluid retention or personality change in women of this age group who have primary dysmenorrhoea, the use of diuretics or amphetamine was equally inappropriate.

The knowledge that prostaglandin synthesis and release from a progestational endometrium is involved in dysmenorrhoea has led to a more scientific approach to treatment. Most cases of spasmodic dysmenorrhoea will respond to treatment with prostaglandin antagonists or to the suppression of ovulation which inhibits prostaglandin synthesis. The use of prostaglandin synthetase inhibitors (aspirin, fenamates and naproxen) offers considerable relief.

Acetylsalicylic acid, which reduces prostaglandin synthesis, is moderately effective in mild cases, but for more severe dysmenorrhoea, drugs which reduce prostaglandin synthesis and oppose its action in the tissues are more effective. Several drugs are available. They include the fenamates (mefenamic acid, 500mg 8-hourly; flufenamic acid 200mg 8-hourly); the proprionic acid derivates (ibuprofen 400mg 8-hourly; naproxen 500mg initially, 250mg 6-hourly) and indomethacin 25mg 8-hourly. A literature review suggests that the fenamates are more effective in relieving pain, with excellent relief in over 85 per cent of patients. The drugs are usually started at the onset of the pain, but may be started earlier if the woman has severe dysmenorrhoea. The side-effects of dizziness, heartburn and intestinal upset affect less than 20 per cent of women, and the drugs relieve the dysmenorrhoea in 85 to 95 per cent of cases.

If the woman has a normal or heavy menstrual loss a low dose oral contraceptive may be preferred; and this regimen is preferable if the woman is sexually active. If the periods are scanty, progesterone alone, in the form of dydrogesterone 10 to 20mg daily from day 5 to 25 is preferable on theoretical grounds at least. The hormones should be given for 3 to 4 cycles, then stopped for 2 to 3 cycles. Thyroid and testosterone should not be used, nor have narcotics any place in the treatment of dysmenorrhoea.

In a few very severe cases which fail to respond to medical treatment, dilatation of the cervix may be required, but presacral neurectomy should be regarded as of doubtful value and avoided. Why dilatation of the cervix relieves dysmenorrhoea is unknown, and, unfortunately, the relief lasts for only about 6 to 9 months.

OVARIAN TUMOURS

Ovarian tumours are relatively uncommon in adolescence as they are in childhood, and the majority of the tumours are either functional cysts (which are not strictly tumours) or benign tumours. Malignant tumours account for only 7 per cent of the total (Table 28/4). They are usually disgerminomas or malignant teratomata.

In most cases the complaint of abdominal discomfort or distension leads to an abdominal examination, when a tumour may be felt; but in one-third of cases the main complaint is of menstrual irregularity, particularly menorrhagia. Before making a firm diagnosis, pregnancy must be excluded. Treatment is surgical, ovarian cystectomy being the preferred procedure, except in the case of malignant tumours.

	Per cent of cases
Functional Cysts	21.0
Benign Tumours	72.0
Teratoma	31
Serous cystadenoma	18
Pseudomucinous cystadenoma	12
Parovarian cysts	5.5
Solid tumours	5.5
Malignant Tumours	7.0
	100.0

Table 28/4 Ovarian tumours in adolescence

Chapter 29

The Climacteric and After

At a time variable from individual to individual, but usually occurring early in the 6th decade of life, the remaining primordial follicles, which number about 8000, begin to disappear. Although the pituitary gland continues to secrete FSH, the follicles become increasingly less responsive, and develop less readily. The changes are not abrupt, and there is a gradual transition from ovulatory cycles to ovarian quiescence.

These alterations signal the climacteric, and the changes in endocrine secretions affect the whole body profoundly. The climacteric can be defined as the period of waning ovarian function which signals the end of the reproductive life-span. During this period, which usually extends over some years, the outstanding biological event is the cessation of menstruation – the menopause. This occurs in Caucasian women at a median age of 50 ± 5 years.

ENDOCRINOLOGY OF THE CLIMACTERIC

The earliest endocrine change presaging the climacteric is an alteration in the ratio of the pituitary gonadotrophins, FSH and LH. This occurs at a time when the woman is still menstruating regularly. Between the ages of 35 and 40, the FSH levels begin to rise. The altered FSH/LH ratio, affects the oestrogen feedback mechanisms, with the result that ovarian follicular function is disturbed, although not consistently. The altered ovarian response is marked by irregular or infrequent ovulation, and consequently the absence, or marked reduction of progesterone production by the theca-lutein cells. During this phase, follicle growth and oestrogen secretion continue, but the amount of oestrogen secreted fluctuates considerably. This, and the absence or defects of luteinization, causes the menstrual irregularities commonly found at this time of life.

As the patient nears the climacteric, the responsiveness of the ovaries to the pituitary gonadotrophins diminishes further, and the oestrogen secreted by the thecal cells of the follicles begins to diminish. This in turn disturbs the oestrogen feedback mechanism which exists between the hypothalamus-pituitary and the ovaries. The result is that the secretion of gonadotrophins increases, with a further alteration in the FSH:LH ratio, FSH secretion increasing to a high level. The LH levels also rise, and the raised gonadotrophin levels remain elevated during the rest of the woman's life. But fewer ovarian follicles are stimulated, so that oestrogen secretion is reduced still further until oligomenorrhoea or amenorrhoea signal the menopause. During the climacteric the follicles disappear from the ovaries which are no longer able to synthesize oestrogen, although they continue to contribute precursors in their stromal cells which undergo some degree of hyperplasia and produce variable quantities of androgenic steroids (usually androstenedione).

The fluctuating, but generally declining levels of oestrogen, and the frequent absence of the regulatory effect of progesterone, alters menstrual patterns in many women. Some women continue to menstruate regularly (and often to ovulate) until the menses cease. Other women develop oligomenorrhoea, the menstrual interval increasing until menstruation finally ceases. Some women have marked fluctuations in oestrogen secretion, leading to episodes of menorrhagia, metrorrhagia, oligomenorrhoea and normal menstrual loss. Women with this pattern of menstrual irregularity require diagnostic curettage to exclude uterine pathology, particularly endometrial carcinoma. During the climacteric most of the remaining follicles disappear from the ovary and the few which remain become unable to respond to gonadotrophin stimulation. The lack of an oestrogen feedback alters circulating hormone levels.

After the menopause both oestradiol and oestrone continue to be secreted in varying, but generally declining, amounts. Oestrone becomes the predominant oestrogen, but its level falls to about 20 per cent of that found in the mid-follicular phase. Oestradiol levels also fall to about 20 per cent of the level found in the mid-follicular phase of women aged 25 to 35.

As the ovary has no follicles, or no functional follicles, oestrogen (predominantly oestrone) is synthesized by aromatization in the stromal cells of adipose tissue of androstenedione, principally secreted by the adrenal cortex, although some ovarian androstenedione is contributed. As the aromatization takes place in adipose tissue, fat women are likely to have higher circulating levels of oestrogens.

The serum levels of oestrone and the more active oestradiol (which mainly results from peripheral oestrone conversion) fall to about 50 per cent of the level found in the follicular phase of the menstrual cycle in younger women, and remain at this level into old age.

Testosterone levels fall to about 60 per cent of their premenopausal values, within a year of the menopause, and then remain unchanged for 30 years or longer. The plasma levels of both oestrogens and androgens have circadian and day to day fluctuations, which makes any attempted correlations between hormone levels and symptoms difficult to interpret.

Pituitary gland

Although there is an increase in the interstitial connective tissue of the pituitary gland after the climacteric, the function of the gland and the secretion of the trophic hormones is unaltered, apart from changes in gonadotrophic secretion. The secretion of gonadotrophins increases just prior to the menopause, and more particularly after that event. At this time the controlling 'feedback' by the ovarian steroids no longer operates, and the quantity of circulating gonadotrophins is tenfold higher than that found in the childbearing years. Only many years (on average 30) after the climacteric, does gonadotrophic secretion begin to fall, together with a reduction in the secretion of all the pituitary hormones, reflecting a generalized tissue senility.

Ovaries

In the early climacteric years the ovaries usually decrease in size and any remaining follicles either disappear or become non-functional. In a few women the ovaries do not atrophy, the stromal cells become hyperplastic and hypertrophic and synthesize androstenedione and testosterone.

Adrenocortical function

The excretion of 17-ketosteroids decreases slowly in the postmenopausal years, as does that of the 17-hydroxycorticosteroids. These reflect a slowly decreasing secretion of corticosteroids by the adrenal gland, which is balanced by a diminished peripheral utilization of the hormone. The gland, however, responds normally to ACTH.

Thyroid function

A slight increase in thyroid function occurs at the time of the climacteric, and in the postclimacteric years a slight diminution of function occurs. The changes are variable and small in amount, and most marked in very old age.

SOMATIC CHANGES IN AND AFTER THE CLIMACTERIC

The somatic changes which occur during the climacteric are related to the reduction in circulating oestrogen and the increased production of gonadotrophins. Since the diurnal secretion of oestrogen varies from woman to woman, the changes which occur are variable in severity, and are slowly progressive in nature, merging after a number of years into the somatic changes associated with old age.

Breasts

During the premenopausal phase, the breasts may show an increase in subcutaneous fat and some proliferation of the lobular buds. Later, with the reduction in circulating oestrogen, the subcutaneous fat is reabsorbed and the gland tissue atrophies. The nipples decrease in size, and eventually the breasts become flattened and pendulous.

Ovaries

The ovaries decrease in size, and any remaining follicles disappear or become non-functional, unable to respond to the circulating gonadotrophins. The

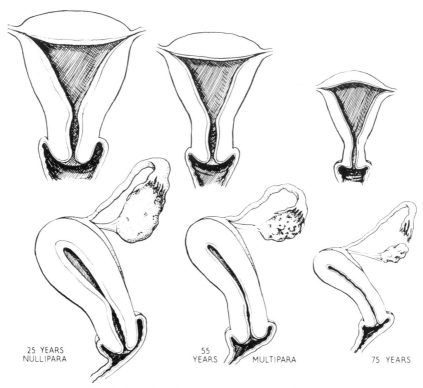

25 YEARS
NULLIPARA

55
YEARS   MULTIPARA

75 YEARS

Fig. 29/1 To show the reduction in the size of the uterus in old age

theca cells and other elements in the stroma provide androstenedione and testosterone.

Uterus and tubes

The endometrium becomes progressively atrophic as oestrogen secretion diminishes, and the myometrium diminishes in size by loss of fluid and transformation of the muscle fibres into fibrous tissue. Myomata, if present, atrophy at a similar rate. The degree of atrophy depends on the quantity of circulating oestrogen and the ability of the uterus to respond (Fig. **29/1**).

Vagina

The mucosa is thinned and the rugae are lost, so that the mucosa is more easily abraded and can be easily irritated. The degree of mucosal atrophy is related to the amount of circulating oestrogen and androgen, and the ratio is reflected by the vaginal exfoliative cytology, the absence of superficial cells indicating lack of circulating oestrogen. The vaginal

secretions diminish, as does the vaginal acidity, so that pathogenic organisms can develop more easily.

The atrophy of the vaginal epithelium, due to oestrogen deficiency, may cause dyspareunia, particularly if the woman only has coitus at infrequent intervals, or vaginal 'burning'. A woman who enjoys regular, frequent coitus is less likely to complain of dyspareunia. Treatment is for the woman to use a vaginal cream containing oestrogen.

Urethra

The urethral mucosa is also oestrogen-dependent to some extent, and may become atrophic. This occurs in about 20 to 30 per cent of women over the age of 55, the prevalence increasing with advancing age. In most cases vaginal and urethral cytology mirror each other. A few women with urethral mucosal atrophy develop symptoms suggestive of cystitis and urethritis, although no bacteria are grown. The symptoms of urgency, frequency, and dysuria can be treated with vaginal suppositories containing oestrogen for 7 to 10 days. There is also a sound rationale for treating elderly women who have a true cystitis with oestrogen pessaries, in addition to giving antibiotics.

The pelvic floor

As hypo-oestrogenism develops, the muscles of the pelvic floor lose their tone and the connective tissue its elasticity, so that relaxation of tissues damaged in childbirth is likely, with varying degrees of prolapse of the organs. To the effect of withdrawal of the hormonal support is added the effect of ageing, but the part played by each is not yet clear. The changes may lead to cystocele, to stress incontinence, to rectocele and to uterine prolapse. Since the vulval orifice also loses much of its elastic tissue, and gapes, the prolapse may appear more severe than it really is.

Vulva

Until old age, few changes occur, but such as do are slowly progressive. There is a slow reabsorption of fat and elastic tissue from the labia majora so that the external genitalia become smaller. With old age, the process is accelerated and in extreme cases a narrow cleft indicates the vaginal orifice. This is called kraurosis, or atrophic or senile 'vulvitis'. However, a simple, more descriptive term is vulval atrophy. Once again the time of onset, and the degree of the change varies between individuals.

Cardiovascular system

VASOMOTOR DISTURBANCES

These are a common accompaniment to the climacteric. The most frequent are hot flushes, but sweating, headaches, fainting and palpitations are also encountered. Hot flushes usually start with a feeling of heat centred on the face, which spreads to the neck and chest and may become generalized. Each flush lasts between 1.5 and 3 minutes and is often accompanied by perspiration. They are associated with peripheral vasodilatation (the finger temperature increases about 3.5°C) and an increase in the heart rate by a mean of 15 b.p.m.

The aetiology of hot flushes has not been established but may be related to the withdrawal of oestrogen, perhaps mediated through changes in oestrogen-sensitive neurones in the hypothalamus linked to the control of GnRH pulsatile release. The phenomena may be due to a sudden transient increase in sympathetic output (drive), and a possible release of a 'vasodilator factor'. This would account for the frequent association of hot flushes, with sweating, headache and with insomnia. Hot flushes are a manifestation of vasomotor instability, and are triggered off by excitement, warmth and emotions, a blush spreading from the neck and over the face.

ATHEROSCLEROSIS

There is some evidence that endogenous oestrogens (and perhaps progesterone) protect *young* women against atherosclerosis. This opinion is based upon the finding that atherosclerosis is about 20 times more common amongst men under the age of 40 than amongst women of similar age in the USA. This difference is much less noticeable, however, in other parts of the world, and the contemporary way of life in developed countries with limited exercise and excessive eating, probably plays a major part in the development of the disease. Although the evidence is that the incidence of atherosclerosis rises with age (and in the 50 to 59 age group in the USA the incidence in men is only twice that in women), there is some evidence to suggest that the administration of exogenous oestrogens will protect post-menopausal women. However, a careful study has shown that there was no greater chance of coronary atherosclerosis developing amongst women castrated in their forties than amongst non-castrated women of similar age. A further problem is that the administration of exogenous oestrogen may, in certain women, predispose them to venous thrombosis, pulmonary embolism and possibly to endometrial carcinoma.

PSYCHOLOGICAL CHANGES

Cultural and emotional influences, as well as hormonal tides, affect the perimenopausal woman considerably, and the dissociation of the effects of the soma from those of the psyche is inexact and liable to biased interpretation. Thus it is difficult to determine whether the depression, insomnia and lassitude commonly complained of are due to altered hormonal ratios, or to a deeper disturbance in the psyche as children grow up, the aspirations of earlier life dissipate into a routine 'suburban' existence, and the woman has to accept, reluctantly, a different social role. Equally, the irritability often encountered amongst perimenopausal women may be due more to psychological factors, than to a postulated fluid retention due to altered steroid production.

Sexual responsiveness is unaltered by the cessation of menstruation in at least 60 per cent of women; 20 per cent have increased sexual urges; and 20 per cent feel diminished urges. This pattern agrees with the concept that coital capacity is not related to sex hormone production once physiological maturation has occurred.

Few studies have been made which analyse the symptoms declared by perimenopausal women, and only four are free from methodological defects.

These four studies suggest that menstrual irregularities, hot flushes (with associated sweats, usually at night, and occasional insomnia) and vaginal 'dryness' can be related to the declining oestrogen secretion at this time. Hot flushes, causing marked physical discomfort affect over half of women during the climacteric, and between one half and two-thirds of them seek medical help. The flushes continue for more than one year in about two-thirds of affected women.

Vaginal discomfort, burning or dryness tend to occur later in the climacteric years, and seem to be more common when the woman is in her late 50s. Vaginal dryness is mainly a problem when coitus is attempted only occasionally. The more often a woman has sexual intercourse, the less likely is she to complain of vaginal dryness.

The complaints of depression, irritability, headache, palpitations and frequency of micturition, and mental 'imbalance' are no more common during the climacteric than at other periods in life when adjustment to a different life-style is needed.

Three phases of psychological adjustment to the climacteric have been defined: (1) a period of *impact*, during which feelings of anxiety and turmoil are experienced. This phase usually merges in a few weeks into (2) a period of *recoil*. In this phase, which may last months, irritation, depression and mood changes are common, and feelings of rejection noticeable. (3) The third and last phase is one of *readjustment*. Usually this phase leads to a firm adjustment to the new role, but in about 1 per cent of women involutional melancholia develops. Many of these women will be found to have exhibited depressive reactions to stress prior to the menopause.

MANAGEMENT OF THE CLIMACTERIC

It must first be remembered that fewer than one-third of women passing through the climacteric have symptoms sufficiently distressing to seek medical aid.

The predominant symptoms of the climacteric have already been discussed and relative proportions of each are seen in Table **29/1**. Only the vasomotor symptoms of hot flushes, hot tingling sensations over the entire body ('flashes'), the accompanying sweats and insomnia can be ascribed to the declining oestrogen production. Oestrogen deprivation also accounts for the atrophic changes which occur in the vagina and vulva leading to the spotting of blood per vaginam, to dyspareunia and to pruritus. However, these symptoms are not common at the time of the climacteric, and occur later, unless the patient has been castrated.

	Percentage with the symptom
Flushes	70.0
Depression	40.0
Sweating	30.0
Irregular menstruation	25.0
Insomnia	25.0
Fatigue	20.0
Hair or skin changes	15.0
Headache	10.0

Table 29/1 Predominant menopausal symptoms of 500 patients who sought medical aid

The objectives of treatment are (1) to provide sympathetic understanding for, and a reasoned explanation of, the changes which are occurring, (2) to provide symptomatic therapy designed to carry the patient over the disturbed period of biological and social readjustment, and (3) in certain cases to provide hormonal therapy, designed to smooth over the endocrine adjustments.

The provision of sympathetic understanding

Women at the time of the climacteric frequently develop feelings of inadequacy and an exaggerated view that the physiological changes occurring will render them neuter, unattractive and useless. Such women first and foremost need a sympathetic hearing, especially as they frequently present with a variety of non-specific symptoms. The sympathetic understanding should be reinforced with an explanation of the changes which are occurring. This treatment is often more effective than the prescription of drugs. The patient must be helped to realize that the climacteric is a period of change and the beginning of a new life, not the end of all life.

Hormone therapy

In the past few years increasing numbers of women seek to continue with replacement oestrogen therapy from the time of the climacteric until they die. Encouraged by articles and books, the women wish to remain 'forever feminine', and to avoid the inevitable changes which occur with ageing. There are no data to indicate that long-term oestrogen replacement therapy promotes vitality, increases femininity, reduces fatigue or prevents ageing, except through psychological mechanisms. Replacement ocstrogen therapy will cure atrophic vaginitis when given in short courses, and may reduce the appearance of skin wrinkles by its fluid retaining effect. Its main value is to control hot flushes if they are severe, disabling and frequent and to delay the onset of osteoporosis. It should be remembered that, despite much unsubstantiated newspaper reporting, oestrogens are only effective in treating vasomotor symptoms. Unfortunately, oestrogens have no rejuvenating effect except on the psyche, nor do they consistently and regularly relieve the symptoms of depression, dizziness, headache and fatigue.

The objectives of therapy are to give the smallest dose which relieves the symptoms and prevents osteoporosis. The reason for this is that exogenous oestrogen (unopposed by progestogens) given to relieve climacteric symptoms is a factor in the development of endometrial carcinoma. Investigations have shown that postmenopausal women who are prescribed unopposed oestrogen therapy for periods longer than 6 months appear to have a 3- to 5-fold risk of developing endometrial carcinoma, compared with women who do not take oestrogens. The longer the duration of the therapy, and the larger the dose of oestrogen used, the greater is the risk: women who take oestrogens for 3 or more years, have a risk 3 to 6 times that of women who do not take the drug.

It should be pointed out that the actual risk is quite small. The probability of an untreated postmenopausal woman developing endometrial carcinoma is 1 per 1000 each year. If oestrogen therapy increases this risk 4-fold, 996 of each 1000 oestrogen treated women will *not* develop endometrial carcinoma each year.

There is evidence that the risk of developing endometrial carcinoma is prevented if a progestogen is given in addition to oestrogen. The progestogen increases the ability of the endometrium to convert oestradiol to the weaker oestrone by increasing the dehydrogenase activity and by decreasing the number of oestrogen receptors. In these ways the stimulatory effect of oestrogen on the endometrial cell is inhibited. A disadvantage of the oestrogen: progestogen regimen is that a number of women on this regimen develop withdrawal bleeding from time to time, which may cause anxiety.

Several oestrogen formulations are available, which are effective in equipotent doses in relieving symptoms. However they differ in their effect on liver enzymes. Piperazine oestrone sulphate raises SHBG and other liver enzyme levels less than conjugated equine oestrogen, which in turn causes less alteration to them than does ethinyl oestradiol.

The route of administration is also important. Most of the available oestrogens are designed to be given by mouth and have to make a first pass through the enterohepatic circulation. The effect on the liver can be avoided if a transdermal system is used. Small doses of oestradiol (50 or 100μg) in a skin patch is applied to the abdomen or the buttocks. The oestradiol is slowly released and absorbed through the skin. The patch is replaced every 3 or 4 days.

When an oral preparation is used the dose is adjusted depending on the number of hot flushes reported by the woman. The aim is to reduce them to two or less per day. The effect is not immediate, so that an increased dose is delayed for about 7 days.

Many gynaecologists start with piperazine oestrone sulphate 0.625mg, or its equivalent if another oestrogen is preferred (see p. 282). If the desired reduction in hot flushes has not been obtained in 7 days the dose is doubled.

The oestrogen can be taken continuously, but a progestogen should be added for the first 12 to 14 days of each month. The dose of progestogen is: northisterone 0.7–1.5mg; levonorgestrel 0.07–0.15mg; medroxyprogesterone acetate 5–10mg. When the new progestogens become readily available (e.g. desogestrel) they will probably replace the older progestogens as they do not alter blood lipids. The addition of progestogen to the regimen is to prevent the

Day	Hormone
1–13	Oestrogen alone
14–27	Oestrogen *plus* progestogen
28–35	No treatment – bleeding may occur
1–13 etc	Repeat sequence

Table 29/2 A regimen of hormonal supplementation for 'menopausal' symptoms

stimulatory effects of oestrogen on the endometrium and the glandular tissue of the breasts. The progestogen often provokes a withdrawal bleed which may occur between the 5th day after starting the drug up to 5 days after the course is completed. If bleeding occurs before the 11th day of progestogen administration, the dose is probably insufficient to 'protect' the endometrium and should be increased. Regular withdrawal bleeds are reassuring and obviate the need for annual curettage, which is the practise of some gynaecologists. However irregular bleeding occurring during treatment needs to be investigated.

Dyspareunia, due to atrophic vaginitis and infrequent coitus, typically develops rather later in a woman's life, but may occur amongst climacteric women.

The treatment is to use an oestrogen cream applied to the vagina through an applicator. As the vaginal cells contain large numbers of oestrogen receptors, the oestrogen is taken up by them, and smaller doses can be used than if oestrogens are given orally. This has the advantage of reducing the uptake of oestrogen into the general circulation, and consequently reducing the possibility of endometrial hyperplasia.

Symptomatic therapy

In some 20 per cent of patients the severity of the symptoms of depression, irritability and mood changes may be relieved by an antidepressant. If vasomotor symptoms occur, but are not severe, and are associated with mood changes, the use of a complex containing phenobarbitone (a central sedative) 40mg, belladonna (a parasympathetic inhibitor) 0.2mg, and ergométrine tartrate (a sympathetic inhibitor) 0.6mg (marketed as Bellergel Retard) given twice a day often helps.

An alternative form of therapy is to use clonidine in a dose of 25 to 75µg twice daily. The drug reduces the sensitivity of small blood vessels to various stimuli, but is not very effective in controlling the symptoms. However, hormone treatment is to be preferred to these treatments, and should be continued for at least 10 years. In general these treatments are indicated only if the woman cannot or does not wish to take oestrogens.

POSTMENOPAUSAL BLEEDING

Bleeding from the genital tract occurring a year or more after the menopause should be considered as due to malignant disease until this has been excluded. The main causes of postmenopausal bleeding are shown in Table **29/3**, and it can be seen that in 20 per cent a malignancy of the genital tract was detected. In 25 per cent of cases investigation showed no cause, and it must be assumed that emotional stimuli initiated a hypothalamic-pituitary response which led to an altered release of FSH. In 20 per cent of cases the cause was iatrogenic, oestrogen having been given as replacement therapy. In susceptible women such unopposed oestrogen supplementing the endogenous oestrogen secreted by the adrenal gland will cause endometrial proliferation and its subsequent irregular shedding.

	Percentage
No demonstrable lesion	25
Oestrogen therapy	20
Atrophic vaginitis	15
Endometrial carcinoma	15
Endometrial polyp or hyperplasia	15
Cervical carcinoma	4
Benign cervical lesions (polyp)	4
Ovarian tumour (most malignant)	1
Bleeding from urinary tract	1

Table 29/3 Causes of postmenopausal bleeding (800 reported cases)

DIAGNOSTIC METHODS

Even the slightest degree of postmenopausal bleeding demands a careful examination of the patient. The general examination should include blood pressure estimations and a urinary examination to exclude glycosuria. A careful examination of the vagina and cervix follows, and smears are taken from the cervix, the cervical canal and the posterior fornix of the vagina to detect the presence of abnormal exfoliated cells. Even if an atrophic vaginitis or a cervical polyp is found, a careful examination under anaesthesia and diagnostic curettage is mandatory.

The curettage will show a proliferative endometrium in about one-third of cases; and an atrophic endometrium in a similar proportion. Endometrial polyps are found in about 10 per cent and endometrial hyperplasia in 20 per cent of cases. Endometrial carcinoma is found in between 5 and 15 per cent of curettings.

TREATMENT

Treatment depends on the cause of the bleeding. If the diagnostic curettage reveals endometrial hyperplasia, particularly adenomatous or atypical hyperplasia, progestogens (such as norgestrel or norethisterone) should be prescribed for 3 months, when a further curettage is performed. In over 95 per cent of cases, progestogen therapy will cause a reversal of the endometrial hyperplasia to a proliferative or an atrophic pattern. However if hyperplasia persists, hysterectomy should be considered. If the curettage reveals endometrial adenocarcinoma, treatment is urgent and is discussed on page 196.

Atrophic vaginitis responds rapidly to the local application of small doses of oestrogen, either as a cream used with an applicator (Dienoestrol cream containing dienoestrol 0.01 per cent); or as pessaries; or as a cream containing oestrogen and progesterone in a ratio of oestrogen 1mg to progesterone 5mg per 30ml. The applications usually produce a cure within 7 to 14 days. Alternatively ethinyl oestradiol 0.02mg, or quinestradol (Pentovis) 0.25mg may be given orally daily for 21-day periods.

OSTEOPOROSIS

Osteoporosis is a common and disabling condition, in which, over the years, the total skeletal mass, including its mineral content, is reduced. The condition has no symptoms, per se, and is usually only detected when a fracture occurs. Osteoporosis commonly affects elderly women (over the age of 65) and some younger women who have been castrated. Approximately 25 per cent of these women develop spinal compression fractures or a fracture of long bones, usually a Colles fracture, or in old women a hip fracture. The predominant symptom is backache, as the vertebrae are involved early. Later a decrease in height occurs, and in the aged, osteoporosis is probably responsible for the high prevalence of fractures of long bones. It is known that after the menopause, and more particularly after an artificial menopause, a rise in plasma calcium (and potassium) level is found. This has been related to increased bone resorption which occurs at this time, bone formation continuing unchanged, although there is an associated reduction in the collagenous matrix of the bone. Recently it has been shown that the renal threshold is the ultimate regulator of the serum (or plasma) calcium level, and if it is altered, calcium is lost in the urine.

Bone is remodelled constantly. About 10 per cent of cortical bone is remodelled each year, and up to 40 per cent of trabecular bone is remodelled in the same period. Up to the age of 35 the bone mass of both cortical and trabecular bone increases, then after an interval of 5 years or so, more bone is lost each year than is formed. At first the rate of loss is about 0.5 per cent each year, but for the 5 to 10 years after the menopause the rate increases to between 3 and 8 per cent, in different women. After this time the bone loss again slows down to about 0.5 per cent. A major factor in the increased rate of bone loss in the post-menopausal years is the decline in endogenous oestrogen but raised gonadotrophin levels may be involved.

In the reproductive years, oestrogen opposes the bone resorption action of parathyroid hormone (PTH) or other agents (especially $1,25(OH)_2D_3$). Oestrogen also regulates calcitonin secretion, increasing the concentration of the hormone which reduces bone resorption. After the menopause, oestrogen levels fall and bone resorption increases. The plasma calcium level is maintained at about 2.4mmol/l (96mg/l) and, on a 'normal' diet urinary calcium excretion rarely falls below 3.75mmol/l (150mg/l). If inadequate amounts of calcium are ingested to maintain these levels, calcium is removed from the bone by the action of PTH to maintain homeostasis. During the reproductive years, action of bone resorbing agents is reduced by circulating oestrogen, but after the menopause, this protection is removed and bone becomes a readily accessible source of calcium.

Many postmenopausal women ingest inadequate amounts of calcium and, with ageing, faecal calcium loss is increased. At the same time the plasma oestrogen levels fall, and a slow but progressive resorption and demineralization of bone occurs leading, in some women after a number of years, to osteoporosis. Spinal osteoporosis, showing as wedging of the vertebrae or as a fracture, affects about 20 per cent of women and becomes clinically detectable 20 to 25 years after the menopause.

PREVENTION

In view of the physiology of bone resorption, several approaches to preventing osteoporosis are possible. These include not smoking, taking more exercise and increasing the daily intake of calcium. Recent work has cast a doubt about the last, but at present the concensus is that calcium intake should be increased to 1500mg daily, in food or as a supplement. These measures should start from the age of 40 and younger women should be encouraged to increase their calcium intake to build up bone mass.

The most effective preventive measure is for women who have reached the menopause to take small doses of an oestrogen each day. The dose seems critical: ethinyl oestradiol 0.02mg (or equivalent) being needed to prevent bone loss.

TREATMENT

The treatment of established osteoporosis is controversial, but most experts use a combination of increased activity, calcium supplements and oestrogen therapy.

Oestrogen is given in the regimen described previously, but the quantity is increased each cycle until the woman is taking conjugated equine oestrogens 5mg daily, (or the equivalent), or a response is obtained. As the oestrogen causes hypertrophy of the breasts and uterus, therapy should only be started after a full examination has been performed. It should include cervical smears and uterine curettage. The patient should be told that the breasts may become tender and uterine bleeding occur. Oestrogen should be continued for the rest of the patient's life.

Chapter 30

The Sex Hormones in Gynaecology

The isolation of the natural sex steroids, and their subsequent synthesis, has given to gynaecologists potent therapeutic agents, which in many cases can replace surgery in the treatment of gynaecological disorders, and in other cases offer a means of alleviating considerable distress in women. One of the results of this is that gynaecology is now predominantly a medical discipline, although surgical skill and expertise will always be required to treat a minority of disorders.

OESTROGENS

Natural oestrogens are steroid hormones produced principally by the ovary but also by the adrenal cortex, and in the male by the testis. During the reproductive years, 90 per cent of oestrogens are synthesized in the ovary, but after the menopause oestrogens are synthesized in the adrenal gland and the subcutaneous fat, and the total secreted is reduced considerably. Oestrogens are closely related to androgens, and to progesterone, and there is clear evidence that oestrogen is derived from the latter steroid (Fig. **30/1**). This close relationship between the sex steroids is of considerable importance.

Oestrogenic production by the theca-lutein cells of the maturing follicles in the ovaries is dependent upon the cyclic secretion of the pituitary gonadotrophins, which does not normally occur until puberty, although the ovary is capable of responding from the 36th week of fetal life on. At the other end of reproductive life the ovaries become incapable of responding to gonadotrophins at a time specific for each individual, when all the remaining follicles disappear.

Although at least twenty oestrogenic compounds have been isolated, the two main forms produced are oestradiol and oestrone. They are secreted into the blood and transported to the target organs bound to serum proteins. The genital tract epithelium possesses specific receptor proteins which have an affinity for oestradiol 17 beta, the most active circulating oestrogen. The specific receptor proteins take up oestradiol from the blood because their affinity is about 100 000 times greater than the protein molecules to which it is bound in the blood.

Once in the cytoplasm of the 'target' cell oestradiol is transferred to the cell nucleus where it is bound to a new receptor. Progesterone interferes with this transfer. In the cell nucleus, oestradiol exerts its effects by gene activation with the resulting appearance of a new RNA species, including specific messenger-RNA. This is then returned to the cell cytoplasm where new proteins are synthesized on cytoplasmic ribosomes.

Following gene activation oestradiol is converted into oestrone and both are quickly inactivated so that the target cells may respond to the next surge of oestrogen. This inactivation is effected by their conversion into the relatively inactive oestriol which is then returned to the blood. In the liver, oestriol is conjugated with glucuronic acid. The conjugates are excreted partly in the bile and partly in the urine. The bile fraction drains into the gut and most of the biliary oestrogens are reabsorbed from there and returned to the liver, where once again they are partly excreted in the bile and partly in the urine.

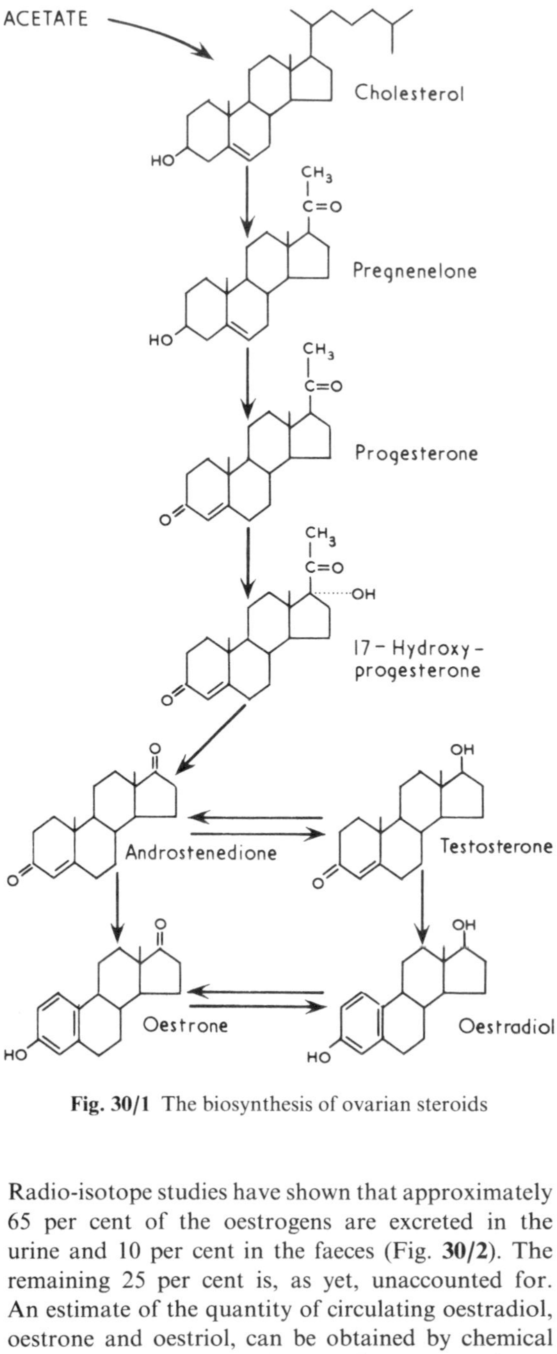

Fig. 30/1 The biosynthesis of ovarian steroids

Radio-isotope studies have shown that approximately 65 per cent of the oestrogens are excreted in the urine and 10 per cent in the faeces (Fig. **30/2**). The remaining 25 per cent is, as yet, unaccounted for. An estimate of the quantity of circulating oestradiol, oestrone and oestriol, can be obtained by chemical methods, particularly using gas chromatography or radio-immuno-assay.

Synthetic analogues of natural oestrogen have been available since 1938, and have the advantage that they are not only active when injected, but are highly active when given by mouth, a property denied to most natural oestrogens. The main synthetic (or semi-synthetic) oestrogens in use today are diethylstilboestrol (stilboestrol), ethinyl oestradiol and its 3-methyl ether, mestranol. Stilboestrol was the original synthetic oestrogen and has largely been replaced by ethinyl oestradiol. Mestranol should probably not be used, as it only binds to target organ receptors after being demethylated and converted into ethinyl oestradiol in the liver. Mestranol has a further disadvantage when used in combination with a 19-nortestosterone derivative (as in certain formulations of 'The Pill'). In combination, its demethylation to ethinyl oestradiol is inhibited to some degree depending on the particular 19-nortestosterone derivative used. Ethynodiol diacetate and norethynodrel produce inhibitions of 40 to 50 per cent; lynoestrenol an inhibition of 20 to 30 per cent, whilst norethisterone only provokes a weak inhibition. There is a difference in the metabolism of stilboestrol (and other synthetic oestrogens) and natural oestrogens, as the former are not so rapidly detoxicated in the liver. Consequently they linger longer in the body and are excreted without having been inactivated. They are then destroyed by the bacteria in the urinary tract. This observation may explain the higher incidence of 'side-effects' associated with the use of synthetic oestrogens.

Several 'natural' oestrogens are currently available, which are either produced in the laboratory or extracted from animals. Those currently used are conjugated equine oestrogens (which contain a high proportion of oestrone sulphate); oestradiol valerate, oestriol succinate and oestrone sulphate.

There is a good deal of controversy whether semi-synthetic and 'natural' oestrogens are to be preferred. The differences (apart from expense) are more apparent than real. Originally it was thought that semi-synthetic oestrogens were more likely to alter blood clotting factors (particularly Factors VII and X) than 'natural' oestrogens; recent studies show that both types have the same effect, nor are there any significant differences between the two types of oestrogen on lipid metabolism.

Although the effect of endogenous oestrogens upon the target organ is rapid, a delay of at least 12 hours occurs before the organ is affected if exogenous oestrogens are administered, and the duration of the effect is 24 hours. It also appears that the oestrogens are more effective, weight for weight, if given in intermittent spaced divided doses, rather than in a single large dose. As far as intramuscular injections are concerned, the effect of a sustained

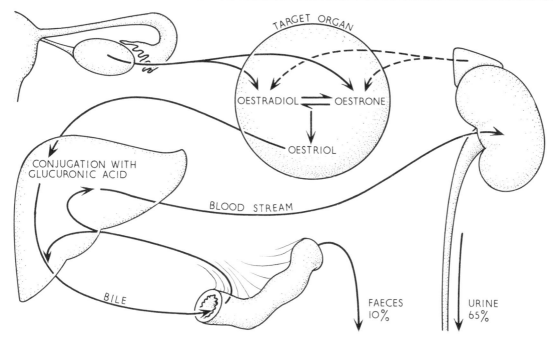

Fig. 30/2 The metabolism of oestrogen, as determined by J. B. Brown

release can be obtained by using a benzoate or di-propionate ester of the oestrogen.

OESTROGEN PRODUCTION DURING THE MENSTRUAL CYCLE

The cyclic production of oestrogens during the normal menstrual cycle has been discussed in Chapter 5, and is shown in Figure **30/3**. In the 1st week the output of oestrogen is low and may fall to values found in the post-climacteric woman. In the 2nd week a fairly rapid rise leads to a marked peak (the 'ovulatory peak') after which it falls, rising again in the 3rd week to a second lower peak (the 'luteal peak'). In the last few days of the cycle the level falls once more. If ovulation fails to occur, the ovulatory peak is not seen, and in most anovulatory cycles there is a relatively constant daily secretion of oestrogens, although in a few women a rise occurs in the later stages of the cycle. In endometrial cystic hyperplasia much higher daily levels are found, which may be constant throughout the cycle, or may show a bell-shaped curve of excretion in the later stages, which is higher than the 'luteal peak' found in the normal cycle (Fig. **30/3**). Amenorrhoea during the reproductive period may be associated with an oestrogen secretion similar to that found in post-climacteric women (hypo-oestrogenism) or else with high levels similar to those found in women with endometrial cystic hyperplasia (hyper-oestrogenism). These conditions are considered in greater detail in Chapter 7.

The variations in the secretion of endogenous oestrogen influence, to a considerable extent, the effect of administered synthetic or semi-synthetic oestrogens, and probably account for the variable severity of side-effects associated with oestrogen therapy.

OESTROGEN THERAPEUTICS

Currently, at least eight oestrogens are available for medication. These are: (1) the semi-synthetic oestrogens, ethinyl oestradiol, mestranol and diethylstil-boestrol, (2) the 'natural' oestrogens, conjugated equine oestrogens (Premarin), and (3) the esterified oestrogens, oestradiol valerate (Progynovera): oestriol succinate or hemisuccinate (Synapause) and piperazine oestrone sulphate (Harmogen, Ogen).

Conjugated equine oestrogens (of which the main components are oestrone sulphate and equilin sulphate) are widely used. In the body, oestrone sulphate is rapidly converted into unconjugated

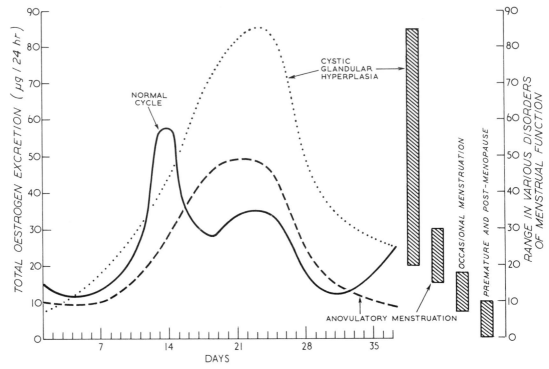

Fig. 30/3 Urinary oestrogen excretion (in μg/24 hours) in certain gynaecological conditions related to the menstrual cycle

oestrone and to oestradiol. The drug is quickly absorbed when given orally or vaginally. Blood levels of oestrone and oestradiol are higher if the latter route is chosen, probably because conjugated equine oestrogen given by mouth has to pass through the enterohepatic circulation before entering the peripheral circulation.

Equilin sulphate tends to be excreted slowly so that it remains in the circulation for longer than oestrone sulphate. The effect of this is not known.

In addition to these oestrogens, two other oestrogens are sometimes prescribed. They are quinestrol and chlortrianisene. Quinestrol is the 3 cyclopentyl ether of ethinyl oestradiol. The drug has a prolonged action and is effective when given weekly, in a dose of 2mg, which may be an advantage in some cases. Chlortrianisene (or TACE) is a prooestrogen, which is stored in body fat and is released slowly to be converted into an active oestrogen. The relative potency of the oestrogens available today is not easy to assess accurately because their biological activity varies according to the route of administration, the dosage adopted and the esterification of the hormone. The approximate potency of

commonly used oestrogens related to stilboestrol is shown in Table **30/1**.

	Approximate equivalent dose
Ethinyl oestradiol	0.01mg
Mestranol	0.02mg
Conjugated equine oestrogens	0.625mg
Piperazine oestrone sulphate	0.625mg
Oestradiol valerate	2mg
Oestriol hemisuccinate	4mg

Table 30/1 Commonly used oestrogens, giving the approximately equivalent dose of each

SIDE-EFFECTS OF OESTROGENS

The side-effects of oestrogenic therapy have been mentioned in Chapter 11, but for convenience are summarized here.

1. Nausea. One quarter of patients initially experience some degree of nausea, feeling 'off colour' or dizzy whilst taking oestrogens. These symptoms depend on the dose and potency of the oestrogen, and tend to be more severe with synthetic hormones. Tolerance usually develops fairly quickly, and by the 3rd month of therapy only 5 per cent of patients are affected.

2. Water and salt retention. Weight gain, due to salt and water retention, is a frequent concomitant, and in susceptible women may be marked.

3. Inhibition of hypothalamus/pituitary. The administration of exogenous oestrogen suppresses the release of FSH and LH in the doses normally used, but the total effect is dose-dependent (Chapter 5).

4. Genital organs. Oestrogens, unless opposed by progestogens given simultaneously, cause thickening in the vaginal mucosa, eversion of the cervical columnar epithelium (which may cause an increased vaginal discharge) and endometrial hyperplasia. This last effect can occur at any age, even in the post-climacteric woman, and may lead to uterine bleeding. In addition the action of unopposed oestrogen at this age increases the woman's risk of developing endometrial carcinoma. It is not clear whether oestrogen is a true carcinogen or a 'tumour promoter'. The latter seems more likely, as the changes appear reversible (in many cases) if oestrogen is withdrawn. The breasts respond to oestrogenic stimulation by enlargement and tenderness. This effect is dose-dependent and occurs in children, old woman and men; it is less noticeable amongst women in the reproductive era. Patients who have benign mammary dysplasia often note an aggravation of the condition when given exogenous oestrogens.

5. Venous thrombosis and thrombo-embolism. These conditions are seven-fold and three-fold respectively as common amongst women taking oestrogen as amongst other women. However, the incidence is relatively low, and fewer than 1 per 2000 women per year will develop the conditions. This is discussed in greater detail in Chapter 11.

6. Biochemical disturbances. Oestrogens increase the level of circulating globulins in the plasma, which bind with iron, cortisol and thyroxine, leading to raised plasma levels of these substances. The raised thyroxine level causes a rise in circulating protein-bound iodine, and tests for thyroid function are altered. Glucose tolerance is diminished and plasma insulin levels raised. Liver function, as judged by enzyme tests, is altered but in the absence of pre-existing liver damage, the change is not deleterious and function returns to 'normal' on withholding the hormone. Platelet adhesiveness, and increases in the blood levels of Factors VII and X, have been reported consistently, and these changes may be of importance in the known increased incidence of thrombo-embolic phenomena occurring amongst women ingesting oestrogens.

THERAPEUTIC USES OF THE OESTROGENS

In the past oestrogens have been prescribed excessively. Today with the introduction of potent synthetic progestogens, and combinations of oestrogens and progestogens, the value of oestrogen therapy is more clearly defined.

1. Genital tract hypoplasia and atrophy

Oestrogens can cause the growth of the uterus, and can mature the vaginal mucosa *provided the genital tract is hormone-sensitive.* The success of oestrogenic therapy is therefore limited in these conditions, and its most useful place is in the local treatment of vulvovaginitis in infancy (p. 259) and atrophic vaginitis (p. 276).

2. The climacteric

The value of oestrogenic therapy in the management of 'hot flushes' is undoubted, but two principles govern hormone therapy. First, as oestrogen may stimulate endometrial (and perhaps breast) cells, a progestogen should be prescribed for at least 12 days each month, and second, the object of treatment is to convert an abrupt drop in circulating oestrogen into a slow decline in level. It follows that in the treatment of the climacteric, oestrogens should be given in a dose sufficient to abolish *all* symptoms. This matter is discussed further in Chapter 29. A few gynaecologists believe that oestrogens, either alone or in combination with progestogens, should be given indefinitely to post-climacteric women, in order to prevent coronary thrombosis and osteoporosis.

3. Dysmenorrhoea

Although oestrogens in adequate dosage will suppress ovulation and prevent spasmodic dysmenorrhoea, the oestrogenic withdrawal bleeding tends to be prolonged, and oestrogen alone has largely been replaced by the use of the antiprostaglandins or of oral contraceptive pills.

4. Breast conditions

Growth of the breasts

Oestrogens given systemically or by local application will cause mammary enlargement, provided the tissues are sensitive to them. The use of oestrogen finds its greatest application in intersex states, and especially in cases of ovarian dysgenesis (see p. 36). If the girl is otherwise normal, and is menstruating regularly, oestrogens will have no effect. But if she is deficient in endogenous oestrogens, oestrogen therapy will increase the size of the breasts. Unfortunately the effect is only temporary and further courses of exogenous oestrogens are required to maintain the mammary enlargement.

Suppression of lactation

Until the prolactin antagonist, bromocriptine, became available, oestrogens were extensively used to inhibit or to suppress lactation. Compared with a placebo, they were significantly more effective, lactation being suppressed in over 90 per cent of women. Unfortunately 'rebound' filling occurred 7 to 14 days after ceasing to take the drug in about 25 per cent of women. There was also some concern that as the dose required was fairly large, increased thrombo-embolism was a possibility. They should not be used to supress lactation.

5. Growth control

Tall parents tend to have tall children, and if the growth in childhood appears to be proceeding too fast, oestrogens have been used in an attempt to obtain premature closure of the epiphyses of long bones, and so prevent abnormal linear growth. The rationale appears to be that the oestrogen 'feeds back' to the hypothalamus and reduces the release of human growth hormone (HGH). This effect is more marked if progestogens are given simultaneously with the oestrogen, and the hormone is given to the pre-pubertal girl. There is some doubt whether administration in this way is entirely harmless.

CONDITIONS IN WHICH OESTROGEN IS OF LITTLE OR NO VALUE

These conditions include: infertility; frigidity (unless the condition is associated with severe hypo-oestrogenism); abortion, whether isolated or recurrent; the induction of abortion or labour; skin diseases (except for adolescent acne); the prevention of coronary thrombosis; and the treatment of benign mammary dysplasia. Oestrogens are contra-indicated in cases of carcinoma of the breast in premenopausal women, and in endometrial carcinoma.

ANDROGENS

Since the introduction of the synthetic progestogens into clinical gynaecology, the use of pure androgens has declined considerably. An androgen is a substance having the capacity to produce masculinization, and is consequently anti-oestrogenic in nature. Although the female produces small amounts of androgen in the adrenal cortex and ovarian stroma as intermediate products in the synthesis of oestrogen from progesterone, its action is masked by the large quantities of oestrogen produced, and its role is obscure.

In the absence of oestrogens, androgens will reverse the oestrogenic changes in the organs of the genital tract, and cause atrophy of the lining epithelia. In larger amounts they suppress feminine body characteristics and attitudes, and may produce frank virilism, such as hirsutes of the face and limbs, en-largement of the clitoris, deepening of the voice, acne and occasionally alopecia. There is a marked individual susceptibility to the dose of androgen which produces these signs, but obviously their frequent occurrence limits the use of androgens in the female.

THERAPEUTIC USES

1. Debility and psychosomatic asthenia

Occasionally androgens are used to increase weight and bring about a feeling of well-being, but the newer non-androgenic anabolic steroids are being used increasingly for this purpose, and it is open to argument whether androgens have any real value.

2. Menopausal symptoms

Androgens, either alone or in combination with oestrogen, are generally contra-indicated in the treatment of certain menopausal symptoms, which respond far better to small doses of oestrogen. The exception is the patient who has previously had a carcinoma of the breast, in whom oestrogens are contra-indicated.

3. Suppression of lactation and prevention of breast engorgement

The use of oestrogens to suppress lactation is not entirely successful, and better results are claimed for the injection of testosterone enanthate 360mg with oestradiol valerate 16mg in 2ml of an oily vehicle (Primodian Depot, Schering; Deladumone OB, Squibb). For the best results, the injection is made in the second stage of labour. This has been replaced by the use of bromocriptine in most centres.

CONDITIONS IN WHICH ANDROGENS HAVE NO VALUE

In the past androgens have been given to treat frigidity, dysmenorrhoea, stress incontinence of urine, benign mammary dysplasia of the breasts, endometriosis and dysfunctional uterine bleeding. There is no evidence that androgens correct frigidity; and other drugs, particularly the progestogens, are available for the management of the other conditions.

PROGESTERONE AND PROGESTOGENS

The term progestogen includes pure progesterone and the synthetic substances derived from 19-nortestosterone or 17-acetoxyprogesterone which have progesterone-like actions. A progestogen is any substance which can produce progestational, or secretory, changes in an oestrogen-primed endometrium.

METABOLISM

Natural progesterone is synthesized in the corpus luteum, by the theca-lutein cells of the follicle (90 per cent of the total secreted), and by the adrenal cortex (10 per cent of the total secreted). In the first half of the menstrual cycle the adrenal cortex is the main source, but after ovulation the corpus luteum produces large amounts; whilst in pregnancy the placenta is the main source of progesterone production. The progesterone secreted remains only a short time in the blood before it is excreted or diffuses into the body tissues, principally the fat, from which it is released as needed. Only small quantities are found in the tissues of the genital tract at any given time. Studies with radioactive progesterone show that 40 to 70 per cent is excreted in the urine, 13 to 20 per cent in the faeces, and 10 to 15 per cent is taken up by the fatty tissues of the body. The proportion which is excreted is inactivated in the liver, and excreted in a variety of forms, the main one being pregnanediol, which can be detected by a fairly simple laboratory investigation. The urinary pregnanediol represents only 13 to 33 per cent of the progesterone produced, and plasma progesterone is now measured.

Natural progesterone is only weakly active when given by mouth, and is not easily soluble, so that it must be given vaginally or by intramuscular injection. Even by this route the effect is transient, and the injection painful. This has severely limited the use of natural progesterone in clinical gynaecology.

SYNTHETIC PROGESTOGENS

The limitations in the use of natural progesterone led to the search for synthetic agents with a progesterone-like action, which were effective orally. Some of the compounds available today are shown in Table **30/2**, and it can be seen that although all have progesterone-like properties, some are more androgenic than others, so that selection is important. It has been agreed internationally that these progesterone-like substances will be called 'progestogens'. Four main groups are in use today, (1) those derived directly from progesterone, (2) those

Parent substance	Trivial name or derivative	Chemical name	Remarks
(I) Progesterone	Dydrogesterone	6-Dehydro-9β, 10α-proges-terone	Weak activity in inhibiting ovulation. Little androgenic effect. Not metabolized to oestrogen. Not very effective in dysfunctional uterine bleeding, but relatively effective in treatment of dysmenorrhoea
(II) 17-Acetoxy-progesterone			
(a) Pregnanes	Hydroxyproges-terone caproate	17α-Hydroxyprogesterone caproate	Not metabolized to oestrogen. Said to be less haemostatic than Group III – but this as yet undecided
	Medroxyproges-terone acetate	17α-Acetoxy-6-methyl-4-pregnene-3,20-dione	
	Chlormadinone acetate	17α-Acetoxy-6-chloro-4,6-pregnadiene-3,20-dione	
(III) 19-Nortestos-terone			
(a) Estranes	Norethisterone Norethisterone acetate	17α-Ethinyl-17β-hydroxy-4-estren-3-one	Metabolized in part to oestrogen. Shorten clotting time. Increase PBI by 40 per cent. ?Reduce 17-oxyketosterol excretion. Suppress gonadotrophin and endogenous ovarian hormone production. All these substances are converted in the body to norethisterone, which is the only estrane which binds with receptors in the target tissues
	Lynestrenol	17α-Ethinyl-17β-hydroxy-4-estrane	
	Norethynodrel	17α-Ethinyl-17β-hydroxy-5(10)-estren-3-one	
	Ethynodiol diacetate	17α-Ethinyl-3β-17β-diacetoxy-4-estrane	
(b) Gonanes	Norgestrel	dl & d 18-Ethyl-17α-ethinyl-17β-hydroxy-4-gonen-3-one	Gonanes bind directly to target tissue receptors. d-norgestrel binds twice as strongly to target tissue receptors as does dl-norgestrel
	Desogestrel Gestodene Norgestimate		These new-generation progestogens are 18-homologated steroids related to 19-nortestosterone. They are similar to natural progesterone in their receptor-binding properties.

Table 30/2 Progestogens in use today

derived from 17-acetoxyprogesterone, called pregnane-progestogens, and (3) those derived from 19-nortestosterone which are either estranes or gonanes. The main drugs available are shown in Table **30/2**. One way of comparing the effectiveness of the different progestogens is by determining the dose required to produce secretory changes in an oestrogen-primed endometrium of a castrated woman. Hydroxyprogesterone caproate in a dose of 250mg will produce this change, and the drug has the advantage that this dose is freely soluble in oil, and if given intramuscularly has an action which persists for longer than 8 days. Medroxyprogesterone acetate is five times as potent as hydroxyprogesterone acetate, and has an action lasting 16 to 30 days. Norethisterone (and its acetate) is derived from 19-nortestosterone, and is metabolized in the body in part to oestrogen (3 per cent) and in a small part to androgen. All the available 19-nortestosterone (estrane) derivatives are converted into

Product	Relative potency	Dose in mg
Medroxyprogesterone	1/10	10
Norethisterone	1	1
Norethisterone acetate	0.75	1.5
Ethynodiol	0.75	1.5
Norgestrel	5–10	0.125
Levonorgestrel	10–20	0.075

Table 30/3 Relative potency of progestogens (tested by (1) delay of menses, (2) endometrial subvacuolization (i.e. secretory change), (3) change in blood lipids)

norethisterone in the body before they are attached to progesterone receptors in the target tissue. The importance of these observations is that the 'potency' of the available progestogens varies, depending on the degree and speed of the conversion into norethisterone (Table 30/3). This suggests that, in general, the only estrane derivative used should be norethisterone.

Norgestrel binds directly to receptors, as do the 17-acetoxyprogesterone (pregnane) derivatives. Dydrogesterone is a 'pure' progestogen, and does not metabolize to oestrogen or to androgen as far as is known. Several other progestogens are available, but only in combination with small doses of oestrogen.

The three main groups of progestogens have slightly different metabolic effects. Pregnane progestogens cause raised triglyceride levels but do not alter glucose carbohydrate tolerance. Estrane-progestogens cause some degree of impairment of glucose tolerance, some degree of insulin resistance and raised triglyceride levels. Gonane progestogens do not alter triglyceride levels significantly but increase the level of insulin secretion relative to the current glucose level (i.e. increase insulin resistance) and reduce HDL-cholesterol. The new generation progestogens do not alter lipid metabolism. Their equivalent doses are: gestodene 75µg; desogestrel 150µg; norgestimate 250µg.

SIDE-EFFECTS OF SYNTHETIC PROGESTOGENS

The side-effects of progestogens have been discussed to some extent in Chapter 11, and are unusual unless the drugs are taken over a prolonged period. The main ones complained of are increase in weight, breast tenderness, 'placidity' and occasionally, a decrease in libido.

THERAPEUTIC USES OF THE PROGESTOGENS

1. Dysfunctional uterine bleeding

(a) *Menorrhagia; metrorrhagia; polymenorrhoea.* The emergency control of an episode of 'flooding' can be obtained by the injection of hydroxyprogesterone caproate 250mg, or by the oral administration of norethisterone 30mg, in divided doses. The patient must be warned that a withdrawal bleed will occur 3 to 5 days after discontinuing the drug, and told to start a further 20 day course of the progestogen in a dose of 5 to 10mg a day on the 4th day of the flow. Thereafter regular cyclic bleeding of normal amount can be re-established by giving norethisterone 5 to 10mg daily from day 20 for 5 days, or from day 15 for 10 days, depending on the individual case. Alternatively, hydroxyprogesterone caproate 125mg on day 15 and 22, or one of the oral contraceptive pills (containing a 19-nortestosterone progestogen) from day 5 can be used for this purpose. The treatment should continue for from 3 to 9 months, depending on the endometrial pathology.

(b) *Oligomenorrhoea and hypomenorrhoea.* When these two symptoms are found together, or if oligomenorrhoea is the only symptom, investigations should be carried out to exclude pathological lesions. The majority of cases will be found to have a hypothalamic cause, probably in turn due to psychogenic factors. With reassurance the woman may accept her bleeding pattern, but if she wishes for predictable regular 'menstruation', this can be provided if progestogens are given following an oestrogen 'priming'. Usually ethinyl oestradiol 10µg twice daily is given for 20 days, and norethisterone 5 to 10mg daily added from day 15 for 10 days. It should be understood that the underlying defect is not corrected, but as the cause is psychogenic in many instances, the therapy over a period of 3 to 6 months often permits a spontaneous cure. The alternative is to give an oral contraceptive pill from day 5.

2. Amenorrhoea

The commonest cause of secondary amenorrhoea during the reproductive period is pregnancy. Pregnancy should be excluded by the use of immunological pregnancy tests before hormone therapy is contemplated as reports have appeared indicating that masculinization of female fetuses may occur if potent progestogens derived from 19-nortestosterone are used.

Once pregnancy has been excluded, a progestogen is often given in the course of the investigation of secondary amenorrhoea, as described in Chapter 8.

3. Dysmenorrhoea

As has been noted earlier, dysmenorrhoea can be largely eliminated by the use of an ovulation-suppressant dose of oestrogen, but since an oestrogen 'withdrawal bleed' tends to be prolonged and irregular, progestogens should be given in the last 10 days of the cycle, as described in the treatment of oligomenorrhoea. A better method is to give a low dose oral contraceptive. A pure progestogen (dydrogesterone), which is thought not to inhibit ovulation, has also been used with some success, although the rationale of its mode of action is unclear. If chosen, dydrogesterone is given from day 5 of the cycle for 20 days in a dose of 10 to 20mg daily.

4. Endometriosis

The introduction into therapeutics of potent orally-administered progestogens has altered considerably the management of endometriosis, and has permitted surgery to be avoided in many instances. The condition can be treated by producing a 'pseudo-pregnancy' using a 19-nortestosterone progestogen or an oral contraceptive over a period of 6 to 9 months, or by producing a 'pseudomenopause' using a 17-acetoxyprogesterone type of progestogen. If the patient desires to have a monthly bleed, intermittent administration of an oral contraceptive (containing a 19-nortestosterone progestogen) may be substituted, but the results are not so good. Recent experience shows that danazol is to be preferred to the progestogens in the treatment of endometriosis (see Chapter 19).

5. Miscellaneous conditions

The *time of a menstrual period* can be advanced or delayed by administering progestogens. Progesterone and progestogens are often recommended in the treatment of *premenstrual tension* although there is doubt about their value, except as a placebo. *Endometrial hyperplasia* in the perimenopausal woman can be suppressed, and endometrial atrophy obtained, if fairly high doses of a 17-acetoxyprogesterone progestogen are given over a period of 6 months. Usually medroxyprogesterone acetate is chosen in a dose of 5 to 10mg orally daily, or 50mg intramuscularly each week. Advanced, inoperable *endometrial carcinoma* may be palliated by giving even larger doses of progestogens.

CONDITIONS IN WHICH PROGESTOGENS ARE OF NO VALUE

These include threatened abortion, recurrent abortion, premature labour and idiopathic infertility (see Chapters 10 and 12).

Bibliography

I have kept the bibliography short because the literature is being up-dated constantly, computer searches are available and because individual teachers may prefer to indicate to students the references they consider important.

GENERAL REFERENCES

COPPLESON MJV. *Gynaecological Oncology*. 2nd ed. Churchill Livingstone, Edinburgh, 1990.

JONES HW, JONES GS (eds). *Novak's Textbook of Gynaecology*, 11th ed. Williams and Wilkins, Baltimore, 1988.

MACDONALD RR (ed.) *Scientific Basis of Obstetrics and Gynaecology*. Churchill Livingstone, Edinburgh, 1985.

CHAPTER REFERENCES

Chapter 1

GATH D *et al.* Psychiatric disorder and gynaecological symptoms in middle aged women: a community study. *Brit Med J*, 1987; **294**, 213–18.

Chapter 2

HAMILTON WJ, BOYD JD, MOSSMAN HW. *Human Embryology*, 3rd ed. Heffer, Cambridge, 1962.

PLENTL A, FRIEDMAN EA. *Lymphatic System of the Female Genitalia*. WB Saunders, Philadelphia, 1971.

SMOUT CFV, JACOBY F, LILLIE EW. *Gynaecological and Obstetrical Anatomy*, 4th ed. Lewis, London, 1969.

Chapter 3

GRUNDMAN E. *General Cytology* I. Arnold, London, 1967.

HSU LYF, KLINGER HP, WEISS J. *Cytogenetics*, 1967; **6**, 371.

JONES HW, HELLER RH. *Pediatric and Adolescent Gynecology*. Williams and Wilkins, Baltimore, 1966.

KLINGER HP, LUDWIG KS. *Stain tech*. 1957; **32**, 235.

Chapter 4

BROOK CGD. Turner's syndrome. *Arch Dis Child*, 1986; **61**, 305–9.

EDITORIAL, Klinefelters Syndrome, *Lancet*, 1988, **1**, 1317–18.

GRIFFIN JG, WILSON JD. Syndromes of androgen resistance. *New Eng J Med*, 1980; **302**, 198–209.

SAENGAR T. Abnormal sex differentiation. *J Paediatrics*, 1984; **104**, 1–17.

SHORT RV. Sex determination and differentiation. *Brit Med Bull*, 1979; **35**, 121–7.

SIMPSON JL. Diagnosis and management of the infant with genital ambiguity. *Amer J Obst Gynec*, 1977; **128**, 137–45.

Chapter 5

GARNER PR. Menstrual abnormalities at the extremes of body-weight. *J Obst Gynaec*, 1982; **3**, 52–61.

MOGHISSI KS *et al*. Composite picture of the menstrual cycle. *Amer J Obst Gynec*, 1972; **11**, 405.

RUBINOW DB et al. Changes in plasma hormones across the menstrual cycle. *Amer J Obst Gynec*, 1988; **158**, 5–11.

SCHALLY AV *et al*. The hypothalamus and reproduction. *Amer J Obst Gynec*, 1974; **122**, 857.

Chapter 6

ABRAHAM SF. Premenstrual or postmenstrual syndromes. *Med J Aust*, 1984; **2**, 327–8.

FISHER HW (ed). The premenstrual syndrome. International Congress and Symposium Series, Royal Society of Medicine; 1987.

HOLMES KHM, SALTER RH. Irritable bowel syndrome – a safe diagnosis? *Brit Med J*, 1982; **285**, 1533–4.

REID RL, YEN SCC. Premenstrual syndrome. *Amer J Obst Gynec*, 1981; **139**, 85–103.

VAITUKAITIS JL. Premenstrual syndrome. *New Eng J Med*, 1984; **311**, 1371–3.

Chapter 7

ELDER M. Prostaglandins and menstrual disorders. *Brit Med J*, 1983; **287**, 703.

Chapter 8

BLACKWELL PE, CHANG RJ. National symposium on the clinical management of prolactin related reproductive disorders. *Fertil and Steril*, 1986, **15**, 607–10.

DEWHURST CJ. Primary amenorrhoea. *Proc Roy Soc Med*, 1970; **63**, 291.

JACOBS HS. Amenorrhoea in athletes. *Brit J Obst Gynaec*, 1982; **89**, 498–9.

KNUTH UA *et al*. Amenorrhoea and loss of weight. *Brit J Obst Gynaec*, 1977; **84**, 801–7.

MASON P *et al*. Induction of ovulation with pulsatile luteinizing releasing hormone. *Brit Med J*, 1984; **288**, 181–5.

TAN SL, JACOBS HL. Management of prolactinomas. *Brit J Obst Gynaec*, 1986; **93** 1025–9.

Chapter 9

DE BEAUVOIR, SIMONE. *The Second Sex*. Jonathan Cape, London, 1963.

GREEN R (ed). *Human Sexuality*. Williams and Wilkins, Baltimore, 1976.

HASTINGS DW. *Sexual Expression in Marriage*. Little, Brown and Co, Boston, 1966.

KAPLIN HS. *The New Sex Therapy*. Baillière Tindall, London, 1974.

KINSEY AC (ed). *Sexual Behaviour in the Human Female*. WB Saunders, Philadelphia, 1953.

MASTERS W, JOHNSON V. *Human Sexual Response*. Little, Brown and Co, Boston, 1966.

MATHEWS A *et al*. Testosterone in the treatment of sexual dysfunctions. *Psych Med*, 1983; **13**, 88–92.

NADELSON C, MARCOTTE DB. *Treatment Interventions in Human Sexuality*. Plenum, New York, 1983.

Chapter 10

BEHRMAN SJ, KISTNER RW. *Progress in Infertility*, 3rd ed. Little, Brown and Co, Boston, 1987.

JEQUIER AM. *Infertility in the Male*. Churchill-Livingstone, Edinburgh, 1986.

MACLEOD J. Human male infertility. *Obstet Gynae Surv*, 1971; **26**, 335.

PEPPERELL RJ, HUDSON B, WOOD C. *The Infertile Couple*, 2nd ed. Churchill Livingstone, Edinburgh, 1987.

Chapter 11

BROSENS L, WINSTON R. *Reversibility of Female Sterilization*. Academic Press, London, 1978.

Family health international. Breast Cancer, *Network* 1989, 10, 3.

GUILLEBAUD J. *The Pill*, 2nd cd, OUP, Oxford, 1983.

KLEINMANN RC (ed). *Family Planning Handbook for Doctors*. 6th ed, IPPF, London, 1988.

LLEWELLYN-JONES D. *Getting pregnant – a guide for an infertile couple*. Ashwood House Medical, Melbourne, 1989.

MCEWEN J. Intrauterine conception. *Brit J Fam Plan*, 1983; **9**, 3–11.

GEORGE WASHINGTON UNIVERSITY. '*Population Reports*' – published bi-monthly (these reports give up-to-date information on various contraceptive methods.

WHO *Steroid Contraception and the Risk of Neoplasia*, Geneva, 1982.

Chapter 12

BENNETT MJ, EDMUNDS DK. *Spontaneous and Recurrent Abortion*, Blackwell, Oxford, 1987.

SARGENT IL *et al*. Maternal immune responses to the fetus in early pregnancy and recurrent miscarriage. *Lancet*, 1988; **2** 1099–1107.

STABILE I *et al*. Ultrasonic assessment of complications during the first trimester of pregnancy. *Lancet*, 1987; **2**, 1237–40.

Chapter 13

WESTROM L, MARDH PA. Current views on pelvic inflammatory disease. *Aust NZ J Obstet Gynaec*, 1984; **24**, 98–105.

Chapter 14

JEFFCOATE TNA. Chronic vulval dystrophies. *Amer J Obstet Gynec*, 1966; **95**, 61.

LANGLANDS AO. Management of advanced gynaecological cancer. *Aust NZ Obstet Gynaec*, 1984; **24**, 162–5.

LAVERY HA. Vulval dystrophies. *Clinics in Obstet. Gynec*, 1984; **11**, 155–69.

LAWSON JB, STEWART DG. Granulomatous infections of the vulva. In *Obstetrics and Gynaecology in the Tropics*, 1st ed. Arnold, London, 1967.

RIDLEY CM (ed.) *The Vulva*. Churchill Livingstone, Edinburgh, 1988

WAY S. Carcinoma of the vulva. *Amer J Obstet Gynec*, 1960; **79**, 692.

Chapter 15

BENEDICT JL *et al*. Vaginal carcinoma. *Obstet Gynec*, 1983; **62**, 715–19.

EDITORIAL COMMENT. Squamous metaplasia of the vagina. *Obstet Gynae Survey*, 1976; **31**, 62.

MORLEY GW. Various types of vaginitis. *Inter Surg*, 1966; **45**, 249.

SOBEL J. Vaginal candidiasis. *New Eng J Med*, 1986; **315**, 1455–8.

Chapter 16

BRUDENELL M *et al*. Cervical dysplasia, carcinoma in situ and microcarcinoma. *J Obstet Gynae Brit Cwlth*, 1973; **80**, 673.

COLEMAN DV, EVANS DMD. Biopsy, *Pathology and Cytology of the cervix*, Chapman and Hall, London, 1988.

COPPLESON M, PIXLEY E, REID B. Colposcopy, 3rd ed. Thomas, Springfield, 1986.

FOX H. Cervical smears: new terminology and new demands. *Brit Med J*, 1987; **294**, 1307–8.

KITCHENER HC. Does HPV cause cervical cancer? *Brit J Obst Gynaec*, 1988; **95**, 1089–91.

KOLSTAD P, STAFL A. *Atlas of Colposcopy*. Univ Park Press, Baltimore, 1972.

SINGER A, MCCANCE D. The wart virus and genital neoplasia. *Brit J Obst Gynaec*, 1985; **92**, 1083–4.

TATTERSALL MHN. The integration of surgery, radiotherapy and chemotherapy in the treatment of advanced gynaecological cancer. *Aust NZ J Obstet Gynaec*, 1984; **24**, 158–61.

WORTH AJ. Cervical cancer screening programs. *Obstet and Gynaec*, 1984; **63**, 135–9.

Chapter 17

EIFEL PJ et al. Adenocarcinoma of the endometrium. *Cancer*, 1983; **52**, 1026–36.

GAMBRELL RD et al. Role of estrogens and progesterone in the etiology and prevention of endometrial cancer. *Amer J Obstet Gynec*, 1983; **146**, 696–706.

GUSBERG SB (ed.) *Female Genital Cancer*. Churchill-Livingstone, Edinburgh, 1988.

Chapter 18

BUTTRAM VC, REITER RC. Uterine leiomyomata (a review). *Fertil and Steril*, 1981; **36**, 433–45.

Chapter 19

American Fertility Society. Classification of endometriosis. *Fertil and Steril*, 1985, **43**, 351–2.

BUTLER L *et al*. Collaborative study of pregnancy rates following danazol therapy of Stage 1 endometriosis. *Fertil and Steril*, 1984; **41**, 373–81.

HENZEL M *et al*. Administration of nasal naferalin compared with oral danazol for endometriosis. *New Eng J Med*, 1988; **318**, 485–9.

RIDLEY JH. Histogenesis of endometriosis. *Obstet Gynec Surv*, 1968; **23**, 1.

SCHENKEN RS, MALINAK LR. Conservative surgery versus expectant management for the infertile patient with mild endometriosis, *Fertil and Steril*, 1982; **37**, 183–6.

Chapter 20

BAGSHAWE KD. *Choriocarcinoma*, 2nd ed. Arnold, London, 1973.

GOLDSTEIN D *et al*. A rapid immuno-assay for HCG. *Amer J Obstet Gynec*, 1975; **45**, 527.

HRESHCHYSHYN MM (ed). Trophoblastic disease. *Clin Obstet Gynec*, 1967; **10**, 267.

KOHORN EI. Criteria toward the definition of non-metastatic gestational trophoblastic disease. *Amer J Obstet Gynec*, 1982; **142**, 416–19.

LLEWELLYN-JONES D. Management of benign trophoblastic tumours. *Amer J Obstet Gynec*, 1967; **99**, 589.

LURAM JG *et al*. Natural history of hydatidiform mole after evacuation. *Amer J Obstet Gynec*, 1983; **145**, 591–5.

STONE M, BAGSHAWE KD. An analysis of influences on patients with hydatidiform moles. *Brit J Obstet Gynaec*, 1979; **86**, 782–92.

Chapter 22

ESCHENBACH DA, DALING JR. Ectopic pregnancy. *J Amer Med Assn*, 1983; **249**, 1759–60.

Chapter 23

BARBER HRK. Ovarian tumours. *Clin Obstet Gynaec*, 1972; **12**, 929.

GRADY HG, SMITH DE (eds). *The Ovary*, 1st ed. Williams and Wilkins, Baltimore, 1963.

LI MC, HSU K. Drug therapy for ovarian carcinoma. *Clin Obstet Gynae*, 1970; **13**, 807.

NEIGT JD *et al*. Randomized trial comparing two combination chemotherapeutic regimens in advanced ovarian carcinoma. *Lancet*, 1984; **2**, 594–9.

WHARTON JT, EDWARDS CL, RUTLEDGE FN. Long-term survival after chemotherapy for advanced ovarian carcinoma. *Amer J Obstet Gynec*, 1984; **148**, 997–1005.

Chapter 24

MOIR JCM. *The Vesico-Vaginal Fistula*, 2nd ed. Baillière Tindall, London, 1967.

Chapter 25

KOMAROFF A. Acute dysuria in women. *New Eng J Med*, 1984; **310**, 368–74.

KRANTZ KE. The anatomy of the urethra. *Amer J Obstet Gynec*, 1951; **62**, 374.

MUNDY AR. The unstable bladder. *Clin Obst Gynec*, 1985; **12**, 43.

NEU HC, PARRY M. Urinary tract infections. *Bull NY Acad Med*, 1983; **59**, 288–99.

STANTON S. *Clinical Gynaecological Urology*. Blackwell, Oxford, 1983.

SUTHERST J, BROWN M. The fluid bridge test for urethral incompetence. *Acta Obstet Gynec Scand*, 1983; **62**, 271–3.

THEIDE HA, SAINI V. Urogynaecology. *Amer J Obst Gynec*, 1987; **157**, 563–8.

Chapter 26

DEWITT JE. Benign tumours of the breast. *Lancet*, 1976; **1**, 793.

LLEWELLYN-JONES D. The breast In *Reproductive Endocrinology* (Shearman, RP (ed)). Churchill Livingstone, Edinburgh, 1985.

MACDONALD I. In *Christopher's Textbook of Surgery*, 6th ed. Saunders, Philadelphia, 1965.

EDITORIAL. Management of early cancer of the breast. *Brit Med J*, 1976; **1**, 1035.

Chapter 27

COWELL CA (ed). Pediatric and adolescent gynaecology. *Ped Clin N Amer*, 1981; **28**, 245–330.

WHITE PC *et al*. Congenital adrenal hyperplasia. *New Eng J Med*, 1987; **316**, 1519–24, 1580–6.

Chapter 28

DEWHURST J. *Female Puberty and its Abnormalities*. Churchill Livingstone, Edinburgh, 1984.

HALBERT DR *et al*. Dysmenorrhoea and prostaglandins. *Obstet Gynec Survey*, 1976; **31**, 77.

HUFFMAN JW. Gynaecology of adolescence, *Clin Obstet Gynae*, 1971; **14**, 961.

OWEN PR. Prostaglandin synthetase inhibitors in the treatment of primary dysmenorrhoea. *Amer J Obstet Gynec*, 1984; **148**, 96–103.

Chapter 29

BUCHBAUM HJ (ed). *The Menopause*. Springer-Verlag, Berlin, 1984.

CONSENSUS DEVELOPMENT CONFERENCE. Prophylaxis and treatment of Osteoporosis. *Brit Med J*, 1987; **295**, 914–15.

LLEWELLYN-JONES D. *Menopause*. Penguin Books, Melbourne, 1988.

RIGGS BL, MELTON LJ. Involutional osteoporosis, *New Eng J Med*, 1986; **314**, 1676–86.

Index